IACM
Clinical Medicine
Update 2025

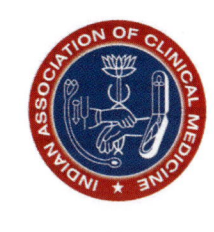

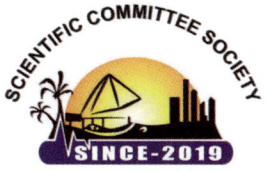

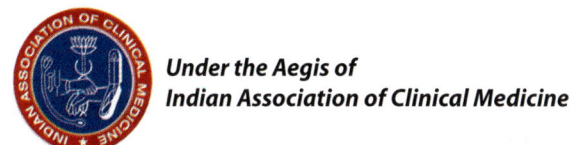

Under the Aegis of
Indian Association of Clinical Medicine

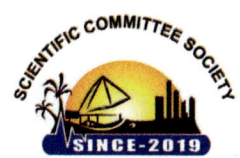

IACM
Clinical Medicine Update 2025

Editor-in-Chief

BL Bhardwaj
MD FIACM MACP FICP FIMSA FGSI MAMS
Pro Vice-Chancellor, Desh Bhagat University, Fatehgarh Sahib, Punjab
Former Professor and Head, Department of Medicine and
Principal, Government Medical College, Patiala, Punjab,
Vice-Chancellor, MMU Sadopur, Ambala, Haryana, India

Executive Editors

RPS Sibia
MD FICM
Professor and Head
Department of Medicine
Director Principal
Government Medical College
Patiala, Punjab, India

Prashant Prakash
MD(Medicine) MD(Respiratory Medicine)
MAMS FICP FIACM
Professor and Head
Department of Pulmonary and
Critical Care Medicine
SN Medical College
Agra, Uttar Pradesh, India

Associate Editors

Kanchan Bhardwaj
MD MAMS FIMSA FIAC
Former Vice Principal
Government Medical College
Patiala, Punjab, India

Gurinder Mohan
MD(Medicine) FIACM
Professor and Head
Department of Medicine
SGRDIMSR, Amritsar, Punjab, India

Forewords

Gurcharan Lal Avasthi   **MM Singh**   **KK Pareek**

A Publication of the Indian Association of Clinical Medicine

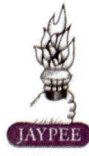

JAYPEE BROTHERS MEDICAL PUBLISHERS
The Health Sciences Publisher
New Delhi | London

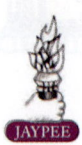 **Jaypee Brothers Medical Publishers (P) Ltd**

Headquarters
EMCA House, 23/23-B
Ansari Road, Daryaganj
New Delhi 110 002, India
Landline: +91-11-23272143, +91-11-23272703
+91-11-23282021, +91-11-23245672
e-mail: jaypee@jaypeebrothers.com

Corporate Office
4838/24, Ansari Road, Daryaganj
New Delhi 110 002, India
Phone: +91-11-43574357
Fax: +91-11-43574314
e-mail: jaypee@jaypeebrothers.com

Overseas Office
JP Medical Ltd.
83, Victoria Street, London
SW1H 0HW (UK)
Phone: +44-20 3170 8910
e-mail: info@jpmedpub.com

EU GPSR Authorised Representative
Logos Europe, 9 rue Nicolas Poussin
17000, La Rochelle, France
Phone: +33 (0) 6 67 93 73 78
e-mail: contact@logoseurope.eu

Website: www.jaypeebrothers.com
Website: www.jaypeedigital.com

© 2026, Jaypee Brothers Medical Publishers

The views and opinions expressed in this book are solely those of the original contributor(s)/author(s) and do not necessarily represent those of editor(s) or publisher of the book.

All rights reserved. No part of this publication may be reproduced, stored or transmitted in any form or by any means, electronic, mechanical, photocopying, recording or otherwise, without the prior permission in writing of the publishers.

All brand names and product names used in this book are trade names, service marks, trademarks or registered trademarks of their respective owners. The publisher is not associated with any product or vendor mentioned in this book.

Medical knowledge and practice change constantly. This book is designed to provide accurate, authoritative information about the subject matter in question. However, readers are advised to check the most current information available on procedures included and check information from the manufacturer of each product to be administered, to verify the recommended dose, formula, method and duration of administration, adverse effects and contraindications. It is the responsibility of the practitioner to take all appropriate safety precautions. Neither the publisher nor the author(s)/editor(s) assume any liability for any injury and/or damage to persons or property arising from or related to use of material in this book.

This book is sold on the understanding that the publisher is not engaged in providing professional medical services. If such advice or services are required, the services of a competent medical professional should be sought.

Every effort has been made where necessary to contact holders of copyright to obtain permission to reproduce copyright material. If any have been inadvertently overlooked, the publisher will be pleased to make the necessary arrangements at the first opportunity.

Inquiries for bulk sales may be solicited at: jaypee@jaypeebrothers.com

IACM Clinical Medicine Update 2025 / BL Bhardwaj
First Edition: **2026**
ISBN: 978-93-7202-810-2

Printed in India

DEDICATION

Dedicated to my beloved parents
**Late Smt Maya Devi and
Late Shri Lajpat Rai Bhardwaj**
Who taught me the value of hard work and dedication.

EDITORIAL BOARD

MPS Chawla
Suresh Kushwaha
Pritam Singh
Gurinder Mohan
RPS Sibia
Kanchan Bhardwaj
Prashant Prakash

EDITORIAL ADVISORY BOARD

MM Singh
HS Pathak
AK Agarwal
GL Avasthi
KK Pareek
AK Gupta
Subash Chander Gupta
Dipanjan Bandyopadhyay
S Chandershekhar
Bharat Bhushan Rewari
DG Jain
Smarajit Banik
Vikas Loomba
MP Singh
Sanjay D Cruz
Vipin Mediratta
Amit Aggarwal
Sumit Singla
HK Aggarwal
DP Aggarwal
Rajesh Bhawani

CONTRIBUTORS

Aastha Takkar MD DM(Neurology)
Associate Professor
Department of Neurology
Postgraduate Institute of Medical
Education and Research (PGIMER)
Chandigarh, India

Abhishek Raj MD(Medicine) FIACM
Professor
Department of Medicine
SN Medical College
Agra, Uttar Pradesh, India

Ajay Bhaskar MD
Assistant Professor
Department of Medicine
Government Medical College
Patiala, Punjab, India

Amandeep Kaur MBBS DGO MD MBA
Professor (Associate)
Department of Community Medicine
and Family Medicine
AIIMS
Kalyani, West Bengal, India

Aman Sharma MD FAMS FIACM FICP
FACR FRCP(London)
Professor
Clinical Immunology and
Rheumatology Wing
Department of Internal Medicine
Postgraduate Institute of Medical
Education and Research
Program Director
COE in HIV Care
Chandigarh, India

Amit Aggarwal DNB MNAMS FIACM FICP
Senior Specialist
Department of Medicine
ABVIMS and Dr Ram Manohar Lohia
Hospital
New Delhi, India

Amit Chakraborty MBBS MD(General Medicine)
Medical Officer (Specialist)
Department of General Medicine
Jalpaiguri Government Medical College
and Hospital
Jalpaiguri, West Bengal, India

Ankan Pathak MD(Medicine)
DNB(Cardiology)
Assistant Professor
Consultant Interventional Cardiologist
Department of Medicine
Jagannath Gupta Institute of
Medical Sciences
Kolkata, West Bengal, India

Aparna Tewari MD(Anesthesia and
Critical Care Medicine)
Senior Resident
Department of Anesthesia
Barasat Government Medical College
and Hospital
Kolkata, West Bengal, India

Aradhana Sharma MBBS MD(Medicine)
FICP
Associate Professor
Department of Medicine
SMS Medical College
Jaipur, Rajasthan, India

Contributors

AR Balamurugan MD DTCD FDiab
Senior Assistant Professor
Department of Internal Medicine
Government Stanley Medical College
Senior Consultant Physician and
Pulmonologist
Chennai, Tamil Nadu, India

Ashish Bhagat MBBS MD
Professor
Department of Medicine
Government Medical College
Patiala, Punjab, India

Ashutosh Kumar Karn MD
DM(Neurology)
Chief Medical Officer
Department of Neurology
ABVIMS and Dr Ram Manohar Lohia
Hospital
New Delhi, India

Asra Brar MBBS
Junior Resident (Final Year)
Sri Guru Ram Das University of
Health Sciences
Amritsar, Punjab, India

Ayush Agarwal MD(General Medicine)
Department of Endocrinology and
Metabolism
Institute of Postgraduate Medical
Education and Research
Kolkata, West Bengal, India

Ben Cherian Mathew MD
Assistant Professor
Department of Medicine
Christian Medical College and Hospital
Ludhiana, Punjab, India

Bimal K Agrawal FIACM FICP FACP
Professor
Department of Medicine
Principal and Dean
MM Institute of Medical Sciences and
Research
Mullana, Haryana, India

BL Bhardwaj MD FIACM MACP FICP FIMSA
FGSI MAMS
Pro Vice-Chancellor, Desh Bhagat
University, Fatehgarh Sahib, Punjab
Former Professor and Head
Department of Medicine and
Principal, Government Medical College
Patiala, Punjab
Vice-Chancellor, MMU Sadopur,
Ambala, Haryana, India

Chandrapaul Gupta MBBS
Postgraduate Trainee
Department of General Medicine
KPC Medical College and Hospital
Kolkata, West Bengal, India

Debaprasad Chakrabarti MBBS MD
Professor and Head
Department of General Medicine
Tripura Medical College
Agartala, Tripura, India

Debasis Chakrabarti MD(Medicine)
FACP FICP FIACM FDI
Head
Department of Medicine
North Bengal Medical College
Siliguri, West Bengal, India

Deepak Jain MBBS MD(General Medicine)
Senior Professor and Unit Head
Department of Medicine
Postgraduate Institute of Medical
Sciences
Rohtak, Haryana, India

Deepak K Jumani ACS(USA) FIAMS
FCSEPI FRCM FISH FRSSDI FDI MBBS(Bom)
PhD(USA) MRCPS(Glasgow) FRCP(Glasgow)
Assistant Professor
Department of Medicine
Sir JJ Group of Government Hospitals
and Grant Medical College
Mumbai, Maharashtra, India
Consultant Sexual Health Physician and
Counselor
Consultant to Mumbai Police

Gagan Priya MD DM(Endocrinology)
Senior Consultant Endocrinologist
Fortis Hospital
Mohali, Punjab, India

Gurinder Mohan MD(Medicine) FIACM
Professor and Head
Department of Medicine
SGRDIMSR
Amritsar, Punjab, India

Harinder K Bali MD DM
Chairman Cardiac Sciences and Dean
Academics and Research
Livasa Hospital
Mohali, Punjab, India

Harnoor Singh MD MAABB MISBTI
Transfusion Safety Officer
University of Iowa Healthcare
Iowa, USA

HK Aggarwal MD FICP FAIMS FIACM
Ex Senior Professor and Head
Department of Medicine
Postgraduate Institute of Medical Sciences
Rohtak, Haryana, India

Jhanvi Pawar MBBS
Postgraduate Student (MD)
Department of Medicine
Government Medical College
Patiala, Punjab, India

Jugal Kishor Sharma Fellow with Distinction of RCPE MD(Medicine) DSc(Honoris Causa) FICP FACP FACE FRCP(London, Edinburgh, Glasgow, Ireland) Founder Fellow IPF
Medical Director
Central Delhi Diabetes and Obesity Centre
New Delhi, India

Kalyan Mitra MD(General Medicine) MRCP(UK) FRCP(Edinburgh)
Consultant and Medical Director
Lila Hospital
Berhampore, West Bengal, India

Kanchan Bhardwaj MD MAMS FIMSA FIAC
Former Vice Principal
Government Medical College
Patiala, Punjab, India

Kapeesh Khanna MD(Medicine)
Senior Resident (Final Year)
Department of Neurology
Sawai Man Singh Hospital
Jaipur, Rajasthan, India

KK Pareek MBBS MD FRCP
Past Dean and National President of the API
Senior Consultant Physician and Director of SN Pareek Memorial Hospital
Kota, Rajasthan, India

Kripa Anna MBBS MD(Medicine)
Assistant Professor
Department of Medicine
Christian Medical College and Hospital
Ludhiana, Punjab, India

K Vengadakrishnan MBBS MD
Professor
Department of Medicine
Sri Ramachandra Medical College and Research Institute
Chennai, Tamil Nadu, India

Lovleen Bhatia MD(Medicine)
Professor
Department of Medicine
Government Medical College
Patiala, Punjab, India

Madhuchanda Kar MBBS MD(General Medicine)
Clinical Director
Department of Oncology
Peerless Hospital
Kolkata, West Bengal, India

MPS Chawla MD FACP FRCP FICP FIACM FISC FIMSA
Professor and Former Head
Department of Medicine
ABVIMS and Dr Ram Manohar Lohia Hospital
New Delhi, India

Navdeep S Sidhu MD DM
Assistant Professor
Department of Cardiology
All India Institute of Medical Sciences
Bilaspur, Himachal Pradesh, India

Pankaj Malhotra MD FRCP
Professor and Head
Department of Clinical Hematology and Medical Oncology
Postgraduate Institute of Medical Education and Research
Chandigarh, India

Pankaj Singhania MD DM(Endocrinology) FICP Double Gold Medalist
Director
Arogyam Health Care
Purulia, West Bengal, India

Paramita Bhattacharya MBBS MD
Assistant Professor
Department of Internal Medicine
College of Medicine and JNM Hospital
Kalyani, West Bengal, India

Partha Sarkar MD(General Medicine) FRCP(Glasgow) WHO Fellow
Professor
Department of General Medicine
KPC Medical College and Hospital
Kolkata, West Bengal, India

Piyush Malik MD(Medicine)
Senior Resident
Department of Medicine
Pandit Bhagwat Dayal Sharma
Postgraduate Institute of Medical Sciences
Rohtak, Haryana, India

Poulami Das MBBS(Honours)
Postgraduate Trainee
Department of General Medicine
KPC Medical College and Hospital
Kolkata, West Bengal, India

Prabhjit Kaur PhD(Neurology)
Project Research Scientist-I
Department of Neurology
Postgraduate Institute of Medical Education and Research (PGIMER)
Chandigarh, India

Prabhpreet Kaur BDS MDS
Fellow – Forensic Odontology
Professor
Department of Oral Pathology
Genesis Institute of Dental Sciences and Research (GIDSR)
Ferozepur, Punjab, India

Pradeep Agarwal MBBS MD FICP FIACM FIMSA FISH FDI
Professor and Unit Head
Department of Medicine
Mahatma Gandhi University of Medical Sciences and Technology
Jaipur, Rajasthan, India

Prashant Prakash MD(Medicine) MD(Respiratory Medicne) MAMS FICP FIACM
Professor and Head
Department of Pulmonary and Critical Care Medicine
SN Medical College
Agra, Uttar Pradesh, India

Contributors | xiii

Priyanka Saha MBBS MD(Pathology)
Medical Officer (Specialist)
Department of Pathology
Mal SSH, Malbazar
Jalpaiguri

Preetkanwal Sibia MD
Professor
Department of Obstetrics and Gynaecology
Government Medical College
Patiala, Punjab, India

Princi Jain MD(Medicine) FICP
Professor
Department of Medicine
Lady Hardinge Medical College
and Smt Sucheta Kriplani Hospital
New Delhi, India

Puneet Rijhwani MBBS MD FACP FRCP(Edinburgh, Glasgow) FICP FIACM FIMSA FISH FDI
Professor and Head
Department of Medicine
Mahatma Gandhi University of Medical Sciences and Technology
Consultant Physician
Rijhwani's Diabetes and Heart Clinic
Federation Lead
MRCP PACES MGUMST
Jaipur, Rajasthan, India

Raghavi Abhilesh Bembey MBBS DNB
Senior Resident
Department of Medicine
ABVIMS and RML Hospital
New Delhi, India

Rajbir Singh BDS MDS
Professor
Department of Periodontics
Genesis Institute of Dental Sciences and Research (GIDSR)
Ferozepur, Punjab, India

Rajesh Kumar MD
Professor
Department of General Medicine
Shri Lal Bahadur Shastri Government Medical College and Hospital
Mandi, Nerchowk, Himachal Pradesh, India

Rajesh Vijayvergiya MBBS MD(Medicine) DM(Cardiology)
Department of Cardiology
Postgraduate Institute of Medical Education and Research
Chandigarh, India

Ram Babu MBBS MD
Senior Consultant and Physician
Department of Medicine
Jaipur Golden Hospital
Rohini, New Delhi, India

Ramesh Kumar MBBS MD(Internal Medicine)
Department of Internal Medicine
Specialist Currently Associated with
Marudhar Hospital
Khatipura, Jaipur, Rajasthan, India

Raminderpal Singh Sibia MD(Medicine)
Director and Principal
Government Medical College
Patiala, Punjab, India

Ram Kishan Jat MBBS MD FICP
Professor, Department of Medicine
Geetanjali Institute of Medical Sciences
Jaipur, Rajasthan, India

Ranjodh Gill MD FACE FACP CCD
Professor
Department of Internal Medicine and Surgery
Division of Endocrinology, Diabetes and Metabolism
Virginia Commonwealth University School of Medicine
Richmond, Virginia, United States

Contributors

RBS Manian DTCD MD(General Medicine)
Senior Assistant
Professor of Medicine
Government Royapettah Hospital
Kilpauk Medical College
Chennai, Tamil Nadu, India

Raman Puri MD DM
Consultant Cardiologist
Department of Cardiology
Apollo Hospital
New Delhi, India

Ritu MBBS MD(Medicine)
Assistant Professor
Department of Medicine
AIIMS Jammu
Jammu and Kashmir, India

RS Bhatia MBBS MD
Visiting Faculty
Department of Respiratory Medicine
MMU, Ambala, Haryana, India

Sandipan Banik MBBS MD(General Medicine)
Assistant Professor
Department of General Medicine
Jalpaiguri Government Medical College
and Hospital
Jalpaiguri, West Bengal, India

Sandipan Mondal MBBS MD(General Medicine)
Medical Officer (Specialist)
Department of General Medicine
Jalpaiguri Government Medical College
and Hospital
Jalpaiguri, West Bengal, India

Satrajit Roy MBBS(Honours) MD CCEBDM
MRCPS(Glasgow) Postgraduate Diploma in
Diabetology University of South Wales UK
Fellow Diabetes India Fellow IDF
Head
Department of Medicine
Central Hospital ECL
Asansol, West Bengal, India

Sayantani Bhadury MBBS
Junior Resident
Department of Medicine
North Bengal Medical College
Siliguri, West Bengal, India

Sehajnoor Singh MBBS
Intern, Sri Guru Ram Das University
of Health Sciences
Amritsar, Punjab, India

S Chandrasekar MD
Head and Professor
Department of Medicine and
Critical Care
In-Charge Rheumatology Department
Government Stanley Medical College
and Hospital
Medical Director
Jayaselvam Diabetes and Heart Center
Chennai, Tamil Nadu, India

Shilpa Atwal MBBS MD(Medicine)
Senior Resident
Department of General Medicine
Shri Lal Bahadur Shastri Government
Medical College and Hospital
Mandi, Himachal Pradesh, India

Shrikant Chaudhary MBBS MD
Associate Professor
Department of Medicine
Mahatma Gandhi University of
Medical Sciences and Technology
Jaipur, Rajasthan, India

S Krupha MBBS
Junior Resident, Stanley Medical College
Chennai, Tamil Nadu, India

Smarajit Banik MD(General Medicine)
FRCP(Glassglow) FACP FICP FIACN
Professor and Head
Department of General Medicine
Jalpaiguri Government Medical College
and Hospital
Jalpaiguri, West Bengal, India

Sonam Spalgais DNB(Respiratory Medicine) MNAMS FIACM
Associate Professor
Department of Pulmonary Medicine
Vallabhbhai Patel Chest Institute
New Delhi, India

Srinivasa Murthy MD(Medicine)
Professor
Department of Medicine
Vardhman Mahavir Medical College and Safdarjung Hospital
New Delhi, India

SS Dariya MD(Medicine) FACP FRCP(Glasgow) FRCP(London) FICP FIACM FGSI FDI FIPA
Associate Professor
Department of Medicine
National Institute of Medical Sciences and Research
Jaipur, Rajasthan, India

Subhash Chandra MD(Honours) SNMC AGRA MRCP(UK) DTM&H(UK) DTCD
Director
Shri Ram Babu Gupta Heart and Medicine Center
Agra, Uttar Pradesh, India

Subhro Jyoti Mukherjee MBBS
Senior Resident
Department of Internal Medicine
College of Medicine and JNM Hospital
Kalyani, West Bengal, India

Sudhir Kumar Atri MD(Medicine) FIACM DM(Clinical Hematology)
Senior Professor and Head
Department of Medicine and Clinical Hematology
Pandit Bhagwat Dayal Sharma Postgraduate Institute of Medical Sciences
Rohtak, Haryana, India

Suman Meyur MBBS MD(Radiation Oncology)
Deputy-in Charge, Medical Oncology,
Saroj Gupta Cancer Center and Research Institute
Kolkata, West Bengal, India

Sumit Sarkar MBBS MD(General Medicine)
Medical Officer (Specialist)
Department of General Medicine
Jalpaiguri Government Medical College and Hospital
Jalpaiguri, West Bengal, India

T Saravanan MD FICP
Professor and Head
Department of Medicine
PSG Institute of Medical Sciences and Research
Coimbatore, Tamil Nadu, India

Vidita Kalra MBBS MD(General Medicine)
Senior Resident
University College of Medical Sciences
New Delhi, India

Vijay Kumar MD(Medicine) FICP FRSSDI FICCMD FIACM FDI FICS PGDH and HM(NIHFW, New Delhi) FGID and AMSP(CMC, Vellore) DFID(CMC, Vellore)
Additional Professor and Unit Head
Department of Medicine
All India Institute of Medical Sciences
Patna, Bihar, India

Vikas Loomba MBBS MD(Medicine) PGDGM FIACM FICP
Professor and Unit Head
Department of Medicine
Christian Medical College and Hospital
Ludhiana, Punjab, India

Vikas Sharma MD
Associate Professor
Department of Medicine
Government Medical College
Patiala, Punjab, India

Vishnu Menon MD(General Medicine)
Junior Resident
Department of Medicine
PGIMS
Rohtak, Haryana, India

Yashraj Saini
2nd Year MBBS Student
Rajasthan University of Health Sciences
Jaipur, Rajasthan, India

FOREWORD

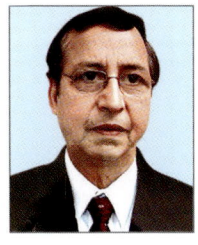

Gurcharan Lal Avasthi MD FICP FIACM FIAMS
Former Professor and Head, Department of Medicine
Dayanand Medical College and Hospital, Ludhiana, Punjab
Senior Consultant and Head, Department of Medicine
Director Medical Services, SPS Hospital, Ludhiana, Punjab, India

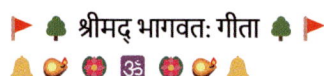

"गुरु शुश्रूषया विद्या पुष्कलेन् धनेन वा।
अथ वा विद्यया विद्या चतुर्थो न उपलभ्यते॥"

From the Shrimad Bhagwad Geeta, this sacred shloka reminds us that true learning arises through service, humility, and mutual respect between the teacher and the learner. Medicine, too, flourishes through this bond—a divine exchange of knowledge, compassion, and experience.

This *"Clinical Medicine Update 2025"* by Dr BL Bhardwaj is a reflection of that very spirit.

Clinical medicine has always been more than the application of facts; it is a living dialogue between knowledge and compassion, observation and understanding, technology and touch. The theme *"Blending Art and Science in Clinical Medicine"* finds its true expression in this book.

To understand the patient as a person is the true art of medicine. While science provides the methods to diagnose and treat, the art teaches us how to apply that knowledge—with empathy, intuition, and respect for human experience.

This compilation beautifully reflects both the facts of science and the grace of clinical wisdom.

I sincerely congratulate Dr BL Bhardwaj and all contributors for their thoughtful and inspiring chapters.

I encourage every reader to explore this book and make the most of the wisdom it offers.

FOREWORD

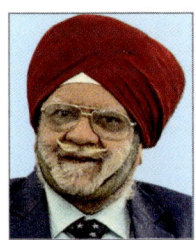

MM Singh MBBS MD(Medicine)
Internal Medicine Specialist
Past President/Founder Secretary
Indian Association of Clinical Medicine
Former Director, Professor, and Head
PG Department of Medicine
SN Medical College, Agra, Uttar Pradesh, India

It is a great pleasure and indeed an honor to write foreword to this *"Clinical Medicine Update 2025"* to be presented on the occasion of the Annual Conference of the Indian Association of Clinical Medicine (IACM).

The field of clinical medicine stands at a remarkable crossroads where tradition meets transformation. Each year, the Association of Clinical Medicine gathers some of the finest minds in their fields to share insights, exchange discoveries, and envision the future of patient care. This year's theme, *"Blending art and Science in Clinical Medicine,"* perfectly captures the evolving spirit of our discipline—one where cutting-edge scientific progress harmonizes with the timeless values of compassion, ethics, and clinical acumen.

Medicine today is no longer confined to the clinic or laboratory; it is a confluence of disciplines—molecular biology, data science, artificial intelligence, genomics, and personalized therapy—all converging to enhance clinical judgment and patient outcomes. As we embrace these advancements, our collective mission remains unchanged, to heal, to relieve suffering, and to uphold the sacred trust between physician and patient. The theme this year reflects a pivotal moment in modern healthcare, where rapid scientific and technological progress merges seamlessly with the art and practice of clinical care.

This volume brought by great efforts of Dr Bachhan Bhardwaj, a clinician par excellence, brings together the intellectual vigor and innovative spirit of our members and contributors. It reflects both the depth of clinical expertise and the dynamism of current research. I hope that readers—whether clinicians, researchers, or students—find in these pages inspiration to explore, learn, and apply knowledge in the service of humanity.

I extend my appreciation to all authors, editors, and organizers for their dedication in bringing this publication to life. May this conference and this book serve as enduring platforms for collaboration, discovery, and the continued advancement of clinical medicine.

FOREWORD

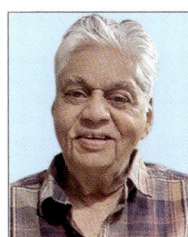

KK Pareek MD FICP FACP(USA) FRCP(London, Glasgow, Edinburgh) FRSSDI
Senior Consultant in Medicine
Past President, API
Past Dean, Indian College of Physicians
Past President, IACM
President, CCDSI
Chief Editor, API Textbook of Medicine

It is indeed a great honor and pleasure to write foreword for *"Clinical Medicine Update 2025"*, the annual publication of the Indian Association of Clinical Medicine (IACM).

The IACM was established 33 years ago in 1992 to establish the primacy of a logical, clinical, and rational approach to medical problems and to save the art and science of clinical medicine and its methodology in the plethora of today's highly advanced scientific investigations and now newly developed artificial intelligence. Keeping this in mind, Dr Bhardwaj has chosen the most appropriate theme *"Blending Art and Science in Clinical Medicine"* for the 31st Annual Conference of IACM.

The enormous responsibility of preparing an educative, meaningful, and exciting scientific agenda and publishing *Clinical Medicine Update* is not a simple task, but with the support of an excellent editorial team, this book becomes a small effort in pursuit of the large motive and movement.

The desire and endeavor of IACM to empower Indian physicians with the creative continue, and significant new knowledge in clinical medicine is being achieved through editing this book.

Professor BL Bhardwaj is a very senior physician, has gained a lot of experience and expertise as a senior professor of medicine, and has been very actively involved in organizing CME programs, conferences, and workshops in the past. The editorial team has made sincere efforts to cover a majority of important clinically relevant topics, which will be of a great help and will serve as ready reckoner for the postgraduates, teaching faculties, and busy practicing clinicians. The chapters in this book contain all the lectures delivered by faculty members of national repute and experts of their subjects. Dr Bhardwaj has expeditiously edited all the chapters and compiled them to this prestigious publication of IACM. He deserves great appreciation and congratulations for the excellent work done by bringing out this prestigious publication.

I wish a great success to the IACMCON-2025, Chandigarh.

FOREWORD

KK Pareek MD FISC FACP FICP FRCP London, Glasgow, Edinburgh, FCCP
MNAMS, Senior Consultant in Medicine
Past President, API
Past Dean, Indian College of Physicians
Past President, IACM
President, CCST
Chief Editor, API Textbook of Medicine

It is indeed a great honor and pleasure to write foreword for Clinical Medicine Update 2025, the annual publication of the Indian Association of Clinical Medicine (IACM). It has truly evolved over the years.

The IACM was established 33 years ago in 1992 to establish the primacy of a logical, clinical and rational approach to medical problems and to save the art and science of clinical medicine and its methodology in the slipstream of today's high-advanced scientific investigations and now newly developed artificial intelligence. Keeping this in mind, Dr Bhardwaj has chosen the most appropriate theme 'Standpoint and Stance in Clinical Medicine' for the 31st Annual Conference of IACM (CMCON 2025) being organized in Lucknow from 14th to 16th February 2025.

The enormous responsibility of preparing an educative, meaningful, and exciting scientific agenda and publishing 'Clinical Medicine Update' is not a simple task, but with the support of an excellent editorial team, this book becomes a small effort in pursuit of the larger theme and movement.

The choice of each article of IACM to empower Indian physicians with the common concerns and significant enhance knowledge in clinical medicine is being represented into enriching this book.

Dr Bhardwaj and his team did a very commendable job in bringing a lot of known and unknown clinical entities and their recent advances in one umbrella. I appreciate the hard work taken by him and his team in bringing out this wonderful book, one of the best publications in the country on clinical medicine.

Looking forward for new horizons of IACM!

Dr KK Pareek
Chief Editor, API Textbook of Medicine
Past President, API, ICP, IACM
President, CCST
Senior Consultant, Department of Medicine, SN Pareek Hospital, Kota, Rajasthan, India
kkpareek@hotmail.com

Dr Pareek, President, IACM 1996-97, Chairman IACM, 2011-12

FROM THE EDITOR'S DESK

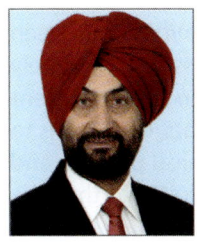

BL Bhardwaj
President-Elect and Chairman, Scientific Committee
IACMCON 2025

It gives me great pleasure to present *"Clinical Medicine Update 2025"* on the occasion of the *31st Annual Conference of the Indian Association of Clinical Medicine (IACMCON 2025)*. I am deeply thankful to all members and office bearers of IACM for entrusting me with the responsibility of publishing this book.

The theme of this year's conference, *"Blending the Art and Science in Clinical Medicine,"* beautifully captures the essence of modern medical practice. With the advent of information technology, social media, smartphones, and artificial intelligence, today's physician is expected to be increasingly techno-savvy. Keeping this in mind, compiling this edition of *Clinical Medicine Update* has been both a challenging and rewarding task. In the rapidly evolving era of medicine, every clinician must stay abreast of the latest developments to provide the best possible patient care.

The responsibility of preparing an educative, meaningful, and engaging scientific program—and publishing this book—has been substantial. However, with the dedicated support of an excellent editorial team and the guidance of our governing body members, we have made this endeavor a reality. This volume represents a humble effort toward IACM's ongoing mission to empower Indian physicians through continuous and creative learning in clinical medicine.

The chapters in this volume include lectures delivered by renowned national and international faculty—experts who have eloquently embodied the conference theme, *"Blending the Art and Science in Clinical Medicine."* Each chapter reflects the authors' vast experience and aims to present the latest advancements in clinical research and practice. The content is designed to meet the practical needs of physicians in their daily work.

As disease patterns and presentations continue to change at a rapid pace, physicians face the constant challenge of keeping up with evolving diagnostic tools and treatment strategies. Education and knowledge thrive through the sharing and dissemination of information. Readers of this book will be able to strengthen their understanding and translate this knowledge into clinical practice. The scientific sessions of the conference further complement this continuous learning process.

In line with our theme, the scientific program emphasizes the inseparable bond between science and clinical practice. To this end, we have included six important workshops and hands-on training sessions on relevant topics such as *Pulmonary Function Testing and Pulmonary Rehabilitation, Basic Life Support (BLS), Point-of-Care Ultrasound (POCUS), Basic Echocardiography for Physicians, Mechanical Ventilation,* and *Neurophysiology*. These workshops will be conducted by leading experts in their respective domains for delegates and postgraduate students.

My journey as *President-Elect and Chairman, Scientific Committee,* has been deeply enriching, offering me new experiences and valuable lessons. I sincerely hope that through this collective effort, our editorial team has been able to present these learnings in a meaningful and practical way for all participants. Our goal is to help delegates transform updated knowledge into improved clinical practice and to ensure that this book serves as a lasting source of learning—fulfilling the core objectives of IACM.

On behalf of the editorial board, I extend heartfelt thanks to the *Governing Body of IACM* for their continuous support and guidance. I warmly welcome all delegates to *IACMCON-2025, Chandigarh*—a conference designed to expand knowledge, refine clinical skills, and foster collaboration and friendship among colleagues and leaders in medicine.

If this book helps our delegates—even in a small way—to enhance their clinical work and knowledge, our efforts will be richly rewarded.

I am deeply indebted to my teacher and guide *Professor HS Dang*, under whose mentorship I learned the true *Art and Science of Medicine*. His meticulous approach to clinical teaching and exemplary humanity left a lasting impression on me. I was equally fortunate to receive training under the mentorship of *Professor JR Sachdeva, Professor Harjit Singh, Professor GP Singh*, and *Professor BK Chopra*.

I also express my heartfelt gratitude to *Dr HS Gill, Chairman, Adesh Welfare Society and Adesh Medical Colleges*, for his invaluable opportunities and encouragement, and to *Dr Guntas Gill, Managing Director*, for unwavering support. My special thanks go to *Professor Arun Kumar Sharma (MMU, Sadopur)* and *Mr Devinder Sharma (GM, Bigtec Labs & Molbio Diagnostics)*, whose assistance was instrumental in publishing this book.

I express my sincere thanks to *Dr Prashant Prakash* and *Dr Kanchan Bhardwaj* for their continued support. I am also very thankful for the assistance provided by *Sandeep Kaur, Ramandeep Sharma*, and *Shikha Shrivastav*.

I remain grateful to our talented editorial team and advisory group for their constructive suggestions and sustained support. Finally, I owe immense gratitude to my colleagues, seniors, and friends for their constant encouragement and insightful feedback.

With the blessings of *God Almighty and my parents*, I humbly present this book—*"Clinical Medicine Update 2025."*

ACKNOWLEDGMENTS

I extend my heartfelt gratitude to the Governing Body of IACM for their continuous support and guidance.

I am deeply indebted to my revered teacher and mentor Professor HS Dang, whose exceptional clinical acumen and humanistic approach shaped my understanding of the true art and science of medicine. I was equally privileged to be guided by Professor JR Sachdeva, Professor Harjit Singh, Professor GP Singh, and Professor BK Chopra.

My sincere appreciation to Dr HS Gill, Chairman, Adesh Welfare Society and Adesh Medical Colleges, for his inspiration, and to Dr Guntas Gill, Managing Director, for steadfast support.

I extend special thanks to Professor Arun Kumar Sharma (MMU, Sadopur) and Mr Devinder Sharma (GM, Bigtec Labs and Molbio Diagnostics) for their invaluable assistance in the publication of this book.

I am grateful to Dr Prashant Prakash and Dr Kanchan Bhardwaj for their constant collaboration and encouragement. My thanks also to Sandeep Kaur, Ramandeep Sharma, and Shikha Shrivastav for their dedicated support.

I sincerely appreciate our editorial team and advisory members for their insights, time, and commitment to excellence.

I remain ever thankful to my seniors, colleagues, and friends for their encouragement, thoughtful suggestions, and unwavering goodwill.

Finally, with profound gratitude, I seek the blessings of God Almighty and my beloved parents, whose guidance and values continue to inspire every step I take.

BL Bhardwaj

CONTENTS

Section 1: Cardiology

1. Reversible Cardiomyopathy: Clinical Insights through Case-based Examples — 3
   Ankan Pathak, Aparna Tewari

2. Unmasking Masked Hypertension — 8
   HK Aggarwal, Deepak Jain, Vishnu Menon

3. The Indian Guidelines for the Management of Dyslipidemia: Evolution and Updates (2016–2023) — 14
   Raman Puri, KK Pareek

4. Ambulatory Blood Pressure Monitoring: Catching What the Clinic Misses — 26
   Debaprasad Chakrabarti

5. ANOCA/INOCA/MINOCA: The Syndromes of Open Artery Ischemia — 31
   Harinder K Bali, Navdeep S Sidhu

6. Life-threatening Findings on Routine Electrocardiogram Screening in Normal Asymptomatic Persons — 39
   Subhash Chandra

7. Primary Percutaneous Coronary Intervention is Superior to Thrombolysis in ST-elevation Myocardial Infarction—Evidence-based Practice — 52
   Rajesh Vijayvergiya

Section 2: Critical Care

8. Current Sepsis Guidelines: A Comprehensive Review — 61
   AR Balamurugan

9. Vasopressors and Inotropes in the Management of Shock — 68
   T Saravanan

Section 3: Dermatology

10. **Dermatological Manifestations of Diabetes: When Glucose Marks the Skin** — 75
    Satrajit Roy

Section 4: Emergency Medicine

11. **Controversies in Snakebite Management: An Indian Perspective** — 81
    Debasis Chakrabarti, Sayantani Bhadury

Section 5: Endocrinology

12. **Male Osteoporosis: An Under-recognized and Growing Health Concern** — 89
    Pankaj Singhania, Ayush Agarwal

13. **Testosterone: Facts and Myths** — 93
    Ranjodh Gill

14. **Sugar in the Shadows: Rare Tales from the Diabetic Spectrum** — 97
    Ram Babu, Raghavi Abhilesh Bembey

15. **A Missed Diagnosis: Why Primary Aldosteronism Deserves More Attention?** — 103
    Bimal K Agrawal

16. **Beyond Blood Glucose: The Multisystem Magic of SGLT-2 Inhibitors** — 107
    Vijay Kumar

17. **Circadian Rhythm Disruption in Endocrinology** — 113
    Gagan Priya

Section 6: Gastroenterology

18. **Gut Microbiota and Its Role in Immunity** — 123
    Princi Jain, Srinivasa Murthy, SS Dariya

Section 7: General Medicine

19. **Artificial Intelligence in Healthcare: Revolutionizing Medicine and Paving the Way for Future** — 135
    Amandeep Kaur

Section 8: Hematology

20. **Hemophilia: Current Approach and Future Outlook** — 143
    Sudhir Kumar Atri, Piyush Malik

21. **Transfusion Practices in Clinical Medicine** — 148
    Kanchan Bhardwaj, BL Bhardwaj, Harnoor Singh

22. **Hemophagocytic Lymphohistiocytosis: An Overview** — 154
    Rajesh Kumar, Shilpa Atwal

23. **Approach to the Patient with Thrombocytopenia** — 162
    Lovleen Bhatia, Vikas Sharma, Jhanvi Pawar

Section 9: Hepatology

24. **Acute-on-Chronic Liver Failure** — 179
    Ashish Bhagat

Section 10: Infectious Disease

25. **Long COVID** — 187
    Pradeep Agarwal, Ramesh Kumar, Yashraj Saini

26. **Tuberculosis and Other Infections in Uncontrolled Diabetes Mellitus** — 203
    BL Bhardwaj, Rajbir Singh, Prabhpreet Kaur, Kanchan Bhardwaj, RS Bhatia

27. **Decoding the Mystery Fever: A Practical Guide to Pyrexia of Unknown Origin: A Simple Approach to Acute Febrile Illness** — 206
    K Vengadakrishnan

28. **Postexposure Prophylaxis for HIV, Hepatitis B, and Hepatitis C** — 210
    Raminderpal Singh Sibia

29. **Complicated Vivax Malaria** — 220
    Kripa Anna, Vikas Loomba

30. **Controversial Updates in Community-acquired Pneumonia** — 225
    Ben Cherian Mathew, Vikas Loomba

Section 11: Nephrology

31. **Clinician's Approach to Secondary Hypertension** — 235
    RBS Manian

32. **Hyponatremia and Hypernatremia: Emergency Management Updates** — 241
    Kalyan Mitra

Section 12: Neurology

33. **Guillain–Barré Syndrome: Expanding Clinical Spectrum** — 253
    Gurinder Mohan, Kapeesh Khanna, Asra Brar, Sehajnoor Singh

34. **Approach to Myelopathy** — 265
    Ashutosh Kumar Karn, Amit Aggarwal, MPS Chawla

35. **Autonomic Dysfunction in Diabetes Mellitus** — 283
    Jugal Kishor Sharma

36. **Neuromyelitis Optica Spectrum Disorder** — 294
    Prabhjit Kaur, Aastha Takkar

Section 13: Oncology

37. **Chronic Lymphocytic Leukemia** — 303
    Madhuchanda Kar, Suman Meyur

38. **Multiple Myeloma: From Incurable to Potentially Curable** — 309
    Pankaj Malhotra

Section 14: Pregnancy

39. **Diabetes in Pregnancy** — 317
    Preetkanwal Sibia, Vikas Sharma, Ajay Bhaskar

Section 15: Pulmonology

40. **Obstructive Sleep Apnea: What a Physician Needs to Know** — 331
    Puneet Rijhwani, Vidita Kalra, Ram Kishan Jat, Shrikant Chaudhary

41. **Bronchial Asthma: Newer Therapies** — 343
    Paramita Bhattacharya, Subhro Jyoti Mukherjee

42. **6-Minute Walk Test** — 350
    Sonam Spalgais, Prashant Prakash

43. **Interpretation of Spirometry** — 356
    Prashant Prakash, Sonam Spalgais, Abhishek Raj

Section 16: Rheumatology

44. **When should We Escalate the Treatment in Rheumatoid Arthritis from the Traditional DMARDS to Biologics?** 367
    SS Dariya, Aradhana Sharma

45. **Diabetes Mellitus–Rheumatology Interface** 370
    Priyanka Saha, Sumit Sarkar, Sandipan Banik, Sandipan Mondal, Amit Chakraborty, Smarajit Banik

46. **Antiphospholipid Syndrome: A Brief Review** 378
    Partha Sarkar, Poulami Das, Chandrapaul Gupta

47. **Immunoglobulin 4-related Disease** 383
    S Chandrasekar, S Krupha

48. **Red Flags in Rheumatology** 390
    Ritu

49. **The Adventure of Systemic Vasculitis: Care and Clinical Research** 396
    Aman Sharma

Section 17: Urology

50. **Erectile Dysfunction Decoded: Diagnosis to Therapy** 403
    Deepak K Jumani

Scan the QR code to access the Index.

SECTION 1

Cardiology

CHAPTER 1

Reversible Cardiomyopathy: Clinical Insights through Case-based Examples

Ankan Pathak, Aparna Tewari

■ INTRODUCTION

Cardiomyopathy is traditionally viewed as a chronic, often progressive disease that results in ventricular dysfunction, adverse remodeling, and eventual heart failure. However, not all forms of cardiomyopathy are irreversible. Certain etiologies, if recognized early and treated promptly, demonstrate remarkable reversibility with near-complete recovery of ventricular function. This concept has significant therapeutic implications, as timely intervention can transform a potentially debilitating condition into a transient illness with a good prognosis.

Reversible cardiomyopathies encompass a spectrum of entities, including stress-induced (Takotsubo) cardiomyopathy, tachycardia-induced cardiomyopathy, PPCM, toxin- or drug-induced cardiomyopathy, and myocarditis-related transient dysfunction. In clinical practice, differentiating these conditions from irreversible causes is essential to avoid premature labeling of patients as having "end-stage heart failure."

This chapter explores reversible cardiomyopathy through illustrative clinical cases, reviews current evidence, and highlights practical lessons for clinicians.

■ CASE 1: STRESS-INDUCED (TAKOTSUBO) CARDIOMYOPATHY

A 62-year-old woman presented with acute chest pain following intense emotional distress. Electrocardiogram (ECG) revealed ST-segment elevation in precordial leads, and troponin levels were mildly elevated. Coronary angiography, however, showed unobstructed coronary arteries. Left ventriculography demonstrated apical ballooning with basal hyperkinesis, consistent with Takotsubo cardiomyopathy. She received supportive therapy with beta-blockers and angiotensin-converting enzyme (ACE) inhibitors. Within 6 weeks, her left ventricular ejection fraction (LVEF) normalized from 30 to 60%.

Clinical Insights

Takotsubo cardiomyopathy is often triggered by catecholamine surge due to emotional or physical stress.

It mimics acute coronary syndrome, but the absence of culprit coronary lesions differentiates it.

Recovery of systolic function typically occurs within 4–8 weeks, underscoring its reversibility.

Recurrence rates are low but not negligible; hence, long-term follow-up is advised.

CASE 2: TACHYCARDIA-INDUCED CARDIOMYOPATHY

A 45-year-old man presented with progressive dyspnea and palpitations. ECG revealed persistent atrial flutter with a ventricular rate of 140 bpm. Echocardiography showed global hypokinesia with an LVEF of 25%. After radiofrequency ablation restored sinus rhythm, repeat imaging at 3 months showed normalization of ventricular size and an LVEF of 55%.

Clinical Insights

Prolonged tachyarrhythmias such as atrial fibrillation, atrial flutter, or incessant supraventricular tachycardia can cause reversible myocardial dysfunction.

The mechanism is believed to involve abnormal calcium handling, neurohormonal activation, and myocardial energy depletion.

Early rhythm control (ablation, cardioversion, and antiarrhythmic drugs) is key to full recovery.

Delay in treatment risks irreversible remodeling despite rhythm correction.

CASE 3: PERIPARTUM CARDIOMYOPATHY

A 32-year-old primigravida developed breathlessness and ankle edema 2 weeks postpartum. Echocardiography revealed a dilated left ventricle (LV) with an ejection fraction (EF) of 30%. She was treated with diuretics, beta-blockers, and bromocriptine under strict obstetric supervision. Over 9 months, her EF improved to 55%.

Clinical Insights

Peripartum cardiomyopathy is a rare but potentially reversible cardiomyopathy occurring in late pregnancy or early postpartum.

Etiology involves oxidative stress, antiangiogenic signaling (prolactin fragments), and genetic predisposition.

Prognosis varies: One-third recover completely, one third stabilize with persistent dysfunction, and one third progress to advanced heart failure.

Early diagnosis and aggressive therapy improve reversibility; subsequent pregnancies carry a recurrence risk.

CHAPTER 1: Reversible Cardiomyopathy: Clinical Insights through Case-based Examples

CASE 4: ALCOHOLIC AND DRUG-INDUCED CARDIOMYOPATHY

A 48-year-old man with chronic alcohol abuse presented with fatigue and heart failure. Echocardiography showed dilated cardiomyopathy with EF 25%. After strict alcohol cessation and optimal heart failure therapy, his EF improved to 50% over 1 year.

Similarly, a 28-year-old woman treated with anthracycline-based chemotherapy for breast cancer developed LV dysfunction (EF 35%). Initiation of cardioprotective therapy with beta-blockers and ACE inhibitors, along with discontinuation of anthracyclines, led to recovery of EF to 55% within 6 months.

Clinical Insights

Chronic alcohol use, anthracyclines, trastuzumab, and recreational drugs (e.g., cocaine and methamphetamines) can cause cardiomyopathy.

Early withdrawal of offending agents coupled with heart failure therapy often restores function.

Surveillance with echocardiography or cardiac magnetic resonance imaging (MRI) is critical in oncology patients.

Irreversibility occurs with delayed recognition or cumulative toxicity.

CASE 5: MYOCARDITIS-ASSOCIATED TRANSIENT DYSFUNCTION

A 26-year-old man presented with chest pain following a viral prodrome. ECG showed diffuse ST changes; troponin was elevated. Echocardiography demonstrated mild LV dysfunction (EF 40%). Cardiac MRI confirmed myocarditis with edema and late gadolinium enhancement. With supportive therapy, EF normalized to 60% within 3 months.

Clinical Insights

- Viral myocarditis can lead to acute LV dysfunction that often recovers spontaneously.
- Cardiac MRI is instrumental in diagnosis and follow-up.
- Management remains supportive, as immunosuppression is reserved for select cases.
- Identifying patients who progress to chronic dilated cardiomyopathy remains challenging.

PATHOPHYSIOLOGICAL UNDERPINNINGS OF REVERSIBILITY

Several mechanisms explain why certain cardiomyopathies are reversible:
- Myocardial stunning without necrosis—as seen in Takotsubo
- Neurohormonal stress and calcium handling abnormalities—as in tachycardia-induced cardiomyopathy

- Toxin withdrawal—as in alcoholic or anthracycline-induced cases
- Resolution of inflammatory injury—as in myocarditis
- Hormonal modulation—as in PPCM

Unlike irreversible cardiomyopathies where myocyte loss and fibrosis predominate, reversible cases demonstrate transient dysfunction without significant scarring, allowing recovery.

MANAGEMENT PRINCIPLES ACROSS REVERSIBLE CARDIOMYOPATHIES

Early recognition: Mislabeling as idiopathic dilated cardiomyopathy may lead to an inappropriate prognosis.

Trigger removal: Stress control, rhythm correction, abstinence from alcohol/drugs, and discontinuation of cardiotoxic agents

Guideline-directed heart failure therapy: Beta-blockers, ACE inhibitors/angiotensin II receptor blockers (ARBs)/angiotensin receptor–neprilysin inhibitor (ARNI), and mineralocorticoid antagonists support recovery.

Close monitoring: Serial echocardiography and biomarkers guide therapy adjustments.

Patient education: Emphasizing abstinence, adherence, and follow-up ensures long-term benefit.

FUTURE PERSPECTIVES

Emerging imaging modalities such as strain echocardiography and advanced cardiac MRI allow earlier detection of subtle myocardial dysfunction. Biomarkers, including microRNAs and circulating inflammatory mediators, are under study for predicting reversibility. Novel cardioprotective agents in oncology and targeted therapies in PPCM may further improve outcomes.

Artificial intelligence-based algorithms that integrate imaging, electrocardiographic, and biomarker data may soon allow clinicians to predict which patients with acute cardiomyopathy are most likely to recover.

CONCLUSION

Reversible cardiomyopathy represents a critical subset of myocardial disease where accurate diagnosis, timely intervention, and elimination of triggers can result in complete recovery of ventricular function. Stress-induced cardiomyopathy, tachycardia-induced dysfunction, PPCM, drug- and alcohol-related cases, and myocarditis-associated dysfunction all exemplify this principle.

For clinicians, awareness of these conditions prevents premature prognostic pessimism and ensures patients receive the opportunity for recovery. Incorporating case-based recognition, pathophysiological understanding, and evidence-guided management transforms the outlook for patients once thought to face inevitable decline.

FURTHER READINGS

1. Lyon AR, Bossone E, Schneider B, Sechtem U, Citro R, Underwood SR, et al. Current state of knowledge on Takotsubo syndrome: a position statement from the Taskforce on Takotsubo Syndrome of the Heart Failure Association of the ESC. Eur J Heart Fail. 2016;18(1):8-27.
2. Shinbane JS, Wood MA, Jensen DN, Ellenbogen KA, Fitzpatrick AP, Scheinman MM. Tachycardia-induced cardiomyopathy: a review of animal models and clinical studies. J Am Coll Cardiol. 1997;29(4):709-15.
3. Sliwa K, Hilfiker-Kleiner D, Petrie MC, Mebazaa A, Pieske B, Buchmann E, et al. Current state of knowledge on aetiology, diagnosis, management, and therapy of peripartum cardiomyopathy: a position statement from the Heart Failure Association of the ESC. Eur J Heart Fail. 2010;12(8):767-78.
4. Armenian SH, Lacchetti C, Barac A, Carver J, Constine LS, Denduluri N, et al. Prevention and monitoring of cardiac dysfunction in survivors of adult cancers: American Society of Clinical Oncology Clinical Practice Guideline. J Clin Oncol. 2017;35(8):893-911.
5. Caforio ALP, Pankuweit S, Arbustini E, Basso C, Gimeno-Blanes J, Felix SB, et al. Current state of knowledge on myocarditis: a position statement of the ESC Working Group on Myocardial and Pericardial Diseases. Eur Heart J. 2013;34(33):2636-48.

Unmasking Masked Hypertension

HK Aggarwal, Deepak Jain, Vishnu Menon

INTRODUCTION

Traditionally, office (clinic) based blood pressure (BP) recording was considered the gold standard for the diagnosis of hypertension. But the reliance on office BP measurements alone often underestimates an individual's true cardiovascular risk. Aynman and Goldshine in 1940 highlighted inconsistencies between clinic BP and home BP recordings obtained prior to the initiation of antihypertensive therapy. These observations underlined the limitations of single-point, office-based measurements of BP and emphasized the potential of home blood pressure monitoring (HBPM) to provide a more representative picture of an individual's usual BP profile, thereby improving diagnostic precision and therapeutic decision-making.

Hinman and colleagues introduced the first device for ambulatory blood pressure monitoring (ABPM) in 1962, which marked a turning point in hypertension research and clinical practice, as it enabled continuous BP measurement over a 24-hour period in real-world settings. Parameters such as daytime BP, nighttime BP, and circadian BP variability derived from ABPM have proven to be superior predictors of left ventricular hypertrophy, chronic kidney disease progression, and cerebrovascular events. As a result, both HBPM and ABPM are now recognized as indispensable tools for the accurate diagnosis, risk stratification, and management of hypertension, moving beyond the inherent limitations of clinic-based BP measurements.

The spectrum of BP values measured through ABPM and HBPM has led to the identification of additional hypertension, i.e., masked hypertension that is often missed in clinical practice. It is the reverse white coat effect, defined as normal office BP but elevated out-of-office BP.

GUIDELINES FOR OUT-OF-OFFICE BLOOD PRESSURE

There are considerable variations among various guidelines regarding the technique of out-of-office measurement of BP and the threshold values for the diagnosis of hypertension **(Table 1)**. In contrast to the National Institute

TABLE 1: Definition of masked hypertension.

	Office BP	Out-of-office measurement	
		Ambulatory BP Measurement	Home BP Measurement (Avg)
NICE UK 2019 guidelines	<140/90 mm Hg	Day/Awake ABPM > 140/90 mm Hg	>140/90 mm Hg
		• Day/Awake ABPM ≥ 135/85 mm Hg	
ESC/ESH 2018 guidelines	<140/90 mm Hg	• Night /Asleep BP ≥ 120/70 mm Hg	≥135/85 mm Hg
		• 24-hour mean BP ≥ 130/80 mm Hg	
ACC 2017 guidelines	≤120–129/80 mm Hg after 3 months lifestyle modification and suspected masked hypertension	Day/Awake ABPM ≥ 130/80 mm Hg	≥130/80 mm Hg

(ABPM: ambulatory blood pressure monitoring; ACC: American College of Cardiology; BP: blood pressure; ESC/ESH: European Society of Cardiology/European Society of Hypertension; NICE UK: National Institute for Health and Care Excellence, United Kingdom)

for Health and Care Excellence (NICE) UK 2019 and American College of Cardiology/American Heart Association (ACC/AHA) 2017 hypertension guidelines, which prefer day BP, the European Society of Cardiology and the European Society of Hypertension (ESC/ESH) 2018 guidelines consider either day, night, or 24-hour mean BP for the diagnosis of hypertension.

PHENOTYPES OF MASKED HYPERTENSION

- *Masked hypertension (MH):* Untreated individuals with normal office BP but elevated out-of-office BP
  - *Daytime/Awake MH*: Normal office BP with elevated daytime ambulatory BP (d135/85 mm Hg)
  - *Nocturnal/Nighttime MH*: Normal office BP with elevated nighttime ambulatory BP [with elevated nighttime ambulatory BP (≥120/70 mm Hg)]
  - *24-hour MH*: Normal office BP with elevated 24-hour average ambulatory BP (≥130/80 mm Hg)
- *Masked uncontrolled hypertension (MUCH):* Treated patients with controlled office BP but uncontrolled out-of-office BP
  - *Isolated daytime MUCH (ID-MUCH)*: Controlled office BP, daytime BP ≥135/85 mm Hg, nighttime BP <120/70 mm Hg
  - *Isolated nighttime MUCH (IN-MUCH)*: Controlled office BP, daytime BP < 135/85 mm Hg, nighttime BP ≥120/70 mm Hg <135/mm Hg
  - *Day-night MUCH (DN-MUCH)*: Controlled office BP, daytime BP ≥135/85 mm Hg and nighttime BP ≥120/70 mm Hg

MERITS VERSUS DEMERITS OF AMBULATORY BLOOD PRESSURE MONITORING AND HOME BLOOD PRESSURE MONITORING IN DIAGNOSIS OF MASKED HYPERTENSION

Table 2 shows the merits and demerits of HBPM and ABPM in masked hypertension.

PREVALENCE

The reported prevalence of MH is highly variable, reflecting differences in study populations, ethnicity, diagnostic definitions, and the measurement modalities employed, including HBPM, ABPM, and distinctions between daytime, nocturnal, and 24-hour recordings. In the general population, prevalence estimates typically range from 8.5 to 16.6%, but rise substantially in individuals with high-normal clinic BP, where rates are as high as 30.4%. When comprehensive 24-hour ABPM, including nocturnal assessment, is employed, prevalence rates may approach 50%. A systematic review by Thakkar et al. further emphasized the influence of ethnicity, demonstrating a markedly higher prevalence among individuals of African descent, with rates up to 52.5% in African Americans, compared to substantially lower values in Koreans (5.7%) and Omanis (6%). Importantly, geographic differences are also apparent, with Asian populations consistently demonstrating higher prevalence than Western counterparts, a finding attributed to greater salt sensitivity, distinctive cardiometabolic risk profiles, and environmental stressors that exacerbate out-of-office BP elevations.

The presence of comorbidities also contributes significantly to variation in prevalence. Prevalence rates of MH include 30% among patients with obstructive sleep apnea, 13.3–66.4% in individuals with diabetes, 7–32.8% in chronic kidney disease, 15% in those undergoing hemodialysis, and 16–39% in renal transplant recipients.

TABLE 2: ABPM versus HBPM in the diagnosis of masked hypertension.		
Feature	ABPM	HBPM
Monitoring period	24–48 hours continuous	Multiple days (5–7), twice daily
Nocturnal BP	Captures sleep patterns of BP	No nocturnal data
Diagnostic standard	Gold standard	Good alternative
Masked HTN detection	Superior	Limited
Patient comfort	Poor—may disrupt sleep	Excellent—convenient
Cost and access	High cost, limited availability	Low cost, widely available
Long-term monitoring	Not suitable	Ideal for titration
Clinical use	Diagnosis and detection	Follow-up and long-term management

(ABPM: ambulatory blood pressure monitoring; BP: blood pressure; HBPM: home blood pressure monitoring; HTN: hypertension)

PATHOPHYSIOLOGY

The pathophysiology of MH is multifactorial, involving dysregulation of autonomic control, circadian rhythm abnormalities, vascular dysfunction, and the influence of behavioral and environmental stressors.

- *Autonomic nervous system dysregulation*: Excessive sympathetic activation during daily activities or at night contributes to elevated out-of-office BP, while attenuated parasympathetic modulation leads to higher heart rate and impaired nocturnal dipping. Some individuals also exhibit "white-coat calmness," wherein a paradoxical reduction of BP occurs in the clinic setting.
- *Circadian rhythm abnormalities*: Nondipping or reverse-dipping nocturnal BP patterns, often linked to obesity, sleep apnea, or high dietary salt intake, play a critical role. Nighttime sympathetic overactivity further drives elevations in nocturnal and early morning BP, which remain undetected by office-based measurements.
- *Vascular dysfunction*: Endothelial dysfunction and increased arterial stiffness, reflected by higher pulse wave velocity, contribute to elevated ambulatory BP. Impaired vasodilatory responses during physical or mental stress amplify real-life BP surges compared to the clinic environment.
- *Behavioral and lifestyle factors*: Smoking, alcohol, caffeine intake, psychosocial stress, poor sleep quality, and physical inactivity are key contributors.
- *Environmental and occupational stressors*: Daily-life stressors such as occupational demands, commuting, and socioeconomic pressures lead to significant daytime elevations in ambulatory BP. These situational influences explain why patients may present with normal office readings yet exhibit hypertension in real-world conditions.

RISK FACTORS

- High-normal office BP (130–139/85–89 mm Hg) has the strongest association with MH.
- Obesity and overweight individuals with a body mass index (BMI) > 25 kg/m^2
- Persons of African ethnicity
- Diabetes mellitus increases the risk of MH via autonomic dysfunction and increased arterial stiffness
- Chronic kidney disease
- *Dietary and lifestyle factors such as*:
  - High sodium diet
  - Irregular meals
  - Alcohol use
  - Smoking

CLINICAL SIGNIFICANCE AND ADVERSE OUTCOMES

Individuals with MH have the highest likelihood of progressing to sustained hypertension compared to those who have normal BP or white coat hypertension. MH is also strongly associated with increased cardiovascular events, target organ damage, and mortality, closely resembling the risks seen in sustained hypertension. Patients with MH demonstrate higher left ventricular mass and increased carotid intima-media thickness, both of which indicate early vascular remodeling and atherosclerotic changes. Observational studies have also shown an increased risk of stroke, greater arterial stiffness, and elevated markers such as cystatin C and urine albumin-to-creatinine ratio in patients with MH independent of traditional cardiovascular risk factors. Collectively, these findings highlight MH as a high-risk condition requiring timely recognition and comprehensive management strategies similar to sustained hypertension.

DIAGNOSTIC APPROACH

Accurate clinic BP measurement remains fundamental to the diagnosis of MH. Healthcare providers must use validated devices, ensure proper cuff sizing according to arm circumference, and perform manual measurements in patients with pulse irregularities like atrial fibrillation, as automated devices may provide inaccurate readings in these conditions. While clinic BP is essential, it is insufficient on its own, and both ABPM and HBPM play a crucial role in the detection and management of MH. ABPM remains the reference standard, offering a comprehensive evaluation of 24-hour, daytime, and nocturnal BP, thereby improving diagnostic accuracy and prognostic value. When using ABPM, at least two measurements per hour should be taken during the person's waking hours, and the average value of at least 14 measured values noted during the person's usual awake hours should be used to diagnose hypertension.

Home blood pressure monitoring, however, is a validated and pragmatic alternative, particularly relevant in resource-limited countries such as India, where ABPM may be limited by cost and accessibility; it supports screening and diagnostic confirmation when ABPM is unavailable or poorly tolerated. When using HBPM, it must be ensured that for each BP recording, two consecutive measurements are taken at least 1 minute apart with the person seated. A practical approach involves screening with well-performed HBPM and reserving ABPM for patients in whom MH or nocturnal hypertension is suspected or where overall cardiovascular risk is high.

EVIDENCE-BASED MANAGEMENT STRATEGIES

Management of MH should pair lifestyle change with guideline-directed therapy. Priorities include reducing dietary sodium to <2.3 g/day (ideally 1.5 g/day) with culturally tailored counseling for Indian cooking and processed foods; achieving BMI under 25 kg/m^2 through traditional diets emphasizing whole grains, legumes, and vegetables; engaging in at least 150 min/week of moderate aerobic activity; practicing stress-reduction (yoga, meditation, and breathing); and limiting alcohol to <2 drinks/day for men and 1 for women. For pharmacotherapy, initiate first-line agents—angiotensin converting enzyme (ACE) inhibitor or angiotensin receptor blocker (ARB), a calcium channel blocker, or a thiazide/thiazide-like diuretic—and favor single-pill combinations to reach <130/80 mm Hg efficiently. Confirm diagnosis with repeat out-of-office measurements within 2 months;

obtain electrocardiogram (ECG), lipids, kidney function, and urinalysis; monitor with regular HBPM and selective ABPM; and adjust treatment based on out-of-office averages rather than clinic readings.

CONCLUSION

Masked hypertension is a prevalent and underrecognized driver of cardiovascular risk, with outcomes comparable to sustained hypertension. Evidence consistently demonstrates its association with increased cardiovascular morbidity, target organ damage, and mortality when compared to sustained normotension or white coat hypertension. MH often remains outside the focus of routine clinical practice, largely due to challenges in detection and the absence of universally standardized diagnostic protocols.

Current international guidance underlines the importance of out-of-office BP measurement as central to identifying MH. ABPM remains the gold standard, particularly for capturing nocturnal BP patterns, while HBPM is a pragmatic, scalable approach for screening and longitudinal follow-up. In practice, integrating both modalities provides an effective pathway, particularly in resource-limited settings such as India, where systematic home-based monitoring supported by selective use of ABPM can enable timely diagnosis.

Prompt screening of high-risk individuals with home BP measurements and ABPM, the diagnosis of MH, and the initiation of treatment may mitigate the adverse cardiovascular effects of MH.

FURTHER READINGS

1. 2025 AHA/ACC/AANP/AAPA/ABC/ACCP/ACPM/AGS/AMA/ASPC/NMA/PCNA/SGIM Guidelines for the prevention, detection, evaluation and management of high blood pressure in adults: a report of the American College of Cardiology/American Heart Association Joint Committee on Clinical Practice Guidelines. Circulation. 2025;152.
2. Penmatsa KR, Biyani M, Gupta A. Masked hypertension: lessons for the future. Ulster Med J. 2020;89:77-82.
3. Parati G, Ochoa JE. White coat and masked hypertension. In: Bakris GL, Sorrentino MJ (Eds). Hypertension: A Companion to BRAUNWALD'S HEART DISEASE, 3rd edition. Philadelphia: Elsevier; 2018. pp. 104-14.
4. Palla M, Saber H, Konda S, Briasoulis A. Masked hypertension and cardiovascular outcomes: an updated systematic review and meta-analysis. Integr Blood Press Control. 2018;11:11-24.
5. Kario K, Hoshide S, Haimoto H, Eguchi K, Iwashima Y, Ishikawa J, et al. Office-masked nocturnal hypertension defined by home blood pressure and cardiovascular risk: the J-HOP Nocturnal Blood Pressure Study. JACC Adv. 2024;3:101352.
6. Huang JF, Zhang DY, An DW, Li MX, Liu CY, Feng YQ, et al. Efficacy of antihypertensive treatment for target organ protection in patients with masked hypertension (ANTI-MASK): a multicentre, double-blind, placebo-controlled trial. EClinMed. 2024;74:102736.

CHAPTER 3

The Indian Guidelines for the Management of Dyslipidemia: Evolution and Updates (2016–2023)

Raman Puri, KK Pareek

INTRODUCTION

India carries one of the highest burdens of premature coronary artery disease globally, with onset nearly a decade earlier compared to high-income countries. This accelerated risk is attributable to a unique lipid profile characterized by lower high-density lipoprotein cholesterol (HDL-C), higher triglycerides, and the predominance of small dense low-density lipoprotein (LDL) particles, which are more atherogenic. Moreover, Indians frequently exhibit metabolic syndrome, insulin resistance, and central obesity, compounding their cardiovascular risk. These factors highlight the inadequacy of applying Western guidelines in their original form to Indian populations. Hence, the Lipid Association of India (LAI) took the initiative to release its first expert consensus statement in 2016, and subsequently in 2020, and 2023, adapting global evidence to local realities.

LIPID ASSOCIATION OF INDIA EXPERT CONSENSUS STATEMENT ON MANAGEMENT OF DYSLIPIDEMIA IN INDIANS 2016: PART 1

A distinctive feature of the 2016 consensus was its emphasis on practical applicability. Rather than relying exclusively on 10-year risk scores such as the Framingham Risk Score or the atherosclerotic cardiovascular disease (ASCVD) risk estimator, which have not been validated for the Indian population, the LAI recommendations incorporated the unique characteristics of the Indian population. This approach considered major risk factors such as smoking, diabetes, hypertension, low HDL, and family history to stratify patients into risk categories. In addition, lifetime risk assessment was encouraged at a younger age, to identify those who may not appear at high short-term risk but are predisposed to early ASCVD events.

For management of lipid disorders, the 2016 consensus statement advocated high-intensity statins as first-line treatment in high and very high-risk groups. Ezetimibe was suggested as an adjunct in patients not meeting targets, while fibrates were reserved for patients with high triglycerides. Non-HDL-C was recognized as a co-primary target, particularly in patients with high triglycerides.

The consensus statement part 2 in 2017 addressed specific clinical groups, patients with acute coronary syndromes (ACSs), familial hypercholesterolemia (FH), chronic kidney disease (CKD), and heart failure (HF), recommending tailored approaches.

KEY HIGHLIGHTS

Risk assessment: The LAI proposed a simpler, more practical risk factor counting approach tailored for use in the Indian population rather than complex risk calculators. The statement also highlighted the importance of considering lifetime risk, especially for younger individuals who might have a low 10-year risk but face a high lifelong burden of disease.

RECOGNITION OF LOW-DENSITY LIPOPROTEIN-C AS PRIMARY GOAL AND NON-HIGH-DENSITY LIPOPROTEIN-C AS A CO-PRIMARY GOAL

Lipid targets: The consensus statement recommended more aggressive LDL-C targets than many international guidelines at the time. For individuals at very high risk in the Indian population, the LDL-C target was set at <50 mg/dL, whereas for those at high risk, the target was <70 mg/dL. The LAI also recognized non-HDL cholesterol as a crucial co-primary target, acknowledging its importance as a part of atherogenic lipoproteins.

JUSTIFICATION FOR LOWER LOW-DENSITY LIPOPROTEIN-C GOALS IN SOUTH ASIAN POPULATIONS

The recommendation for more stringent LDL-C targets in South Asians, including Indian population, is supported by several key factors specific to this population:
- *Distinct cardiometabolic profile*: South Asians exhibit a unique and particularly high-risk lipid profile. This phenotype is characterized by reduced HDL-C and elevated triglyceride levels, with LDL-C being normal or only mildly increased. Importantly, there is a higher prevalence of small dense LDL particles, which are more atherogenic and are frequently seen as part of the metabolic syndrome. Collectively, these features contribute to a significantly increased risk of premature coronary artery disease (CAD) in this population.
- *Epidemiological evidence*: Large-scale studies, such as the INTERHEART study, have demonstrated that the average non-fasting LDL-C level in South Asian populations is approximately 10 mg/dL lower than that observed in Western cohorts. Despite this lower baseline LDL-C, South Asians continue to experience a higher incidence of CAD. This suggests that, at any given LDL-C level, South Asians experience a higher cardiovascular risk than their Western counterparts, highlighting the need for lower LDL-C targets in this population.
- *The "Lower is Better" paradigm*: Multiple large clinical trials have provided compelling evidence for a direct relationship between achieved LDL-C levels and reduction in cardiovascular events. For every 40 mg/dL decrease in

LDL-C, there is an associated 21% reduction in major cardiovascular events, regardless of the starting LDL-C. The absolute reduction in LDL-C is the most critical determinant, rather than the percentage reduction from baseline.

ADDRESSING THE "LOWER BASELINE" CHALLENGE

Because South Asians generally have lower baseline LDL-C yet higher cardiovascular risk than Western populations, achieving the same LDL-C target would still leave South Asians at comparatively greater risk. For example, whereas reducing LDL-C from 100 to 60 mg/dL in a Western individual confers a ~21% reduction in cardiovascular events, a South Asian starting at 90 mg/dL would need to reach 50 mg/dL to achieve a comparable benefit.

Accordingly, LDL-C targets for South Asians are set approximately 10 mg/dL lower to achieve comparable reductions in cardiovascular risk.

COMPREHENSIVE RISK CONSIDERATIONS

Lower LDL-C goals for South Asians also reflect the influence of additional risk factors such as central obesity, insulin resistance, and the tendency toward atherogenic dyslipidemia.

These factors further elevate cardiovascular risk beyond LDL-C alone. Western guidelines may not adequately account for the distinct risk profile of the Indian population, potentially leading to higher residual risk if applied without adaptation. Accordingly, the LAI recommends more aggressive LDL-C targets to address the specific risk landscape and to better prevent premature cardiovascular events through a tailored, population-specific approach.

THERAPEUTIC IMPLICATIONS

In line with these recommendations, statin therapy is affirmed as the first-line treatment for dyslipidemia, with an emphasis on the use of high-intensity statins where indicated. The critical role of lifestyle interventions, including dietary modification, smoking cessation, and increased physical activity, was strongly emphasized. For patients who do not achieve target lipid levels with statin therapy alone, non-statin agents such as ezetimibe were recommended as adjuncts **(Flowchart 1 and Table 1)**.

TREATMENT GOALS AND STATIN INITIATION THRESHOLDS ACCORDING TO ATHEROSCLEROTIC CARDIOVASCULAR DISEASE RISK CATEGORIES

Limitations

While groundbreaking, the 2016 statement had its limitations. It considered non-conventional risk factors such as lipoprotein(a), non-alcoholic fatty liver disease [now termed metabolic dysfunction-associated steatotic liver disease (MASLD)], and environmental factors.

CHAPTER 3: The Indian Guidelines for the Management of Dyslipidemia: Evolution and...

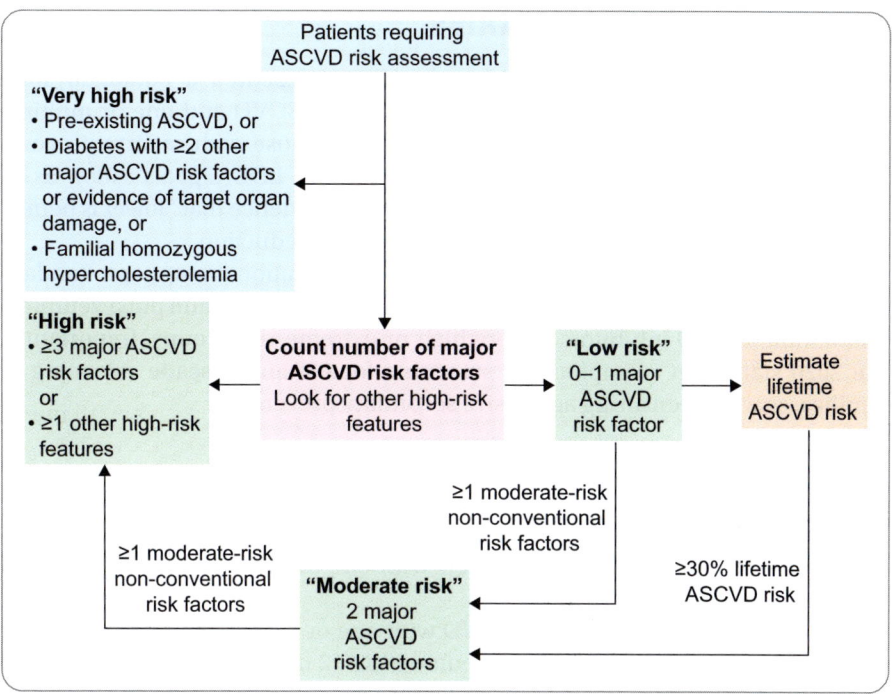

FLOWCHART 1: Recommended approach to atherosclerotic cardiovascular disease (ASCVD) risk stratification in Indians: Consensus Statement Part 1 (2016).

TABLE 1: Recommended approach to atherosclerotic cardiovascular disease (ASCVD) risk stratification in Indians: Consensus Statement Part 1 (2016).

Risk category	Primary goal—LDL-C		Co-primary goal—non-HDL-C	
	LDL-C (mg/dL)	Non-HDL-C (mg/dL)	LDL-C (mg/dL)	Non-HDL-C (mg/dL)
	Treatment goals		Consider drug therapy	
Very high risk	<50	<80	≥50 (preferably in all)	≥80 (preferably in all)
High risk	<70	<100	≥70 (preferably in all)	≥100 (preferably in all)
Moderate risk	<100	<130	≥100	≥130
Low risk	<100	<130	≥130*	≥160*

*After an initial adequate nonpharmacological intervention for at least 3 months.

Additionally, the role of subclinical atherosclerosis detection through imaging (like coronary calcium scoring) was not yet a central part of risk stratification.

It addressed special populations including FH, CKD, NAFLD (MASLD), HF, and others.

PUSHING THE BOUNDARIES

The introduction of "extreme risk" categories represented a paradigm shift. extreme risk A included patients with established ASCVD and one or multiple high-risk features, while extreme risk B included those with recurrent events despite achieving LDL <50 mg/dL. For these groups, LDL-C goals as low as 30 mg/dL were suggested, reflecting mounting global evidence that "lower is better" and possibly "the lowest is best", with respect to LDL reduction.

This consensus statement also highlighted combination therapy as a standard approach in such patients, recommending the routine use of statin plus ezetimibe, and adding PCSK9 inhibitors in very high or extreme risk groups. Importantly, the 2020 statement reemphasized screening for FH and cascade screening in families, as well as ensuring aggressive secondary prevention.

KEY ADDITIONS

- *Extreme risk group:* This new category was divided into two sub-groups:
  - *Category A:* Patients with ASCVD with one or more features of high-risk group.
  - *Category B:* Patients with ASCVD with one or more features of very high-risk group or recurrent ACS events within 12 months despite an LDL-C of less than 50 mg/dL or polyvascular disease.
- *Even lower LDL-C goals:* For this new extreme risk group, the consensus statement proposed even lower LDL-C goals. The recommended goal for category A was an LDL-C of less than 50 mg/dL and optional goal of ≤30 mg/dL, whereas the recommended goal for category B was an LDL-C of ≤30 mg/dL, reflecting the "lower the better" paradigm that was gaining traction in global trials.
- *Non-statin agents:* The role of non-statin therapies was expanded. The guidelines now gave greater recognition to adding agents such as PCSK9 inhibitors for patients who could not reach these more aggressive targets with statin and ezetimibe regimens.
- *Other lipid measures:* While LDL-C and non-HDL-C remained the primary targets and co-primary goals respectively, apolipoprotein B (Apo B) was also recognized as a valuable secondary goal in specific clinical settings.

The 2020 consensus statement directly addressed the need for more intensive treatment strategies for Indians with multiple and complex risk factors, building on the framework established in 2016 **(Flowchart 2 and Table 2)**.

The 2023 Consensus Statement IV

The Latest Revolution

A major innovation in 2023 was the acknowledgment of non-conventional and Indian-specific risk factors. These included non-alcoholic fatty liver disease (renamed MASLD), metabolic syndrome, elevated lipoprotein(a), high triglycerides (>150 mg/dL), and even environmental factors such as air pollution, which has been linked to accelerated atherosclerosis in urban India.

Risk factors/markers

Major ASCVD risk factors:
- Age ≥45 years in males and ≥55 years in females
- Family history of premature ASCVD
- Current cigarette smoking or tobacco use
- High blood pressure
- Low HDL-C

Other high-risk features:
- Diabetes with 0–1 other major ASCVD risk factors and no evidence of target organ damage
- CKD stage 3B or 4
- Familial hypercholesterolemia (other than familial homozygous hypercholesterolemia)
- Extreme of a single risk factor
- Coronary calcium score >300 HU
- Non-stenotic carotid plaque
- Lipoprotein (a) ≥50 mg/dL

Moderate risk non-conventional risk factors:
- Coronary calcium score 100–299 HU
- Increased carotid IMT
- Lipoprotein (a) 20–49 mg/dL
- Impaired fasting glucose*
- Increased waist circumference**
- Apolipoprotein B ≥110 mg/dL
- hsCRP ≥2 mg/L***

Risk group

Low risk	Moderate risk	High risk	Very high risk	Extreme risk	
0–1 major ASCVD risk factor and life-time CVD risk <30%	• 2 major ASCVD risk factors • Low risk group with ≥1 moderate risk nonconventional risk factor • Life-time CVD risk ≥30%	• ≥3 major ASCVD risk factors • 2 major ASCVD risk factors with ≥1 moderate risk nonconventional risk factor • ≥1 other high-risk features	• Preexisting ASCVD • Diabetics with ≥2 other major ASCVD risk factors or evidence of target organ damage • Familial homozygous hypercholesterolemia	Category A	Category B
				CAD with ≥1 feature of high-risk group	CAD with ≥1 feature of very high-risk group or recurrent ACS (within one year) despite LDL-C ≤50 mg/dL or polyvascular decease

* A fasting blood sugar level from 100 to 125 mg/dL. It should be confirmed by repeat testing.

** Waist circumference is to be measured at the superior border of the iliac crest just after expiration. Increased waist circumference is defined as >90 cm in men and >80 cm in women. If increased waist circumference is the only risk factor, it should again be measured after 6 months after initiating heart healthy lifestyle measures.

*** On two occasions at least 2 weeks apart. For reclassifying moderate risk group only.

FLOWCHART 2: Updated Risk Stratification Approach Recommended by Lipid Association of India: Consensus Statement Part III (2020).

Note: Clinical judgment to be used if the patient has atherosclerotic peripheral arterial disease instead of coronary artery disease.

TABLE 2: Newer treatment goals and statin initiation thresholds based on the risk categories proposed by LAI Consensus Statement Part III (2020).

Risk category	Treatment goals		Recommend drug therapy	
	LDL-C mg/dL	Non-HDL mg/dL	LDL-C mg/dL	Non-HDL mg/dL
Extreme risk group	<50 (optional goal ≤30)	<80 (optional goal ≤60)	≥50	≥80
Category A	≤30	≤60	>30	>60
Very high risk	<50	<80	≥50	≥80
High risk	<70	<100	≥70	≥100
Moderate risk	<100	<130	≥100	≥130
Low risk	<100	<130	≥130*	≥160*

*After an adequate nonpharmacological intervention for at least 3 months.

Furthermore, the consensus equated subclinical atherosclerosis, detected by coronary artery calcium (CAC) scoring, carotid intima-media thickness, or femoral plaque ultrasound, with established ASCVD, thus significantly broadening the scope of individuals considered high or very high risk.

The most notable addition was the introduction of the Extreme Risk Category C. This group encompassed patients experiencing cardiovascular events despite maintaining LDL-C ≤30 mg/dL on maximal therapy. For these rare but critical cases, an unprecedented LDL-C goal of 10–15 mg/dL was recommended, emphasizing the relentless pursuit of lower LDL levels. This mirrors global trials such as FOURIER and ODYSSEY, which demonstrated continued benefit at very low-LDL concentrations, without major safety concerns.

The 2023 consensus also advocated for rapid LDL-C lowering in ACS patients, recommending that LDL goals be achieved within 2 weeks of the acute event, rather than the more relaxed timelines previously suggested. Early initiation of combination therapy was thus endorsed.

KEY NEW ELEMENTS

- *Risk stratification*: The 2023 statement places a much stronger emphasis on lifetime ASCVD risk over the 10-year risk. It also formally includes major ASCVD risk factors, high risk conditions, and risk modifiers.
- *Subclinical atherosclerosis*: Detection of plaque by vascular doppler, CAC score, or ABI <0.9 is now treated as equivalent to established ASCVD, warranting similarly aggressive management.
- *Even more aggressive targets:* A new extreme risk category C was added for patients who continue to have CV events despite achieving an LDL-C ≤30 mg/dL despite all guidelines directed medical treatment and required interventions. For this group, the consensus statement recommended ultralow LDL goals of 10–15 mg/dL.
- *Screening:* The consensus statement recommends initiating lipid screening earlier and conducting it more frequently, beginning at age 20 years for the general population and even earlier in individuals with a family history of high cholesterol or premature CAD. It also advocates including lipoprotein(a) in initial risk assessments and for certain populations.

THERAPY TIMING

The consensus underscores the critical importance of promptly achieving LDL-C targets, particularly in high-risk scenarios. For individuals presenting with ACS, it is recommended that LDL-C goals be attained within the first 2 weeks following the event. This accelerated approach reflects the urgent need to reduce cardiovascular risk during the vulnerable post-ACS period.

For patients who do not have clinical evidence of ASCVD, the guidelines advise that LDL-C targets should be reached within three months or sooner. This proactive strategy aims to minimize the progression of risk and ensure that patients receive timely and effective lipid management, tailored to their risk profile **(Flowchart 3)**.

Risk factors/markers		
Major ASCVD risk factors: • Age ≥45 years in males and ≥55 years in females • Current cigarette smoking or tobacco use* • High blood pressure* • Low HDL-C	High-risk features: • Family history of premature ASCVD • CKD stage 3B or 4 • Apolipoprotein B >130 mg/dL • Extreme elevation of a single risk factor† • Lipoprotein (a) ≥50 mg/dL • Metabolic syndrome • Non-alcoholic fatty liver disease with fibrosis grade 2 or 3 fibrosis • CACS 1–99 and <75th percentile	Risk modifiers: • Lipoprotein (a) 20–49 mg/dL • Impaired fasting glucose (fasting blood glucose 100–125 mg/dL)‡ • Increased waist circumference (>90 cm in men, >80 cm in women)§ • hsCRP >2 mg/L¶ • Plasma triglycerides >150 mg/dL fasting or >175 mg/dL. non-fasting • Rheumatoid arthritis, psoriasis, and spondyloarthropathies • Premature menopause, pre-eclampsia, gestational diabetes, PCOS • High polygenic risk score • Air pollution • Human immunodeficiency virus infection

Risk group					
Low risk	Moderate risk	High risk	Very high risk	Extreme risk	
• 0–1 major ASCVD risk factor • LDL-C 100–129 mg/dL • Non-HDL-C 130–159 mg/dL • Life-time CVD risk <30%#	• 2 major ASCVD risk factors • LDL-C 130–159 mg/dL • Non-HDL-C 160–189 mg/dL • Low-risk group with ≥1 risk modifier or lifetime ASCVD risk >30%	• ≥3 major ASCVD risk factors • LDL-C 160–189 mg/dL • Non-HDL-C 190–219 mg/dL • Diabetes with 0–1 major ASCVD risk factors • 2 major ASCVD risk factor + ≥1 risk modifier • Any 1 high-risk feature	• Diabetes with target organ damage • Diabetes with ≥2 major ASCVD risk factors • CACS 100–299 or >75th percentile if CACS 1–99 • ≥2 high risk features • Established ASCVD (obstructive or nonobstructive$) • Heterozygous FH or LDL-C ≥190 mg/dL	Category A ↓ • ASCVD with ≥1 feature of high-risk group • CACS ≥300 • Homozygous FH	Category B ASCVD with: • ≥1 feature of very high-risk group • Recurrent ACS • Polyvascular disease • Homozygous FH
				Recurrent ASCVD event despite LDL-C around 30 mg/dL These patients require special consideration, please see the text for more details. Category C	

*High blood pressure has been defined as office blood pressure ≥140/90 mm Hg or on anti-hypertensive treatment. Tobacco use includes cultural tobacco, such as *bidis, paan, gutka*, etc.

†Extreme of a single risk factor defined as regular smoking >1 pack of cigarettes per day or blood pressure >180/110 mm Hg

‡Should be confirmed by repeat testing

§Waist circumference is to be measured at the superior border of the iliac crest just after expiration. If increased waist circumference is the only risk factor, it should be measured again 6 months after initiating heart-healthy lifestyle measures

¶On two occasions at least 2 weeks apart

#Estimated using the QRISK3-lifetime cardiovascular risk calculator (https://qrisk.org/lifetime/)

$Includes stenotic or non-stenotic carotid, femoral or coronary arterial plaques, as well as an ankle-brachial index <0.9 in either leg.

FLOWCHART 3: Updated 2023 Atherosclerotic Cardiovascular Disease (ASCVD) risk stratification approach recommended by the Lipid Association of India Consensus Statement Part III (2023) **(Table 3).**

(ACS: acute coronary syndrome; ASCVD: atherosclerotic cardiovascular disease; CACS: coronary artery calcium score; CKD: chronic kidney disease; FH: familial hypercholesterolemia; HDL-C: high-density lipoprotein cholesterol; hsCRP: high sensitivity C-reactive protein; LDL-C: low-density lipoprotein cholesterol; non-HDL-C: non-high-density lipoprotein cholesterol; PCOS: polycystic ovary syndrome).

TABLE 3: Treatment goals for low-density lipoprotein (LDL)-C and non-high-density lipoprotein (HDL)-C and initiating threshold of statins and other lipid lowering therapies based on risk categories as proposed by the Lipid Association of India in the Consensus statement IV (2023).

Risk category	Treatment goals		Recommend drug therapy	
	LDL-C mg/dL	Non-HDL mg/dL	LDL-C mg/dL	Non-HDL mg/dL
Extreme risk group	<50 (optional goal ≤30)	<80 (optional goal ≤60)	≥50	≥80
Category A	≤30	≤60	>30	>60
Category C	10–15 mg/dL	40–45 mg/dL	>10–15 mg/dL	>40–45 mg/dL
Very high risk	<50	<80	≥50	≥80
High risk	<70	<100	≥70	≥100
Moderate risk	<100	<130	≥100	≥130
Low risk	<100	<130	≥130*	≥160*

*After an adequate nonpharmacological intervention for at least 3 months.

PRACTICAL IMPLICATIONS FOR CLINICIANS

The 2023 LAI consensus statement recommends that Indian clinicians adopt a proactive, individualized, and intensive approach to dyslipidemia management, which entails:

- *Thinking beyond the 10-year risk:* Assess lifetime risk, especially for younger patients with multiple risk factors.
- *Comprehensive risk assessment and early detection:* The 2023 statement advocates for the use of all available tools in risk stratification and management of ASCVD. This includes the systematic incorporation of major ASCVD risk factors, identification of emerging high-risk features, and the inclusion of new risk modifiers in the risk assessment process. Clinicians are encouraged to take a comprehensive approach that goes beyond traditional risk factors, effectively capturing the full spectrum of patient risk.

  Additionally, where feasible, screening for subclinical atherosclerosis is recommended. Techniques such as vascular Doppler studies, CAC scoring, or ankle-brachial index (ABI) measurements can help detect early plaque formation before clinical disease manifests. Incorporating these advanced diagnostic strategies supports earlier intervention and more personalized risk management.
- *Screening early:* Start lipid screening at age 18–20 and be vigilant in patients with a family history.
- *Setting aggressive targets:* Aim for LDL-C goals of <50 mg/dL for most high-risk patients and consider ultralow goals of 10–15 mg/dL for those in the extreme risk C category.

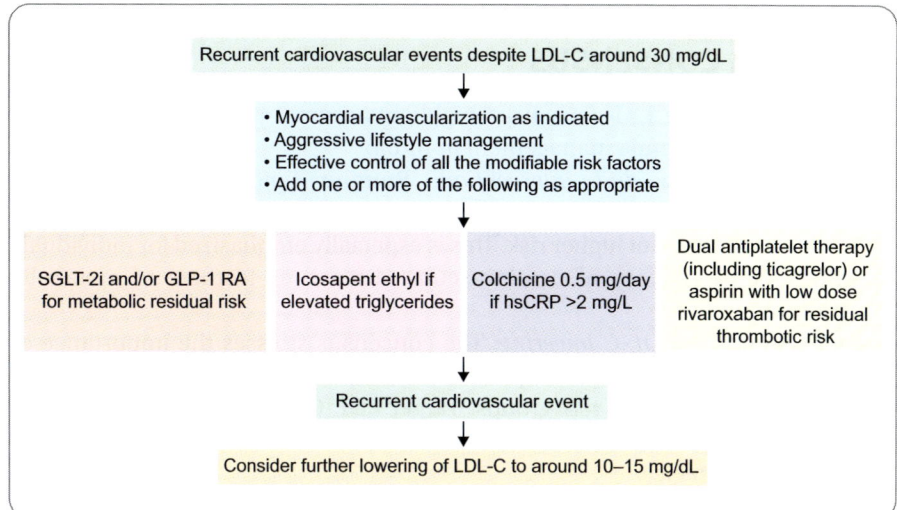

FLOWCHART 4: Management strategy for patients suffering recurrent cardiovascular events despite achieving a very low level of low-density lipoprotein (LDL)-C (extreme risk group-C): Consensus statement IV (2023).

(GLP-1 RA: glucagon-like peptide-1 receptor agonists: hsCRP: high sensitivity C-reactive protein: LDL-C: low-density lipoprotein cholesterol: SGLT-2i: sodium-glucose cotransporter-2 inhibitors)

- *Aggressive LDL-C target setting:* In alignment with the evolving approach to dyslipidemia management, clinicians are encouraged to adopt stringent LDL-C target levels for optimal cardiovascular risk reduction. For very high-risk patients, the goal should be to achieve LDL-C levels below 50 mg/dL. This assertive target is designed to maximize the reduction in atherosclerotic risk and reflects the consensus that lower LDL-C levels yield greater cardiovascular protection.
- Additionally, for individuals classified within the new extreme risk C category, clinicians should consider aiming for ultralow LDL-C levels, specifically in the range of 10–15 mg/dL. This recommendation acknowledges the exceptionally high risk faced by these patients and emphasizes the importance of intensive lipid-lowering strategies to prevent future cardiovascular events **(Flowchart 4)**.
- *Utilizing combination therapy:* Do not hesitate to add ezetimibe or consider PCSK9 inhibitors earlier, especially in high-risk patients, to achieve targets.

While these guidelines present a clear path forward, it is crucial to acknowledge the practical challenges, such as the cost of newer therapies, patient adherence, and the availability of advanced diagnostic tools. Nonetheless, the evolution of the LAI's consensus statements reflects a commendable effort to tailor global scientific evidence to the unique needs of the Indian population, offering a more effective strategy to combat the rising tide of cardiovascular disease.

KEY PRINCIPLES OF THE EVOLVING LIPID ASSOCIATION OF INDIA CONSENSUS

The evolution of the LAI consensus highlights several pivotal changes in the approach to dyslipidemia management in India:

- *Earlier screening and intervention*: Routine lipid screening is now recommended to begin as early as age 18–20 years, with prompt intervention for those identified at higher risk. This is especially emphasized for individuals with a family history of cardiovascular disease or features of metabolic syndrome.
- *More aggressive LDL-C lowering*: The consensus stresses the importance of aggressively lowering LDL-C, particularly in patients classified as very high risk or within extreme risk groups. Target LDL-C levels are set significantly lower than in previous guidelines, reflecting a shift toward more intensive risk reduction strategies.
- *Lower LDL-C and non-HDL-C goals compared to western guidelines*: Indian guidelines advocate for lower LDL-C and non-HDL-C targets than those commonly recommended in Western populations, tailoring recommendations to the unique risk profile of Indian patients.
- *Incorporation of subclinical atherosclerosis and risk modifiers*: The assessment of subclinical atherosclerosis through imaging and the consideration of non-traditional risk modifiers are integrated into risk stratification, enabling more precise and individualized care.
- *Greater reliance on combination therapy*: Combination lipid-lowering therapy is increasingly prioritized, particularly for patients at high or extreme risk, to help ensure that stringent lipid targets are achieved.
- *Low-density lipoprotein-C as the primary goal, with non-HDL-C and Apo B as important co-targets*: LDL-C remains the central focus for lipid management, but non-HDL-C is recognized as a key co-target, especially in patients with elevated triglycerides. Additionally, Apo B is considered an important secondary marker for risk assessment and therapeutic monitoring.

IMPLICATIONS FOR CLINICAL PRACTICE IN INDIA

For clinicians, these evolving recommendations translate into a proactive and preventive approach to cardiovascular risk management. Early and regular screening from young adulthood, particularly in high-risk populations, has become standard practice. LDL-C continues to be the principal target for therapy, but attention to non-HDL-C and ApoB values provides additional granularity and aids in tailoring treatment, especially for individuals with mixed dyslipidemia. The use of combination therapy is increasingly expected, especially for those in extreme risk categories. Collectively, these strategies embody a model of preventive cardiology that is not only aggressive and early but also intended to be lifelong in its application.

CONCLUSION

The evolution of the LAI consensus statements illustrates a progressive transformation in dyslipidemia management for the Indian population. Beginning in 2016, the guidelines established risk models specifically designed for Indian patients, acknowledging the distinct cardiometabolic characteristics prevalent in the Indians. This India-specific approach provided a practical foundation for clinicians to address cardiovascular risk more accurately.

The 2020 consensus marked a significant advancement by introducing extreme risk categories and setting ambitious LDL cholesterol targets, with recommendations for levels as low as ≤30 mg/dL. This bold move signaled a shift toward more aggressive lipid-lowering strategies, prioritizing intensive risk reduction for those most vulnerable to cardiovascular events.

In 2023, the guidelines were further refined to incorporate non-conventional risk factors, advanced imaging techniques, and ultralow LDL cholesterol goals. This comprehensive model enabled a more nuanced assessment of cardiovascular risk, considering subclinical disease and additional risk modifiers beyond traditional measures.

Taken together, these developments underscore the necessity for earlier intervention, more aggressive treatment targets, and highly individualized management strategies in the Indian context. The trajectory of the LAI guidelines—from pragmatic adaptations in 2016 to the adoption of ultralow LDL targets in 2020, and the integration of advanced risk stratification in 2023—highlights the dynamic nature of dyslipidemia management in India. The approach remains statement responsive to global evidence while being carefully tailored to the unique cardiovascular risk profile of Indian patients.

FURTHER READINGS

1. Iyengar SS, Puri R, Narasingan SN, Wangnoo SK, Mohan V, Mohan JC, et al. Lipid Association of India Expert Consensus Statement on Management of Dyslipidemia in Indians 2016: Part 1. J Assoc Physicians India. 2016;64(3 suppl):7-52.
2. Yusuf S, Hawken S, Ounpuu S, Dans T, Avezum A, Lanas F, et al. Effect of potentially modifiable risk factors associated with myocardial infarction in 52 countries (the INTERHEART study): case-control study. Lancet. 2004;364(9438):937-52.
3. Cholesterol Treatment Trialists' (CTT) Collaboration; Baigent C, Blackwell L, Emberson J, Holland LE, Reith C, et al. Efficacy and safety of more intensive lowering of LDL cholesterol: a meta-analysis of data from 170,000 participants in 26 randomised trials. Lancet. 2010;376(9753):1670-81.
4. Iyengar SS, Puri R, Narasingan SN, Nair DR, Mehta V, Mohan JC, et al. Lipid Association of India (LAI) expert consensus statement on management of dyslipidaemia in Indians 2017: part 2. Clin Lipidol. 2017;12(1):56-109.
5. Puri R, Mehta V, Iyengar SS, Narasingan SN, Duell PB, Sattur GB, et al. Lipid Association of India Expert Consensus Statement on Management of Dyslipidemia in Indians 2020: Part III. J Assoc Physic India. 2020;68(11[Special]):8-9.

CHAPTER 4

Ambulatory Blood Pressure Monitoring: Catching What the Clinic Misses

Debaprasad Chakrabarti

■ INTRODUCTION

Ambulatory blood pressure monitoring (ABPM) involves automated, non-invasive measurements taken every 15–30 minutes during the day and hourly at night over a 24-hour period, providing 50–100 readings that reflect true blood pressure behavior during daily activities and sleep.

Ambulatory blood pressure monitoring uses validated oscillometric devices with cuff inflation, allowing patients to maintain normal routines while data is stored for analysis. This method addresses the limitations of office blood pressure, which represents only a snapshot and is prone to observer error or patient anxiety.

Unlike clinic measurements, ABPM minimizes observer bias and provides averages for 24-hour, daytime, and nighttime periods.

Common errors include incorrect cuff size, improper patient positioning, or rushed measurements.

■ METHODOLOGY AND NORMAL VALUES

Ambulatory blood pressure monitoring devices are worn on the upper arm and programmed to take readings at specified intervals, with patients keeping a diary of activities to contextualize data. Valid sessions require at least 70% successful readings, with nighttime defined by patient-reported sleep times or fixed intervals such as 10 PM to 6 AM. The 2025 Thai Hypertension Society guidance recommends at least seven valid nighttime readings for reliable nocturnal assessment.

Normal ABPM values, per 2024 ESC guidelines, include:
- 24-hour averages below 130/80 mm Hg
- Daytime below 135/85 mm Hg, and
- Nighttime below 120/70 mm Hg

These thresholds are lower than office values due to the absence of clinical stress, and deviations indicate hypertension phenotypes. In Indian settings, ABPM helps overcome office measurement inaccuracies common in diverse populations.

CHAPTER 4: Ambulatory Blood Pressure Monitoring: Catching What the Clinic Misses

Hypertension is diagnosed with ABPM if:
- 24-hour averages ≥130/80 mm Hg
- Daytime ≥135/85 mm Hg,
- Nighttime ≥120/70 mm Hg, and
- Morning average ≥135/85

KEY ADVANTAGES OF AMBULATORY BLOOD PRESSURE MONITORING OVER CLINIC MEASUREMENTS

Ambulatory blood pressure monitoring offers superior diagnostic accuracy, with higher sensitivity and specificity for hypertension diagnosis.

It is a better predictor of cardiovascular events and mortality, as it correlates more strongly with organ damage and prognosis.

Cost-effective in the long term, by avoiding misdiagnosis and unnecessary treatment.

LIMITATIONS OF CLINIC BLOOD PRESSURE

Clinic blood pressure measurements provide only 1–2 readings in an artificial environment, often inflating values due to patient anxiety. This leads to overdiagnosis in 10–30% of cases and misses true elevations in daily life, limiting prognostic accuracy.

Office readings fail to capture blood pressure variability, nocturnal dips, or activity-related surges, which are critical for cardiovascular risk prediction. Studies confirm ABPM's better association with left ventricular hypertrophy and stroke risk compared to clinic values.

WHITE COAT HYPERTENSION

White coat hypertension occurs when office blood pressure exceeds 140/90 mm Hg, but ABPM shows less than 130/80 mm Hg, affecting 10–30% of clinic-diagnosed hypertensives. This condition, more common in elderly women and non-smokers. ABPM confirms this phenotype, preventing overtreatment and reducing costs.

Patients with white coat hypertension often lack target organ damage, unlike sustained hypertensives, highlighting ABPM's diagnostic precision. Guidelines recommend ABPM for all with borderline office readings to identify this entity. Long-term follow-up shows 20–40% conversion to sustained hypertension over years.

MASKED HYPERTENSION

Masked hypertension features normal office readings below 140/90 mm Hg but ABPM shows >130/80 mm Hg, present in 15–30% of normotensives and carrying risks similar to sustained hypertension. It is prevalent in diabetics, smokers,

TABLE 1: Contrasting features of WCHTN and MHTN, including blood pressure readings, cardiovascular (CV) risk, and recommended management strategies.

Aspect	WCHTN	MHTN
Office BP	≥140/90 mm Hg	<140/90 mm Hg
ABPM BP	Normal (<130/80 mm Hg)	Elevated (≥130/80 mm Hg)
Prevalence	10–30% of clinic hypertensives	15–30% of normotensives
CV risk	Lower than sustained HTN	Similar to sustained HTN
Management	Lifestyle, monitor annually	Antihypertensive therapy

and those with chronic kidney disease, often involving isolated nocturnal elevation. ABPM detects this hidden risk, enabling timely intervention to prevent cardiovascular events.

In African Americans, masked hypertension reaches 34% prevalence, associated with left ventricular mass increase. The 2025 European guidelines stress ABPM screening for high-normal office pressures to uncover this phenotype. Untreated masked hypertension doubles stroke and heart disease risk compared to true normotension **(Table 1)**.

NOCTURNAL HYPERTENSION AND CIRCADIAN RHYTHMS

Nocturnal hypertension, defined as nighttime ABPM ≥120/70 mm Hg, affects 7–19% and predicts cardiovascular events better than daytime values.
- If BP drops >10% at night, the person is called a "dipper",
- If the nighttime drop is <10%, the person is a "non-dipper",
- If BP is higher at night than during the day, it is called "reverse dipping".

Ambulatory blood pressure monitoring identifies non-dippers and reverse dippers, indicating higher risk of organ damage (heart/kidney).

EARLY MORNING BLOOD PRESSURE SURGE

Heart attacks, strokes, and sudden cardiac deaths often happen in early morning. ABPM identifies whether a sharp BP rise in the morning predicts these events, major studies such as PIUMA and PAMELA did not find it to be an independent risk.

ROLE IN RESISTANT HYPERTENSION

In patients uncontrolled on ≥3 drugs, ABPM identifies true resistance versus white-coat effect (~33% have normal 24-hour BP).

Clinic overestimates resistance, leading to inappropriate escalation; ABPM guides better management and eligibility for procedures such as renal denervation.

True resistant cases show more organ damage and worse prognosis.

CHAPTER 4: Ambulatory Blood Pressure Monitoring: Catching What the Clinic Misses

CLINICAL APPLICATIONS OF AMBULATORY BLOOD PRESSURE MONITORING

Ambulatory blood pressure monitoring evaluates resistant hypertension by confirming true elevations and assessing treatment efficacy over 24 hours. It monitors therapy response, detecting inadequate nocturnal coverage in 40–50% of patients.

In pregnancy and pediatrics, ABPM refines diagnosis where office readings vary.

For elderly patients, ABPM distinguishes white coat effects from true issues, reducing polypharmacy. In clinical trials, ABPM standardizes endpoints beyond office control. It also quantifies variability, a marker for stroke risk.

The 2024 ESC recommends ABPM for all with office hypertension confirmation. In Asia, ABPM aids in metabolic syndrome screening for masked cases. Postural hypotension detection via ABPM prevents falls in vulnerable groups.

COST-EFFECTIVENESS ANALYSIS

A 2023 analysis showed ABPM reduces total costs versus clinic monitoring by avoiding overtreatment of white coat cases and preventing complications. Long-term models (>10 years) demonstrate dominance in women and elderly.

CURRENT GUIDELINES AND RECOMMENDATIONS

The 2024 ESC guidelines mandate ABPM for elevated office readings, with thresholds
<115/65 mm Hg for 24-hour control. AHA/ACC 2017 positions ABPM as the reference for out-of-office assessment. NICE requires ABPM confirmation before therapy initiation.

In 2025 Thai guidance, ABPM classifies phenotypes such as non-dippers for targeted management. Chinese 2020 standards define nocturnal thresholds at ≥120/70 mm Hg. Repeat ABPM every 3–6 months for nocturnal cases.

Guidelines emphasize ABPM in high-risk groups such as diabetics. Integration with home monitoring enhances reproducibility. Global adoption varies, with Europe leading at 50% usage.

TECHNOLOGICAL ADVANCES AND FUTURE DIRECTIONS

Recent ABPM devices feature wireless connectivity and AI for real-time analysis, improving compliance. Cuffless wearables emerge, using optical sensors for continuous monitoring without inflation. The 2025 review highlights smartphone apps for data integration.

Future focuses on home nocturnal devices matching ABPM accuracy, reducing clinic visits. Telemedicine platforms enable remote ABPM review. Validation studies ensure new tech meets prognostic standards.

AI algorithms predict dipping patterns from baseline data. Pediatric and wearable cuffless options expand applications. Challenges include affordability in low-resource settings.

CONCLUSION

Ambulatory blood pressure monitoring transforms hypertension management by revealing clinic-missed dynamics like masked and nocturnal elevations, reducing misdiagnosis by 20–40%. Its integration into guidelines underscores superior risk stratification over office methods. As technology evolves, ABPM will become standard, catching subtle threats to cardiovascular health.

Ambulatory blood pressure monitoring catches critical patterns such as white-coat, masked, nocturnal, and morning hypertension that clinic measurements miss.

It provides superior prognostic value, diagnostic accuracy, and guides more effective treatment.

Essential for accurate hypertension management to reduce CV risks and avoid misdiagnosis.

FURTHER READINGS

1. Anchala R, Kannuri NK, Pant H, Khan H, Franco OH, Di Angelantonio E, et al. Hypertension in India: a systematic review and meta-analysis of prevalence, awareness, and control of hypertension. J Hypertens. 2014;32(6):1170-7.
2. Mohan B, Aslam N, Ralhan U, Sharma S, Gupta N, Singh VP, et al. Office blood pressure measurement practices among community health providers (medical and paramedical) in northern district of India. Indian Heart J. 2014;66(4):401-7.
3. Tocci G, Presta V, Figliuzzi I, Attalla El Halabieh N, Battistoni A, Coluccia R, et al. Prevalence and clinical outcomes of white-coat and masked hypertension: analysis of a large ambulatory blood pressure database. J Clin Hypertens. 2018;20(2):297-305.
4. Turner JR, Viera AJ, Shimbo D. Ambulatory blood pressure monitoring in clinical practice: a review. Am J Med. 2015;128(1):14-20.
5. Sogunuru GP, Kario K, Shin J, Chen CH, Buranakitjaroen P, Chia YC, et al. Morning surge in blood pressure and blood pressure variability in Asia: evidence and statement from the HOPE Asia Network. J Clin Hypertens. 2019;21(2):324-34.

CHAPTER 5

ANOCA/INOCA/MINOCA: The Syndromes of Open Artery Ischemia

Harinder K Bali, Navdeep S Sidhu

■ INTRODUCTION

Cardiovascular diseases (CVDs) are the foremost cause of global mortality and morbidity, accounting for roughly one-quarter to one-third of the adult deaths in most countries of the world including India. Ischemic heart disease (IHD) is responsible for majority of the disease burden related to CVDs and is characterized by myocardial ischemia, either at rest or minimal exertion [leading to acute coronary syndromes (ACS)], or with significant exertion/stress [leading to chronic coronary syndromes/diseases (CCS/CCD)].

The vast majority of cases of myocardial ischemia are related to atherosclerotic obstructive coronary artery disease (CAD) (defined classically as >50% diameter stenosis in one or more major epicardial coronary arteries), which causes limitation to the blood flow either on exertion (as in CCS/CCD), or when more severe/unstable plaque, to limitation at rest as in ACS. However, recently there has been an increased recognition of a growing group of coronary ischemic syndromes which do not fit into this traditional paradigm of epicardial coronary syndromes and are responsible for myocardial ischemia in a sizeable proportion (reaching up to 50–70% in some studies) of IHD patients. This group including angina with nonobstructive coronary arteries (ANOCA), ischemia with nonobstructive coronary arteries (INOCA), and myocardial infarction with nonobstructive coronary arteries (MINOCA) is the focus of present chapter.

Terminology and Definitions

Angina with nonobstructive coronary arteries is characterized by the presence of clinical symptoms of myocardial ischemia (often angina, or its equivalent like dyspnea) in the absence of obstructive epicardial CAD, including functional assessment of intermediate stenosis using physiological measures such as fractional flow reserve (FFR) or instant wave-free ratio (IFR). INOCA is its counterpart with demonstrable evidence of myocardial ischemia using noninvasive stress tests such as stress electrocardiography, stress echocardiography, or nuclear imaging. The terms ANOCA and INOCA are often used interchangeably, but some experts prefer to use ANOCA, as ischemia is often implied but not readily demonstrated on stress testing.

TABLE 1: The spectrum of non-obstructive coronary artery disease.			
Entity	Anginal symptoms	Documented ischemia	Cardiac biomarkers
ANOCA	+	-	-
INOCA	+	+	-
MINOCA	+	+	+

The term MINOCA is used to identify the cases of acute myocardial infarction (AMI) (as evidenced by the rise in cardiac biomarkers such as troponins) in the absence of obstructive CAD **(Table 1)**.

ANGINA WITH NONOBSTRUCTIVE CORONARY ARTERIES/ISCHEMIA WITH NONOBSTRUCTIVE CORONARY ARTERIES

Prevalence

Angina with nonobstructive coronary arteries/INOCA are fairly common, but underappreciated and under-reported. Recent studies have revealed that ANOCA occurs in about 40–70% of the patients undergoing coronary angiography for angina, and INOCA is seen in 20–30% of these patients. Patients with ANOCA/INOCA are often younger with fewer traditional CVD risk factors compared to their counterparts with obstructive CAD. ANOCA/INOCA is more prevalent in women, probably related to differences in hormonal milieu and vascular biology. Asian individuals, particularly of Japanese and Korean ethnicity, have higher susceptibility to vasospastic causes of ANOCA/INOCA.

Pathophysiological Basis (Fig. 1)

Coronary arterial circulation is composed of three major components: Epicardial arteries—500 µm to 5 mm in size, prearterioles—100-500 µm, and intramyocardial arterioles—<100 µm. The epicardial coronary arteries, constituting only 10% of the coronary circulation volume, function mainly as conduits and offer very little resistance to the blood flow in the unobstructed state. The microcirculation (prearterioles and arterioles) makes up for 90% of the coronary vascular bed and is the major site of resistance to the blood flow. These vascular segments adjust the vascular resistance, and therefore, the blood flow, according to the metabolic demands of the myocardial tissue, often leading to demand induced increase in the blood flow to nearly five times in the healthy individuals.

Although often multifactorial, the predominant mechanisms in ANOCA/INOCA include coronary microvascular dysfunction (CMD) or epicardial coronary vasospasm (vasospastic angina).

Coronary microvascular dysfunction may be categorized as structural or functional. The structural form (sometimes known as cardiac syndrome Y) is nonendothelium dependent and is related to structural remodeling of the microcirculation such as arteriolar thickening, rarefaction of the microcirculation,

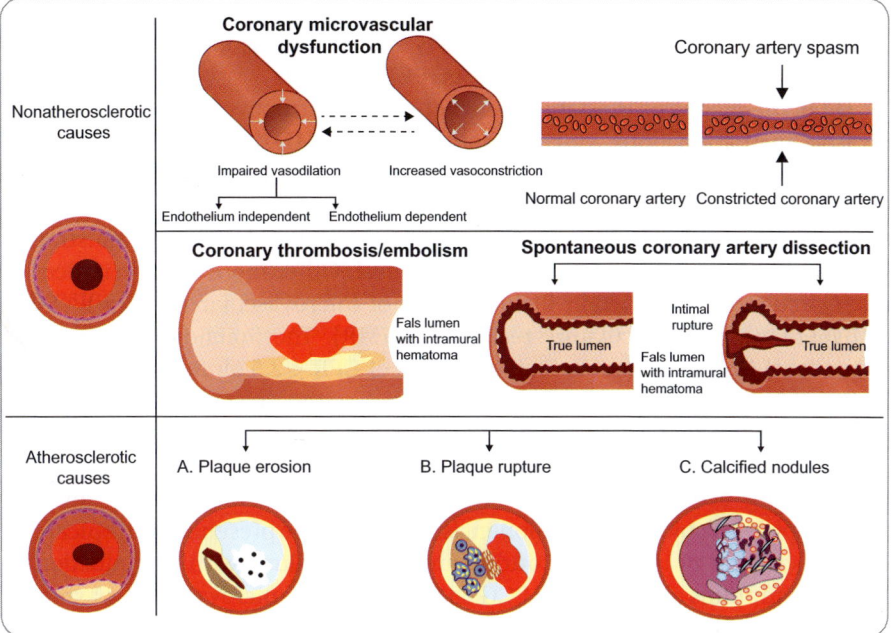

FIG. 1: Pathophysiology of open artery ischemic syndromes.

Source: Tudurachi A, Anghel L, Tudurachi BS, Zăvoi A, Ceasovschih A, Sascău RA, et al. Beyond the Obstructive Paradigm: Unveiling the Complex Landscape of Nonobstructive Coronary Artery Disease. J Clin Med. 2024;13(16):4613.

and perivascular fibrosis, often resulting from long-term interplay of traditional CV risk factors such as hypertension, smoking, dyslipidemia, or diabetes mellitus. These changes lead to increase in the index of microcirculatory resistance (IMR) and impaired coronary flow reserve (CFR). The functional form (sometimes called the cardiac syndrome X or microvascular angina) is often mediated by the endothelial dysfunction in which there is attenuation (or in severe cases reversal) of the physiological microcirculatory vasodilatation in response to a variety of endogenous and exogenous stimuli.

The epicardial coronary vasospasm is related to enhanced vasoreactivity of the vascular smooth muscle cells to a variety of stimuli including smoking, stress, cold exposure, drugs, and hyperventilation.

Less common causes may include atherosclerotic triggers [such as plaque disruption (includes rupture/erosion/calcified nodules) with nonobstructive disease due to activity of intrinsic fibrinolytic system], spontaneous coronary artery dissection (SCAD), coronary thrombosis (as seen in hypercoagulability disorders) or embolism. The events of plaque disruption may lead to vasoconstriction or distal embolization.

Clinical Assessment and Diagnostic Approach

The patients with ANOCA/INOCA often present with angina (or its equivalents such as dyspnea), often indistinguishable from patients with obstructive CAD.

The electrocardiogram may reveal ischemic ST-T changes. Ischemia might be demonstrable on noninvasive stress tests such as stress electrocardiography, stress echocardiography, or nuclear tests (PET/SPECT).

Often the diagnosis is established when a nonobstructive CAD is found on an invasive angiogram along with a demonstration of CMD or vasospasm on further testing. CFR is the ratio of coronary blood flow during hyperemia versus at rest and represents the ability of microcirculation to increase the blood flow in response to an increased demand. It is the most important index for demonstrating CMD and a CFR <2.5 is considered pathological. Other more specific indices of microcirculatory dysfunction include index of microvascular resistance (IMR) or hyperemic microcirculatory resistance (HMR). The functional (endothelial dependent) CMD is characterized by values of CFR < 2.5 along with IMR < 25/HMR < 2.5, whereas structural CMD is implied by the presence of slow flow on angiogram or CFR <2.5 along with IMR > 25/HMR > 2.5.

Coronary vasospastic components may be demonstrated by provocative testing using acetylcholine, ergonovine, or hyperventilation during invasive angiography. An epicardial component is implied by the presence of an epicardial vasoconstriction of >90% seen during angiography along with reproduction of anginal symptoms and ischemic ECG changes, while a microvascular spasmodic component is suggested by the occurrence of ischemic symptoms and ECG changes in the absence of visual epicardial narrowing.

Treatment

In the absence of large, dedicated trials and specific guidelines, the treatment of ANOCA/INOCA includes an individualized management depending upon the underlying pathophysiology and the associated CVD risk factors. Major components of the management are lifestyle changes, control of CVD risk factors (smoking cessation, weight management, control of hypertension, diabetes, and dyslipidemia) along with pharmacotherapy.

Traditional antianginal therapies include beta-blockers, calcium channel blockers (CCBs), and nitrates. The vasodilating (through nitric oxide release) and antioxidant beta-blockers such as nebivolol or carvedilol may be of particular use in these patients. In patients with inadequate response, a CCB or a long-acting nitrate may be added. Second-line antianginals such as ranolazine or trimetazidine may be tried in resistant cases. Ivabradine may be useful to control heart rate in some patients especially that intolerant to beta-blockers or rate lowering CCBs. Also, there is some evidence to suggest that angiotensin-converting enzyme inhibitors (ACE inhibitors), angiotensin II receptor blockers (ARBs), and statins may improve endothelial dysfunction and prevent vasospasm.

In patients with predominant vasospastic components, beta-blockers (especially nonselective) should be avoided, and CCBs are the first-line antianginal agents along with nitrates. Nicorandil may also be useful in some resistant cases.

In patients with evidence of atherosclerosis on angiograms, the use of antiplatelet and lipid-lowering therapy such as statins is indicated.

Newer therapies being investigated include endothelin receptor antagonists (zibotentan), Rho-kinase inhibitors (fasudil), and xanthine derivates (like aminophylline). Also, the use of coronary sinus reducer devices to treat CMD is also being investigated, with dedicated randomized control trials (RCTs) like SERRA-I and A-Flux reducer likely to shed more light on this topic in the near future.

Outcome/Prognosis

The prognosis of patients with ANOCA/INOCA is variable and depends upon the underlying cause and variability of response to the treatment. In general, these patients have lower mortality rates compared to patients with obstructive CAD, but higher than the general population.

MYOCARDIAL INFARCTION WITH NONOBSTRUCTIVE CORONARY ARTERIES

Diagnostic Criteria

Refer to **Figure 2**.

Prevalence

It may be challenging to estimate the true prevalence of MINOCA due to evolving diagnostic criteria, non-uniformity of troponin assay usage in patients with suspected ACS and variability in sensitivity of troponin assay across healthcare systems. The estimated prevalence ranges from 5 to 15% of AMI cases. Compared to patients with AMI due to obstructive CAD, MINOCA patients are younger, more likely to be women and have lower prevalence of dyslipidemia, but similar prevalence of other CVD risk factors.

Pathophysiology

The pathophysiological basis of MINOCA may include a non-obstructive epicardial disease, CMD or miscellaneous causes like Takotsubo or other cardiomyopathies, myocarditis or troponin assay discrepancies **(Fig. 3)**. Many of these overlap with those of ANOCA/INOCA and in general, any ANOCA/INOCA causes when severe and/or persistent may lead to myocardial necrosis, troponin elevation and thus, by definition, MINOCA.

AMI defined by the Fourth universal definition of MI criteria	Nonobstructive coronary arteries on angiography	Absence of other cause of the acute presentation
• Rise and or fall in cTN values with at least one value above the 99° percentile URL • Evidence of myocardial ischemia	Absence of stenotic lesion angiographically 50% or greater in the major epicardial coronary artery	• Myocarditis • Takotsubo syndrome • Pulmonary embolism • Sepsis

FIG. 2: Diagnostic criteria for MINOCA.

Source: Parlati ALM, Nardi E, Sucato V, Madaudo C, Leo G, Rajah T, et al. ANOCA, INOCA, MINOCA: The New Frontier of Coronary Syndromes. J Cardiovasc Dev Dis. 2025;12(2):64.

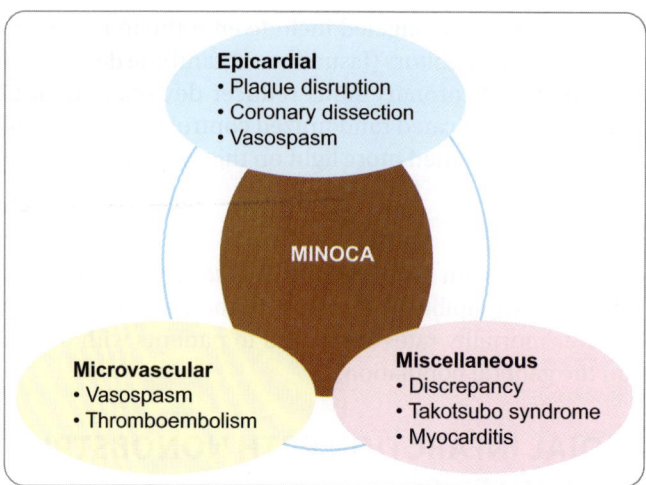

FIG. 3: The mechanisms of MINOCA.
Source: Parlati ALM, Nardi E, Sucato V, Madaudo C, Leo G, Rajah T, et al. ANOCA, INOCA, MINOCA: The New Frontier of Coronary Syndromes. J Cardiovasc Dev Dis. 2025;12(2):64.

Diagnostic Approach: The Traffic Light Approach

Myocardial infarction with nonobstructive coronary arteries is a working diagnosis and emphasizes the need for further evaluation to understand the mechanism of patient's clinical presentation. The traffic light algorithm by American Heart Association (AHA) stresses the red signal, yellow signal, and green signal approach a patient with MINOCA. An initial patient with MINOCA (positive troponin, ischemic background, and nonobstructive CAD) is in red zone and underscores the need to rule out alternative causes of troponin elevation such as sepsis, renal dysfunction, and pulmonary embolism. After this step, the yellow signal zone starts and if the physician still considers the MI as the most probable diagnosis, the angiograms should be reassessed carefully to look for an un-noticed obstructive CAD/coronary thrombus or emboli/SCAD. A functional assessment of the left ventricle (LV) with echocardiography or LV angiography should be done. A cardiac magnetic resonance (CMR) should be considered if available. A CMR, although not compulsory, helps in diagnosing an infract with certainty, besides ruling other causes of clinical presentation such as myocarditis, Takotsubo syndrome, or other cardiomyopathies. After excluding the alternative diagnosis, the clinical reaches the green zone, where if available, further work-up to elicit the mechanism of MINOCA such as intravascular imaging [optical coherence tomography (OCT) and intravascular ultrasound (IVUS)] or coronary functional assessment to diagnose CMD (as detailed above) is considered.

Treatment

There is absence of large dedicated RCTs or consensus guidelines for treatment of MINOCA. Antiplatelet therapy in the form of low-dose aspirin and lipid-lowering therapy (statins, etc.) is recommended (similarly to the patients with AMI due to obstructive CAD) especially in patients with evidence of atherosclerosis on angiography or intravascular imaging. However, the role of dual antiplatelet therapy is disputed and is not generally recommended. Similarly the use of ACE inhibitors or ARBs is not uniformly recommended. In cases with demonstrated CMD/vasospasm, a treatment similar to that adopted for ANOCA/INOCA (as discussed above), may be initiated.

Prognosis

The prognosis of MINOCA patients depends on the underlying mechanism and outcomes may be better than that seen in patients with MI due to obstructive CAD. Active research is going on in this field.

CONCLUSION

Angina with nonobstructive coronary arteries/INOCA/MINOCA are syndromes of myocardial ischemia with nonobstructive CAD and have gained increased attention in recent years. It is an area of active scientific research to unravel its pathophysiology and to guide dedicated management strategies in the future.

FURTHER READINGS

1. Mensah GA, Fuster V, Murray CJ, Roth GA; Global Burden of Cardiovascular Diseases and Risks Collaborators. Global Burden of Cardiovascular Diseases and Risks Collaborators. Global burden of cardiovascular diseases and risks, 1990–2022. J Am Coll Cardiol. 2023;82:2350-473.
2. Rao SV, O'Donoghue ML, Ruel M, Rab T, Tamis-Holland JE, Alexander JH, et al. 2025 ACC/AHA/ACEP/NAEMSP/SCAI Guideline for the Management of Patients With Acute Coronary Syndromes: A Report of the American College of Cardiology/American Heart Association Joint Committee on Clinical Practice Guidelines. Circulation. 2025;151(13):e771-862.
3. Virani SS, Newby LK, Arnold SV, Bittner V, Brewer LC, Demeter SH, et al. 2023 AHA/ACC/ACCP/ASPC/NLA/PCNA Guideline for the Management of Patients With Chronic Coronary Disease: A Report of the American Heart Association/American College of Cardiology Joint Committee on Clinical Practice Guidelines. Circulation. 2023;148(9):e9-119.
4. Byrne RA, Rossello X, Coughlan JJ, Barbato E, Berry C, Chieffo A, et al. ESC Scientific Document Group. 2023 ESC Guidelines for the management of acute coronary syndromes. Eur Heart J. 2023;44(38):3720-826.
5. Vrints C, Andreotti F, Koskinas KC, Rossello X, Adamo M, Ainslie J, et al. ESC Scientific Document Group. 2024 ESC Guidelines for the management of chronic coronary syndromes. Eur Heart J. 2024;45(36):3415-537.
6. Pepine CJ. ANOCA/INOCA/MINOCA: Open artery ischemia. Am Heart J Plus. 2023;26:100260.
7. Parlati ALM, Nardi E, Sucato V, Madaudo C, Leo G, Rajah T, et al. ANOCA, INOCA, MINOCA: The New Frontier of Coronary Syndromes. J Cardiovasc Dev Dis. 2025;12(2):64.
8. Kunadian V, Chieffo A, Camici PG, Berry C, Escaned J, Maas AHEM, et al. An EAPCI Expert Consensus Document on Ischaemia with Non-Obstructive Coronary Arteries in Collaboration with European Society of Cardiology Working Group on Coronary Pathophysiology & Microcirculation Endorsed by Coronary Vasomotor Disorders International Study Group. EuroIntervention. 2021;16(13):1049-69.
9. Samuels BA, Shah SM, Widmer RJ, Kobayashi Y, Miner SES, Taqueti VR, et al. Microvascular Network (MVN). Comprehensive Management of ANOCA, Part 1-Definition, Patient Population, and Diagnosis: JACC State-of-the-Art Review. J Am Coll Cardiol. 2023;82(12):1245-63.

10. Smilowitz NR, Prasad M, Widmer RJ, Toleva O, Quesada O, Sutton NR, et al. Microvascular Network (MVN). Comprehensive Management of ANOCA, Part 2-Program Development, Treatment, and Research Initiatives: JACC State-of-the-Art Review. J Am Coll Cardiol. 2023;82(12):1264-79.
11. Tudurachi A, Anghel L, Tudurachi BS, Zăvoi A, Ceasovschih A, Sascău RA, et al. Beyond the Obstructive Paradigm: Unveiling the Complex Landscape of Nonobstructive Coronary Artery Disease. J Clin Med. 2024;13(16):4613.
12. Vavuranakis M, Bhatt DL. Relieving the Pressure: Evaluating the Coronary Sinus Reducer for Refractory Angina. JACC Cardiovasc Interv. 2025;18(15):1878-80.
13. Tamis-Holland JE, Jneid H, Reynolds HR, Agewall S, Brilakis ES, Brown TM, et al; American Heart Association Interventional Cardiovascular Care Committee of the Council on Clinical Cardiology; Council on Cardiovascular and Stroke Nursing; Council on Epidemiology and Prevention; and Council on Quality of Care and Outcomes Research. Contemporary Diagnosis and Management of Patients With Myocardial Infarction in the Absence of Obstructive Coronary Artery Disease: A Scientific Statement From the American Heart Association. Circulation. 2019;139(18):e891-908.
14. Tognola C, Maloberti A, Varrenti M, Mazzone P, Giannattasio C, Guarracini F. Myocardial Infarction with Nonobstructive Coronary Arteries (MINOCA): Current Insights into Pathophysiology, Diagnosis, and Management. Diagnostics (Basel). 2025;15(7):942.
15. Scalone G, Niccoli G, Crea F. Pathophysiology, diagnosis and management of MINOCA: an update. Eur Heart J Acute Cardiovasc Care. 2019;8(1):54-62.
16. Agewall S, Beltrame JF, Reynolds HR, et al; WG on Cardiovascular Pharmacotherapy. ESC working group position paper on myocardial infarction with non-obstructive coronary arteries. Eur Heart J. 2017;38(3):143-53.

CHAPTER 6

Life-threatening Findings on Routine Electrocardiogram Screening in Normal Asymptomatic Persons

Subhash Chandra

INTRODUCTION

Even minor ECG abnormalities detected with annual checks signal a greater risk of future CVD events, a study of several million working-age people affirms, although questions remain about whether there is a net benefit to such routine screening.

Even one minor abnormal finding was associated with a greater likelihood of developing a major abnormality on a subsequent screening ECG.

BRUGADA SYNDROME

Brugada syndrome (BrS) is a genetic disorder in which the electrical activity within the heart is abnormal. It increases the risk of abnormal heart rhythms and sudden cardiac death. About a quarter of those with Brugada syndrome have a family member who also has the condition. Some cases may be due to a new genetic mutation or certain medications. The most commonly involved gene is SCN5A which encodes the cardiac sodium channel.

Diagnosis is typically by electrocardiogram (ECG), Brugada syndrome is diagnosed by identifying characteristic patterns on an electrocardiogram. The pattern seen on the ECG includes ST elevation in leads V_1-V_3 with a right bundle branch block (RBBB) appearance. There may be evidence of a slowing of electrical conduction within the heart, as shown by a prolonged PR interval. These patterns may be present all the time, but may appear only in response to particular drugs, when the person has a fever, during exercise, or as a result of other triggers **(Fig. 1)**. Three forms of the Brugada ECG pattern have been described as:

Type 1:
- Most commonly gene is *SCN5A* which encodes the cardiac Na^+ channel.
- Diagnosis typically by ECG **(Fig. 2)**
- T1 has a coved type ST elevation with at least 2 mm (0.2MV) J-point elevation.

Type 2:
- Type 2 has a saddle back pattern with 2 mm J-point elevation **(Fig. 3)**

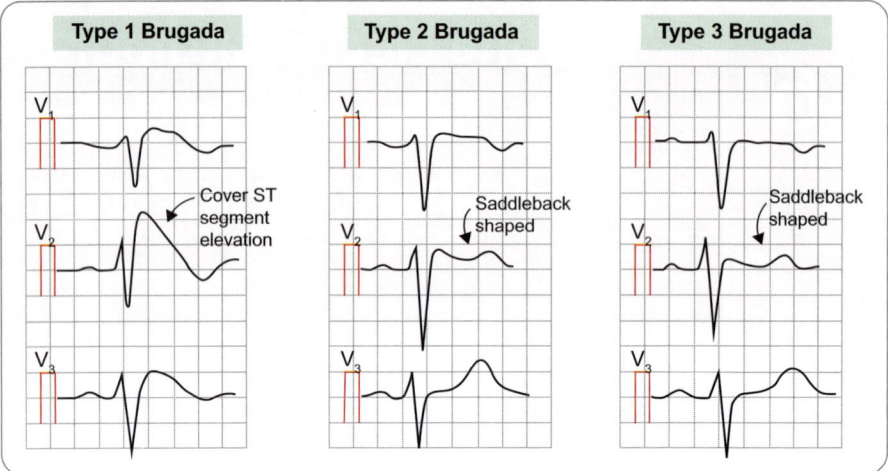

FIG. 1: Three forms of the Brugada ECG pattern.

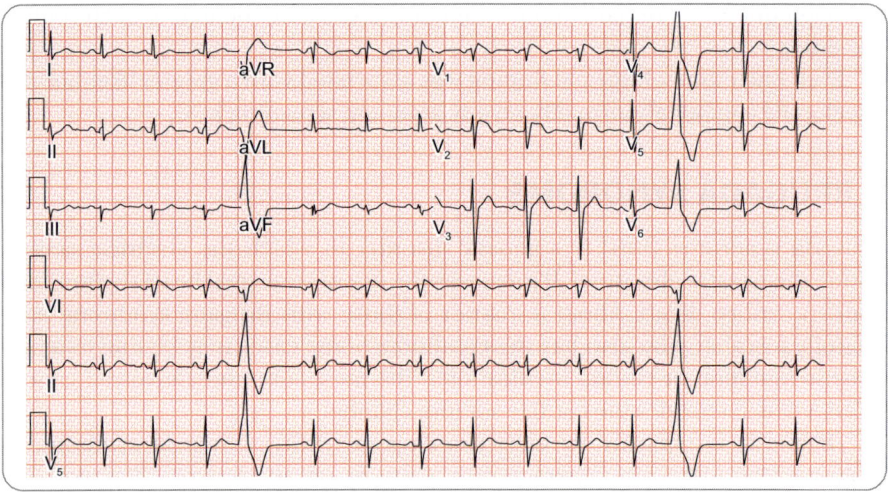

FIG. 2: Type 1 Brugada syndrome.

Type 3:
- Type 3 has either a coved or a saddle back pattern with <2 mm J-point elevation **(Fig. 4)**.

According to a recent consensus document, ECG pattern in Brugada syndrome are Type 1, ST-segment elevation, either spontaneously present or induced with the sodium channel-blocker challenge test, is considered diagnostic. Type 2 and 3 may lead to suspicion, but provocation testing is required for diagnosis. The ECGs in the right and left panels are from the same patient before (right panel, type 3) and after (left panel type 1) administration of Ajmaline.

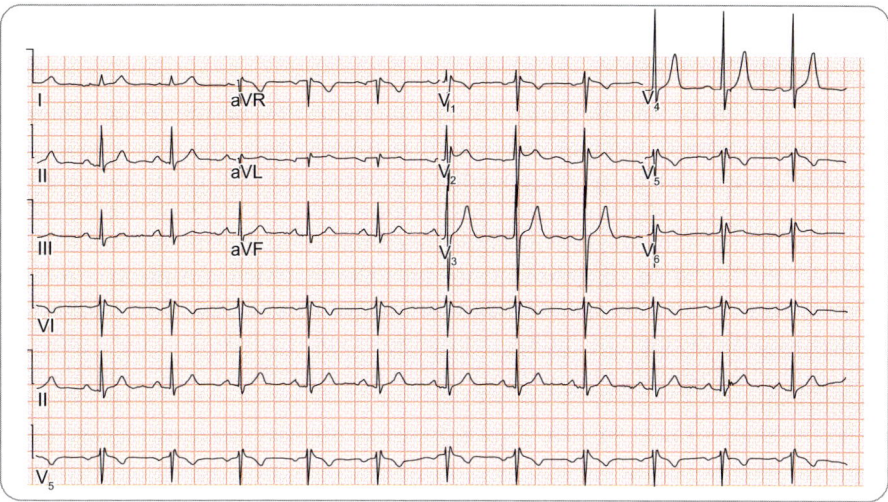

FIG. 3: Type 2 Brugada syndrome.

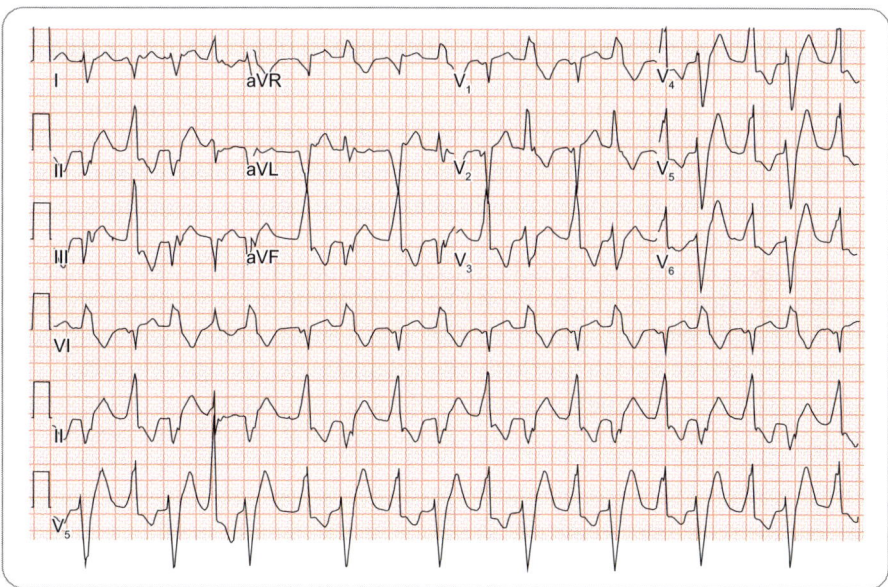

FIG. 4: Type 3 Brugada syndrome.

CATECHOLAMINERGIC POLYMORPHIC VENTRICULAR TACHYCARDIA

Catecholaminergic polymorphic ventricular tachycardia (CPVT) is an inherited genetic disorder that predisposes those affected to potentially life-threatening abnormal heart rhythms or arrhythmias. The arrhythmias seen in CPVT typically occur during exercise or at times of emotional stress, and classically take the form of bidirectional ventricular tachycardia or ventricular fibrillation, those affected may be asymptomatic, but they may also experience blackouts or even sudden cardiac death.

The CPVT is caused by genetic mutations affecting proteins that regulate the concentrations of calcium within cardiac muscle cells. The most commonly identified gene is *RYR2*, which encodes a protein included in an ion channel known as the ryanodine receptor; this channel releases calcium from a cell's internal calcium store, the sarcoplasmic reticulum, during every heartbeat.

The CPVT is often diagnosed from an ECG recorded during an exercise tolerance test, but it may also be diagnosed with a genetic test. The condition is treated with medication including beta-adrenoceptor blockers or flecainide, or with surgical procedures including sympathetic denervation and implantation of a defibrillator.

The resting 12-lead ECG is a useful test to differentiate CPVT from other electrical diseases of the heart that can cause similar abnormal heart rhythms. Unlike conditions such as long QT syndrome and Brugada syndrome, the resting 12-lead ECG in those with CPVT is generally normal. However, approximately 20% of those affected have a slow resting heart rate or sinus bradycardia.

ARRHYTHMOGENIC RIGHT VENTRICULAR DYSPLASIA

Arrhythmogenic right ventricular dysplasia (ARVD), or arrhythmogenic right ventricular cardiomyopathy (ARVC), is an inherited heart disease. ARVD is caused by genetic defects of the parts of heart muscle (also called myocardium or cardiac muscle) known as desmosomes, areas on the surface of heart muscle cells which link the cells together.

The disease is a type of nonischemic cardiomyopathy that involves primarily the right ventricle. It is characterized by hypokinetic areas involving the free wall of the right ventricle, with fibro fatty replacement of the right ventricular myocardium, with associated arrhythmias originating in the right ventricle.

ARVC/D is an important cause of ventricular arrhythmias in children and young adults. It is seen predominantly in males, and 30–50% of cases have a familial distribution.

Up to 80% of individuals with ARVD present have symptoms like syncope and dyspnea. The remainder frequently present with palpitations or other symptoms due to right ventricular outflow tract (RVOT) tachycardia (a type of monomorphic ventricular tachycardia).

Symptoms are usually exercise-related. In populations where hypertrophic cardiomyopathy is screened out prior to involvement in competitive athletics, it is a common cause of sudden cardiac death. The first clinical signs of ARVD are usually during adolescence.

90% of individuals with ARVD have some EKG abnormality. The most common EKG abnormality seen in ARVD is T wave inversion in leads V_1-V_3.

Electrocardiographic features:
- ARVD is associated with characteristic ECG abnormalities
- Epsilon wave (most specific finding, seen in 30% of patients)
- T wave inversion in V_1–V3 (85% of patients)

- Prolonged S-wave upstroke of 55ms in V_1–V_3 (95% of patients)
- Localized QRS widening of 110 ms in V_1–V_3
- Paroxysmal episodes of ventricular tachycardia with left bundle branch block (LBBB) morphology (e.g., right ventricular VT)

Right bundle branch block (RBBB) itself is seen frequently in individuals with ARVD. This may be due to delayed activation of the right ventricle, rather than any intrinsic abnormality in the right bundle branch **(Figs. 5 and 6)**.

The epsilon wave is found in about 50% of those with ARVD. This is described as a terminal notch in the QRS complex. It is due to slowed intraventricular conduction.

Ventricular ectopy seen on a surface EKG in the setting of ARVD is typically of left bundle branch block (LBBB) morphology, with a QRS axis of –90 to +110 degrees. The origin of the ectopic beats is usually from one of the three regions of fatty degeneration (the "triangle of dysplasia") **(Fig. 7)**.

HYPERTROPHIC CARDIOMYOPATHY

Hypertrophic cardiomyopathy (HCM): It is a condition in which a portion of the heart becomes thickened without an obvious cause. This results in the heart being

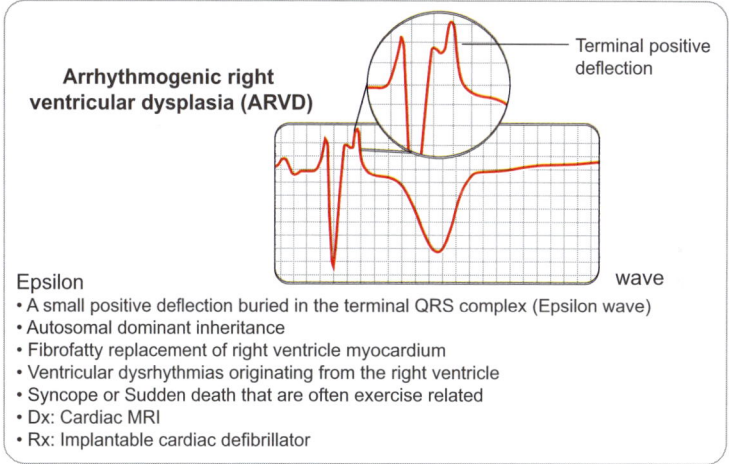

FIG. 5: Arrhythmogenic right ventricular dysplasia (ARVD): Epsilon wave on ECG and associated clinical characteristics, genetics, and management.

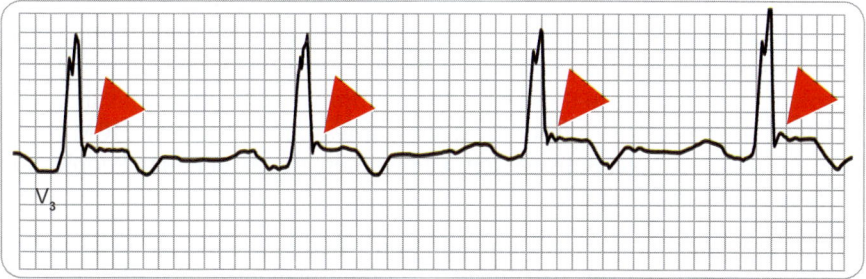

FIG. 6: The epsilon wave (marked by red triangle) seen in arrhythmogenic right ventricular dysplasia (ARVD).

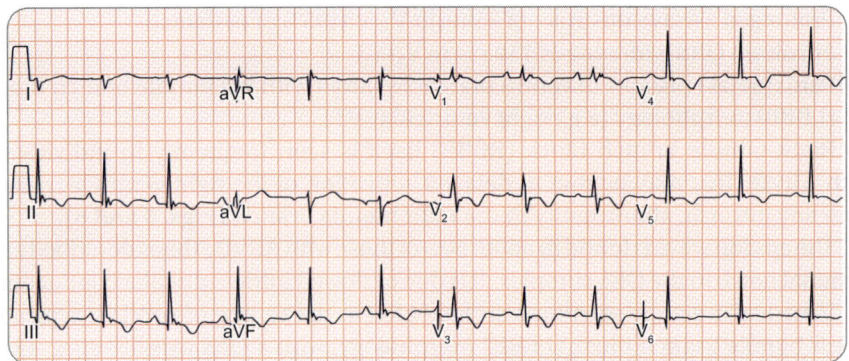

FIG. 7: The RV outflow tract, the RV inflow tract, and the RV apex.

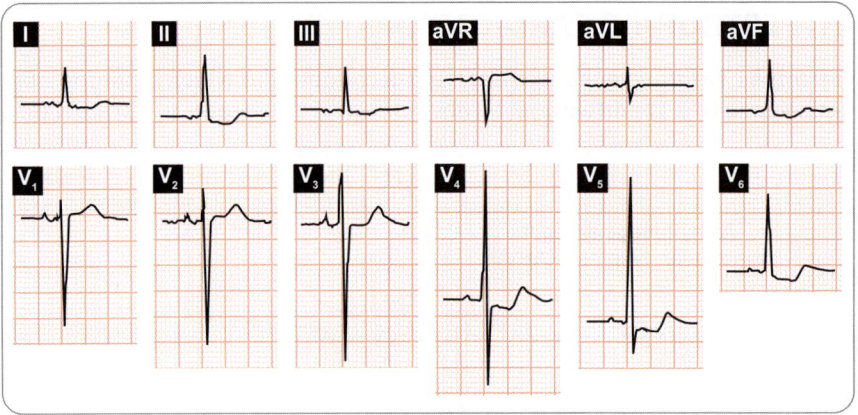

FIG. 8: Hypertrophic cardiomyopathy.

less able to pump blood effectively. Symptoms vary from none to feeling tired, leg swelling, and shortness of breath. It may also result in chest pain or fainting. Complications include heart failure, an irregular heartbeat, and sudden cardiac death.

Hypertrophic cardiomyopathy is most commonly inherited from a person's parents. It is often due to mutations in certain genes involved with making heart muscle proteins.

Treatment may include the use of beta blockers, diuretics, or disopyramide, an implantable cardiac defibrillator may be recommended in those with certain types of irregular heartbeat. Surgery, in the form of a septal myectomy or heart transplant, may be done in those who do not improve with other measures. With treatment, the risk of death from the disease is less than 1% a year. HCM affects about one in 500 people. Rates in men and women are about equal. People of all ages may be affected **(Fig. 8)**.

Obstructive or nonobstructive: Depending on whether the distortion of normal heart anatomy causes an obstruction of the outflow of blood from the left ventricle of the heart, HCM can be classified as obstructive or nonobstructive.

The obstructive variant of HCM, hypertrophic obstructive cardiomyopathy (HOCM), has also historically been known as idiopathic hypertrophic subaortic stenosis (IHSS) and asymmetric septal hypertrophy (ASH). Another, nonobstructive variant of HCM is apical hypertrophic cardiomyopathy, also called Yamaguchi syndrome or Yamaguchi hypertrophy, first described in individuals of Japanese descent.

The classical ECG finding is Large Dragger like "Septal Q wave" in the lateral and sometimes inferior leads due to the abnormally hypertrophied interventricular septum.

The apical variant of HOCM, known as "Yamaguchi syndrome," does not result in septal Q waves, as the septum is normal in thickness in this conduction. The cardiac apex is abnormally thickened, resulting in diffuse T wave changes throughout the precordial leads. This is sometimes referred to as "giant T Wave Inversion" **(Figs. 9 to 11)**.

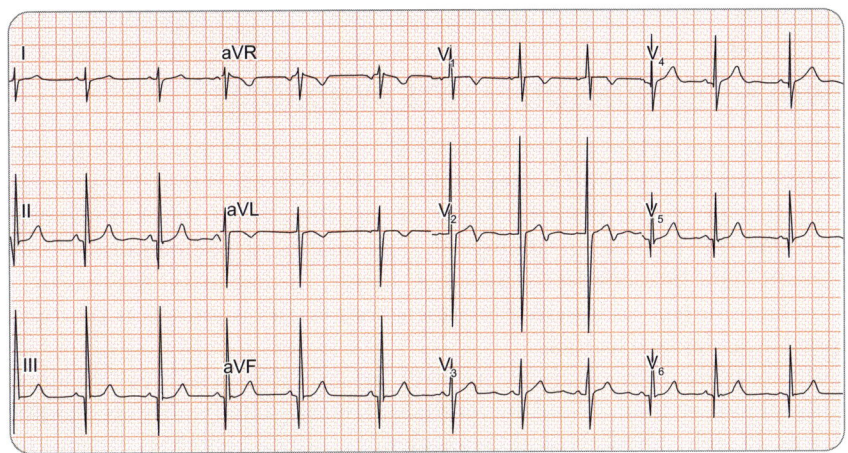

FIG. 9: ECG showing Brugada type 3 pattern (right) converting to type 1 pattern (left) after Ajmaline administration.

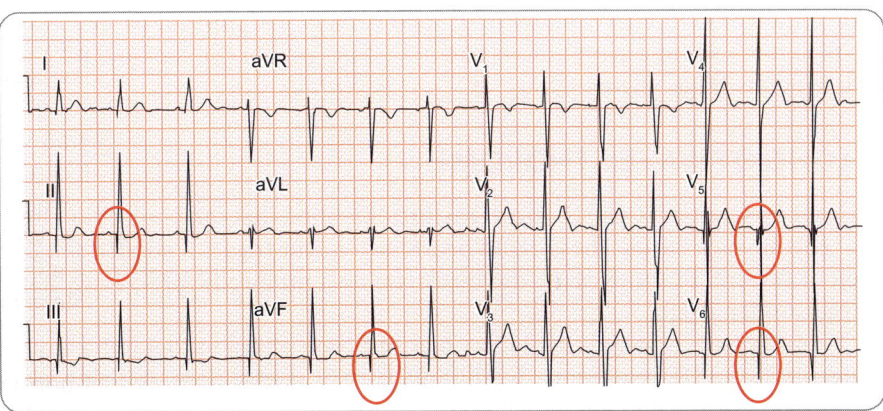

FIG. 10: ECG demonstrating septal Q-waves in leads indicating hypertrophic cardiomyopathy (HCM).

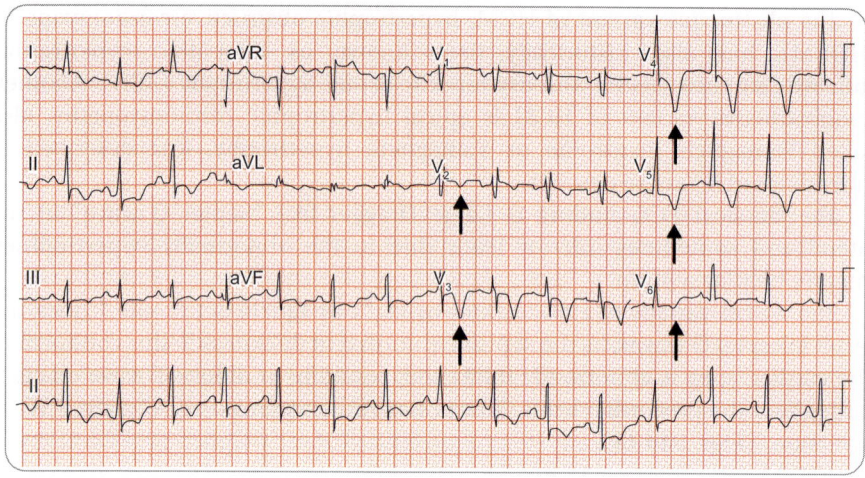

FIG. 11: ECG demonstrating septal Q-waves (circled) characteristic of hypertrophic cardiomyopathy (HCM).

WOLFF–PARKINSON–WHITE SYNDROME

Wolff–Parkinson–White syndrome (WPWS) is a disorder due to a specific type of problem with the electrical system of the heart which has resulted in symptoms. About 40% of people with the electrical problem never develop symptoms. Symptoms can include an abnormally fast heartbeat, palpitations, shortness of breath, light-headedness, or syncope. Rarely, cardiac arrest may occur. The most common type of irregular heartbeat that occurs is known as paroxysmal supraventricular tachycardia.

The underlying mechanism involves an accessory electrical conduction pathway between the atria and the ventricles. It is associated with other conditions such as Ebstein anomaly and hypokalemic periodic paralysis. Diagnosis is typically when an electrocardiogram (ECG) shows a short PR interval and a delta wave. It is a type of pre-excitation syndromes.

The WPW syndrome is treated with either medications or radiofrequency catheter ablation. It affects between 0.1 and 0.3% in the population. The risk of death in those without symptoms is about 0.5% per year in children and 0.1% per year in adults **(Figs. 12 and 13)**.

LONG QT WAVE SYNDROME

Long QT syndrome (LQTS) is a heart rhythm condition that can potentially cause fast, chaotic heartbeats. These rapid heartbeats might trigger a sudden fainting spell or seizure. In some cases, the heart can beat erratically for so long that it causes sudden death.

You can have a genetic mutation that puts you at risk of being born with congenital long QT syndrome. In addition, certain medications, imbalances of the body's salts and minerals (electrolyte abnormalities), and medical conditions might cause acquired long QT syndrome.

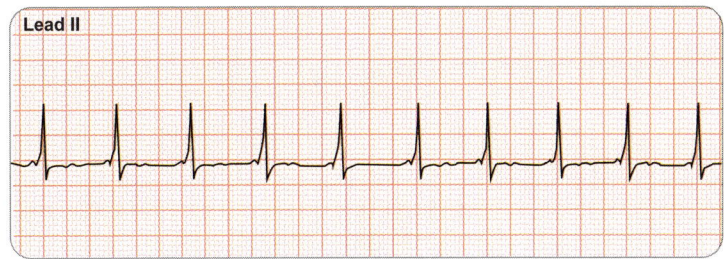

FIG. 12: Classic ECG pattern of Wolff–Parkinson–White (WPW) syndrome in Lead II.

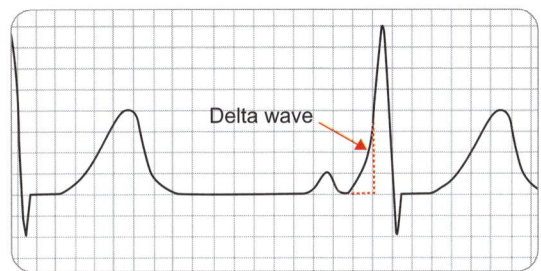

FIG. 13: Magnified QRS complex illustrating the characteristic delta wave in Wolff–Parkinson–White (WPW) syndrome.

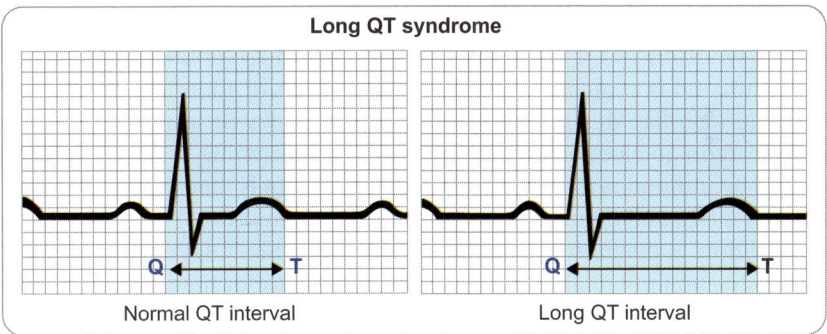

FIG. 14: ECG demonstrating prolonged QT interval.

You will also need to avoid certain medications that could trigger your long QT syndrome. After treatment, you likely can live and thrive, even with this condition. You may be able to continue being active in recreational and even competitive sports **(Fig. 14)**.

Causes:
- Genetic
- *Medications*: Macrolides, quinolones, antidepressants, antipsychotics, and antihistamines
- Thyroid disease
- *Electrolyte imbalance*: Hypomagnesemia, hypocalcemia, and hypokalemia

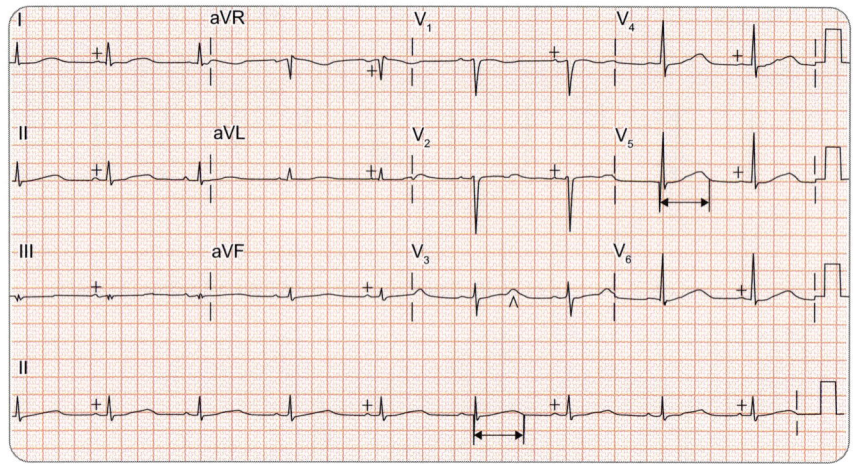

FIG. 15: ECG demonstrating prolonged QT interval.

Many people who have long QT syndrome do not have any signs or symptoms. You might be aware of your condition only because of:
- Results of an electrocardiogram (ECG) done for an unrelated reason
- A family history of long QT syndrome
- Genetic testing results **(Fig. 15)**

■ SHORT QT SYNDROME

Short QT syndrome (SQT) is a very rare genetic disease of the electrical system of the heart, and is associated with an increased risk of abnormal heart rhythms and sudden cardiac death. The syndrome gets its name from a characteristic feature seen on an electrocardiogram (ECG)—a shortening of the QT interval. It is caused by mutations in genes encoding ion channels that shorten the cardiac action potential, and appears to be inherited in an autosomal dominant pattern. The condition is diagnosed using a 12-lead ECG. Short QT syndrome can be treated using an implantable cardioverter-defibrillator or medications including quinidine. Short QT syndrome was first described in 2000, and the first genetic mutation associated with the condition was identified in 2004 **(Fig. 16)**.

The mainstay of diagnosis of short QT syndrome is the 12-lead ECG. The precise QT duration used to diagnose the condition remains controversial with consensus guidelines giving cutoffs varying from 330 ms, 340 ms, or even 360 ms when other clinical, familial, or genetic factors are present. The QT interval normally varies with heart rate, but this variation occurs to a lesser extent in those with short QT syndrome. It is, therefore, recommended that the QT interval is assessed at heart rates close to 60 beats per minute. Other features that may be seen on the ECG in short QT syndrome include tall, peaked T-waves and PR segment depression.

Causes:
- Genetic
- Hypercalcemia

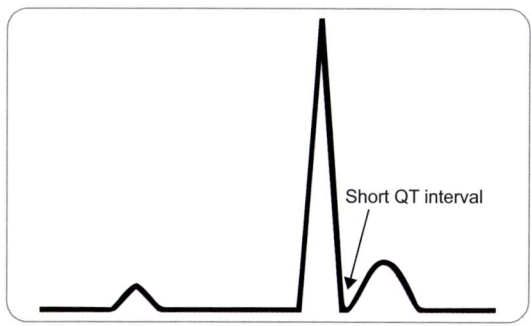

FIG. 16: Magnified QRS complex illustrating a short QT interval.

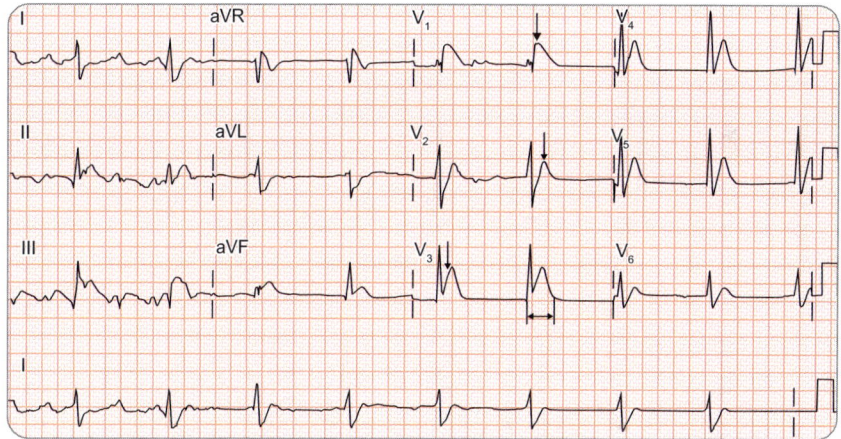

FIG. 17: ECG demonstrating features of short QT syndrome (SQTS).

- Hyperkalemia
- Acidosis
- Hyperthermia

Drugs:
- Mallotoxin
- NS/643 (Both Herg current stimulators)
- Levcromakalim
- Nicorandil

Risk of short QT: Can cause arrhythmias in which you may feel dizziness, fainting, or heart palpitation. They may even cause cardiac arrest and sudden cardiac death **(Fig. 17)**.

EARLY REPOLARIZATION PATTERN AND SYNDROME

Early repolarization syndrome (ERS), demonstrated as J-point elevation on an electrocardiograph was formerly thought to be a benign entity, but the recent studies have demonstrated that it can be linked to a considerable risk of life-threatening arrhythmias and sudden cardiac death (SCD). Early repolarization characteristics associated with SCD include high-amplitude J-point elevation, horizontal and/or down slopping ST segments, and inferior and/or lateral leads location. The prevalence of ERS varies between 3 and 24% depending on age, sex, and J-point elevation (0.05 mV vs. 0.1 mV) being the main determinants. ERS patients are sporadic and they are at a higher risk of having recurrent cardiac events.

ERS is an electrocardiographic (ECG) entity characterized by J-point elevation manifested either as either QRS slurring (at the transition from the QRS segment to the ST-segment) or notching (a positive deflection inscribed on terminal S wave), ST segment elevation with upper concavity and prominent T-waves in at least two contiguous leads **(Figs. 18A and B)**.

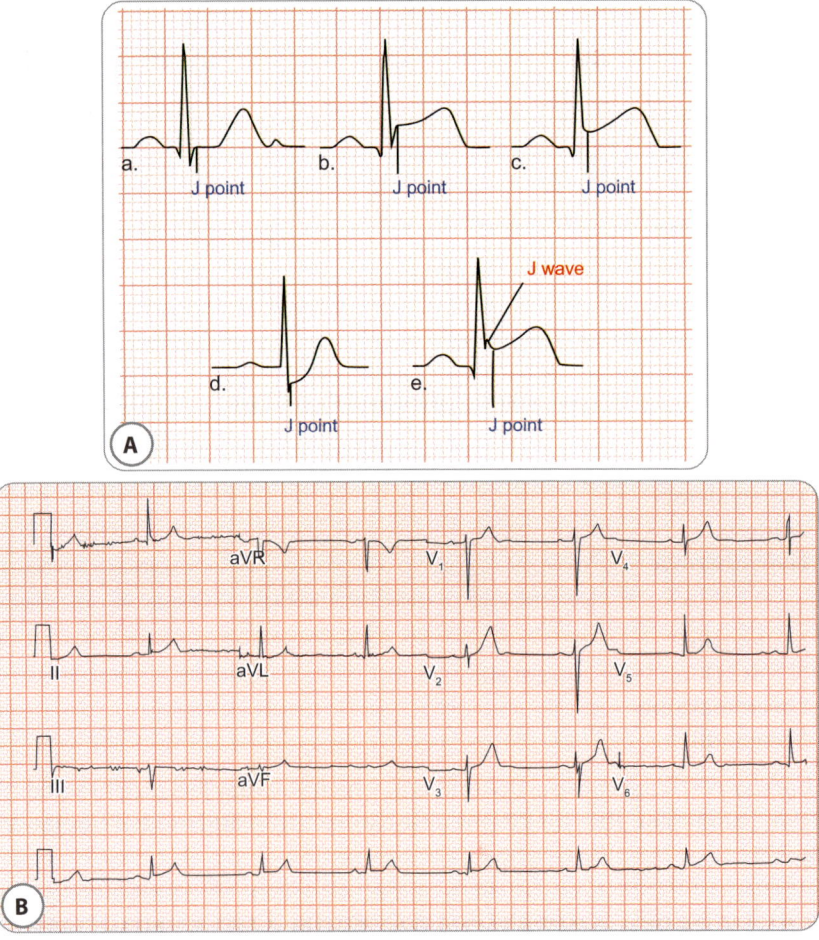

FIGS. 18A AND B: ECG illustrating the J-point elevation and ST segment features of early repolarization pattern.

CONCLUSION

Routine ECG screening in asymptomatic individuals can reveal life-threatening electrical disorders such as Brugada syndrome, CPVT, ARVD, HCM, and Wolff–Parkinson–White (WPW) and long/short QT syndromes. Recognizing characteristic ECG patterns—like the Brugada patterns, epsilon waves in ARVD, septal Q waves in HCM, delta waves in WPW, and prolonged/shortened QT intervals—is crucial for early diagnosis, risk stratification, and implementing life-saving treatments like ICD implantation or medications, ultimately reducing the risk of sudden cardiac death.

FURTHER READINGS

1. Brugada P, Brugada J. Right bundle branch block, persistent ST segment elevation and sudden cardiac death: a distinct clinical and electrocardiographic syndrome. A multicenter report. J Am Coll Cardiol. 1992;20(6):1391-6.
2. Priori SG, Wilde AA, Horie M, et al. HRS/EHRA/APHRS expert consensus statement on the diagnosis and management of patients with inherited primary arrhythmia syndromes. Heart Rhythm. 2013;10(12):e85-108.
3. Zipes DP, Wellens HJ. Sudden cardiac death. Circulation. 1998;98(21):2334-51.
4. Thiene G, Corrado D, Basso C. Arrhythmogenic right ventricular cardiomyopathy/dysplasia.
5. Maron BJ, Maron MS. Hypertrophic cardiomyopathy. Lancet. 2013;381(9862):242-55.

CHAPTER 7

Primary Percutaneous Coronary Intervention is Superior to Thrombolysis in ST-elevation Myocardial Infarction—Evidence-based Practice

Rajesh Vijayvergiya

■ INTRODUCTION

India has the highest burden of acute coronary syndrome (ACS) patients in the world, with >3 million ST-elevation myocardial infarction (STEMI) cases occurring every year. Indian patients are younger (56.3 years) and have a higher proportion (>60.6%) of STEMI than patients in developed countries. The guiding principle—"time is myocardium"—highlights that delayed reperfusion leads to increased myocardial damage, left ventricular dysfunction, and higher mortality. Broadly, the two main approaches for coronary reperfusion are intravenous thrombolytic (fibrinolytic) therapy and primary percutaneous coronary intervention (PPCI). While thrombolysis remains widely accessible and effective in time, accumulating evidence shows that PPCI provides better clinical outcomes in terms of mortality, reinfarction, and stroke risk—primarily when performed promptly by experienced teams.

■ RATIONALE AND EVOLUTION OF REPERFUSION THERAPY

The Fibrinolytic Therapy Trialists (FTT) Collaborative Group meta-analysis showed that early fibrinolytic therapy within 12 hours of symptom onset significantly lowers mortality, especially when started within the first hour (the "golden hour"). Each 30-minute delay raises 1-year mortality by 7.5%, saving 65 lives (0–1 hour), 37 lives (1–2 hours), and 26–29 lives (2–6 hours) per 1,000 treated patients. However, systemic thrombolysis has some limitations, such as incomplete coronary patency (TIMI 3 flow achieved in only 50–60% of patients), reocclusion rates of 10–15%, contraindications due to bleeding risks, and lower effectiveness in elderly or late presenters. In contrast, PPCI offers nearly complete coronary reperfusion (TIMI 3 flow in over 90% of cases), lower reocclusion rates (2–3%), and decreased risk of intracranial hemorrhage; therefore, considered the gold standard for STEMI management.

Few of many randomized controlled trials and meta-analyses, such as the DANAMI-2 trial, compared transfer for PPCI versus on-site thrombolysis in STEMI, revealing a significantly reduced composite endpoint of death, reinfarction, or stroke (8% vs. 13.7%; $p < 0.002$), representing a 40% relative risk reduction and a number needed to treat (NNT) of 17 to prevent one major event. Similarly, the PRAGUE and PRAGUE-2 trials demonstrated consistent superiority of percutaneous coronary intervention (PCI) over thrombolysis, even when PCI required an interhospital transfer within 90 minutes. However, the CAPTIM trial suggests that very early prehospital thrombolysis (<2 hours) may approximate PCI outcomes, but beyond 2 hours, PCI remains superior. The STREAM-2 trial reinforced the concept of a pharmacoinvasive strategy when timely PCI is not feasible: early fibrinolysis followed by routine early PCI yielded outcomes comparable to PPCI. The PPCI is the first choice; pharmacoinvasive therapy is the next best option when PCI cannot be performed promptly **(Table 1)**.

■ IMPORTANCE OF TIME TO REPERFUSION

ST-elevation myocardial infarction is a dynamic process that does not occur instantaneously but rather evolves over hours, and the infarct size remains the most critical determinant of prognosis in patients with STEMI **(Fig. 1)**.

TABLE 1: Comparing various outcomes between the thrombolysis and primary percutaneous coronary intervention (PCI).

Parameters	Thrombolysis	Primary PCI
Initial TIMI 3 flow	30–50%	85–95%
Reocclusion rate	15–30%	<5%
Time to reocclusion	Often within 24–48 hours	Rare with a stent and antithrombotic
Need for rescue PCI	Common (25–30%)	–
30-day mortality	7–9%	4–6%
Stroke risk	Slightly higher	Lower
Major bleeding risk	Higher intracranial bleeding	Lower by transradial approach and tailored anticoagulation

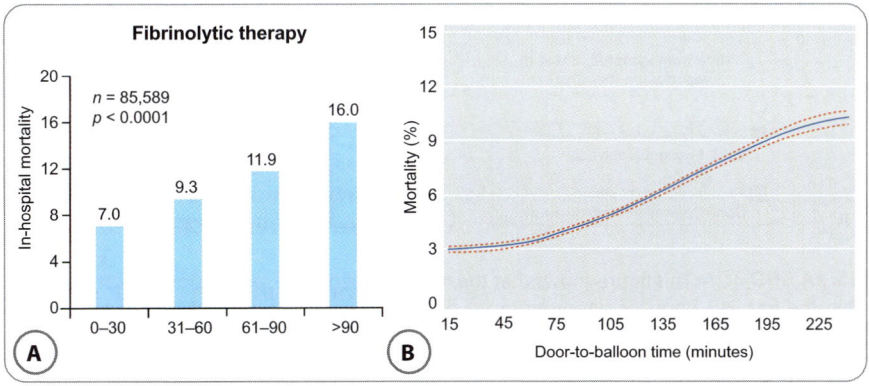

FIGS. 1A AND B: Importance of time to reperfusion in patients undergoing fibrinolysis, (A or B) Primary percutaneous coronary intervention (PCI) for STEMI. Graph based on data from (n = 85,589) patients treated with fibrinolysis. (A) The in-hospital mortality rate increases by 0.5% for every 30-minute delay. (B) Based on data from (n = 43,801) patients, this graph shows the adjusted in-hospital mortality rate as a function of door-to-balloon time. Estimated mortality ranged from 3% with a door-to-balloon time of 30 minutes to 10.3% in patients with a door-to-balloon time of 240 minutes.

As such, evidence supports system-level interventions to reduce time-to-device **(Fig. 2)**, and according to Ibanez B et al., the goals of the system and initial reperfusion treatment for patients with STEMI can be achieved through pharmacologic (fibrinolysis) or catheter-based (PPCI) approaches, which may involve transfer from a non-PCI-capable to a PCI-capable center. The pathway and various metrics, as shown in **Figures 3A and B**, can be adjusted, and reperfusion strategies for patients with STEMI can be tailored, whether they are admitted to a PCI-capable or non-PCI-capable hospital. The best approach depends on the timing of symptom onset, the patient's eligibility for fibrinolysis, and the options for timely transfer to a PCI-capable hospital.

In India, STEMI care is delayed due to long times before hospital admission, as the Indian ACS registry reports median symptom-to-first medical contact times of 6–8 hours, with fewer than 5% of patients reaching the golden hour. However, as shown by the Kerala ACS registry only approximately 40% of STEMI patients in India receive any reperfusion, and median symptom-to-door times often exceed 6 hours. The Tamil Nadu STEMI program demonstrated that a hub-and-spoke model combined with telemedicine can significantly reduce treatment delays and achieve reperfusion rates over 90%. Additional innovations, such as tele-ECG transmission, prehospital thrombolysis, and state-wide AMI networks further decreased door-to-needle times and serve as scalable, cost-effective

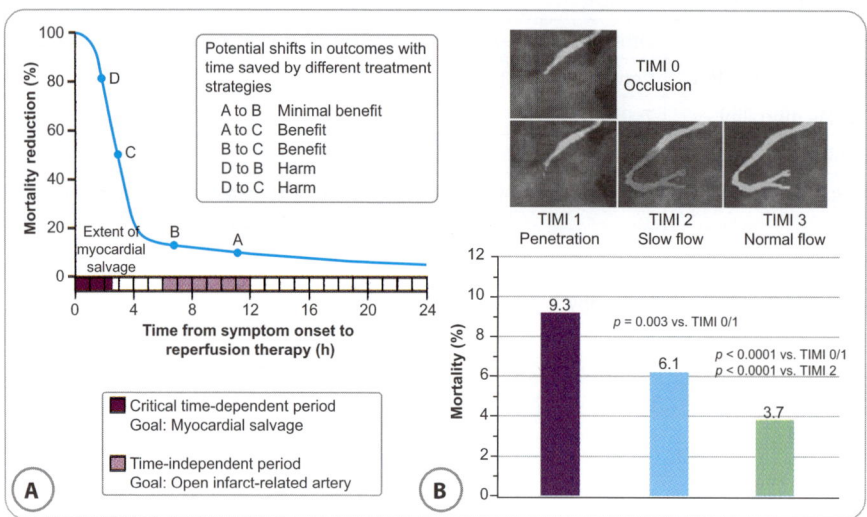

FIGS. 2A AND B: (A) This figure shows that the mortality benefit of reperfusion is most significant within the first 2–3 hours of symptom onset due to maximal myocardial salvage. As the curve flattens beyond this period, benefit declines; hence, transitions from *point A/B to C* yield substantial survival gains, whereas *A to B* offers minimal benefit. Delays in early reperfusion, such as during transfer for percutaneous coronary intervention (PCI), may shift outcomes unfavorably from *point D to C or B*; (B) Correlation of thrombolysis in myocardial infarction (TIMI) flow grade and mortality. A pooled analysis of data from ($n = 5,498$) patients across several angiographic trials of reperfusion for ST-elevation myocardial infarction (STEMI) showed a gradient in mortality when angiographic findings were stratified by TIMI flow grade. Patients with TIMI 0 or TIMI 1 flow had the highest mortality rate, TIMI 2 flow was associated with an intermediate mortality rate, and the lowest mortality rate was observed in patients with TIMI 3 flow.

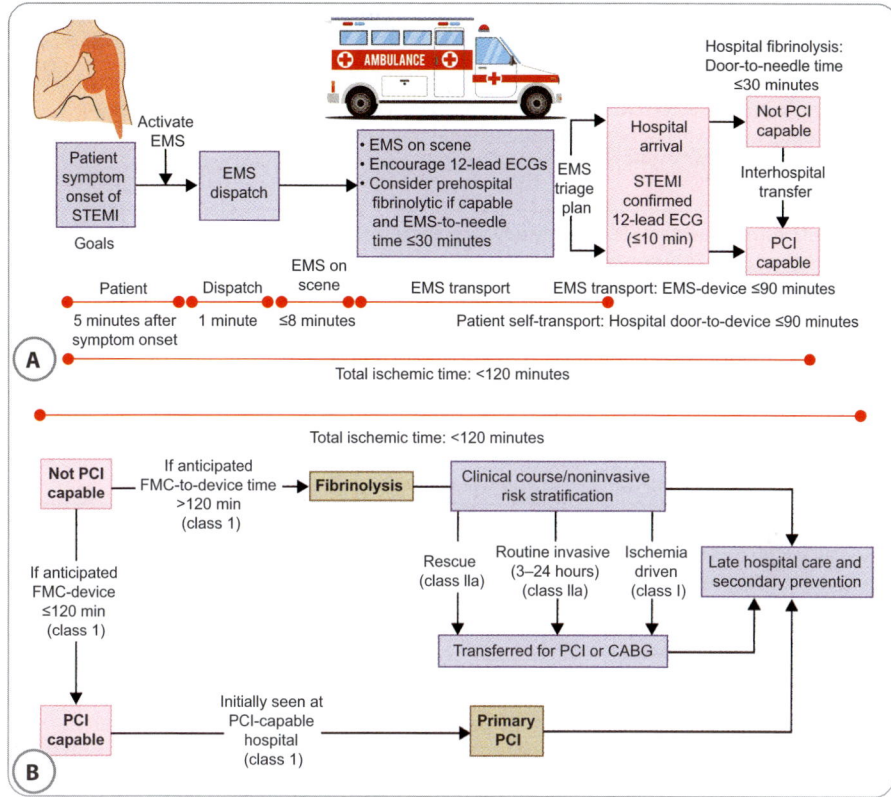

FIGS. 3A AND B: System goals and initial reperfusion treatment of patients with STEMI. (A) Pathway once the patient reaches the emergency medical services (EMS) and the time metrics and the STEMI systems goal is to maintain a network of transportation and destination hospitals so that the total ischemic time is kept to <120 minutes; (B) The reperfusion strategies for patients with STEMI, regardless of whether they go to a PCI-capable or to a non-PCI-capable hospital (denoted class I and class II recommendations are from the ACC/AHA guidelines for the management of STEMI).

(ACC/AHA: American College of Cardiology/American Heart Association; CABG: coronary artery bypass grafting; FMC: first medical contact; PCI: percutaneous coronary intervention; STEMI: ST-elevation myocardial infarction)

TABLE 2: Time metrics and outcomes.		
Time interval	Target duration	Rationale
Symptom onset to FMC	<30 minutes	Early recognition
FMC to ECG	≤10 minutes	Rapid diagnosis
Diagnosis to thrombolysis	≤10 minutes	"Door-to-needle"
Diagnosis to PCI wire crossing	≤90 minutes (transfer), ≤60 minutes (on-site)	"Door-to-balloon"
PCI delay vs. thrombolysis	≤120 minutes	Acceptable threshold
(FMC: first medical contact; PCI: percutaneous coronary intervention)		

strategies to improve STEMI outcomes in India. These models emphasize the critical importance of system-level logistics in optimizing reperfusion therapy **(Tables 2 and 3)**.

TABLE 3: Latest recommendations for STEMI.

Recommendation	COR
In patients with suspected ACS in which the initial ECG is nondiagnostic of STEMI, serial ECGs to detect potential ischemic changes should be performed, especially when clinical suspicion of ACS is high, symptoms are persistent, or the clinical condition deteriorates	1
In patients with suspected STEMI, early advanced notification of the receiving PCI-capable hospital by EMS personnel and activation of the cardiac catheterization team is recommended to reduce time to reperfusion	1
All communities should create and maintain regional systems of STEMI care that coordinate prehospital and hospital-based STEMI care processes with the goal of reducing total ischemic time and improving survival in patients with STEMI	1
In patient with STEMI presenting <12 hours after symptom onset, PPCI should be performed with a goal of FMC to device activation of ≤90 minutes or ≤120 minutes in patients requiring hospital transfer, to improve survival	1
In patients with ACS and cardiogenic shock or hemodynamic instability, emergency revascularization of the culprit vessel by PCI or CABG is indicated to improve survival, irrespective of time from symptom onset	1
In patients with STEMI presenting 12–24 hours after symptom onset, PPCI is reasonable to improve clinical outcomes	2a
In patients with STEMI presenting >24 hours after symptom onset with the presence of ongoing ischemia or life-threatening arrhythmia, PPCI is reasonable to improve clinical outcomes	2a
In patients who are stable with STEMI who have a totally occluded infarct-related artery >24 hours after symptom onset and are without evidence of ongoing ischemia, acute severe HF, or life-threatening arrhythmia, PPCI should not be performed due to lack of benefit	3
In patients with STEMI and an estimated time from FMC to device activation of ≤120 minutes or those with a contraindication to fibrinolytic therapy, transfer to a PCI-capable hospital for PPCI is recommended to reduce MACE	1
In patients with STEMI and symptom onset of 120 minutes from FMC, fibrinolytic therapy should be administered in patients without contraindication to reduce MACE	1
In patients with STEMI and symptom onset of 12–24 hours, transfer to a PCI-capable hospital for PPCI is reasonable to reduce infarct size and MACE	1
In patients with STEMI with suspected failed reperfusion after fibrinolytic therapy, immediate angiography with rescue PCI is recommended to reduce the risk of death or recurrent MI	1
In patients with STEMI treated with fibrinolytic therapy, early angiography between 2 and 24 hours with the intent to perform PCI is recommended to reduce the rates of death or MI	1

(ACS: acute coronary syndrome; CABG: coronary artery bypass grafting; COR: class of recommendation; EMS: emergency medical services; FMC: first medical contact; HF: heart failure; MACE: major adverse cardiovascular event; MI: myocardial infarction; PCI: percutaneous coronary intervention; PPCI: primary percutaneous coronary intervention; STEMI: ST-elevation myocardial infarction)

CONCLUSION

In conclusion, PPCI is the most effective reperfusion strategy for STEMI, offering superior survival and lower complication rates compared with thrombolysis. Its true advantage, however, is realized only within integrated, time-efficient systems of care that ensure rapid diagnosis, coordinated transfer, and timely intervention. Building such network-based STEMI programs remains the cornerstone for achieving universal, equitable, and high-quality cardiac care in India.

FURTHER READINGS

1. Alexander T, Mullasari AS, Kaifoszova Z, Khot UN, Nallamothu B, Ramana RGV, et al. Framework for a National STEMI Program: Consensus document developed by STEMI INDIA, Cardiological Society of India and Association Physicians of India. Indian Heart J. 2015;67(5):497-502.
2. Shen YC, Krumholz H, Hsia RY. Association of Cardiac Care Regionalization With Access, Treatment, and Mortality Among Patients With ST-Segment Elevation Myocardial Infarction. Circ Cardiovasc Qual Outcomes. 2021;14(3):e007195.
3. Jollis JG, Al-Khalidi HR, Roettig ML, Berger PB, Corbett CC, Doerfler SM, et al. Impact of Regionalization of ST-Segment–Elevation Myocardial Infarction Care on Treatment Times and Outcomes for Emergency Medical Services–Transported Patients Presenting to Hospitals With Percutaneous Coronary Intervention: Mission: Lifeline Accelerator-2. Circulation. 2018;137(4):376-87.
4. Indications for fibrinolytic therapy in suspected acute myocardial infarction: collaborative overview of early mortality and major morbidity results from all randomised trials of more than 1000 patients. Fibrinolytic Therapy Trialists' (Ftt) Collaborative Group. Lancet. 1994;343(8893):311-22.
5. Andersen HR, Nielsen TT, Rasmussen K, Thuesen L, Kelbaek H, Thayssen P, et al. A Comparison of Coronary Angioplasty with Fibrinolytic Therapy in Acute Myocardial Infarction. N Engl J Med. 2003;349(8):733-42.
6. Mocova Bilkova D, Motovska Z, Prochazka B, Groch L, Zelizko M, Aschermann M, et al. Transportation to primary percutaneous coronary intervention, compared with on-site fibrinolysis, is a strong independent predictor of functional status after myocardial infarction: 5-year follow-up of the PRAGUE-2 trial. Eur Heart J Acute Cardiovasc Care. 2014;3(2):105-9.
7. Steg PG, Bonnefoy E, Chabaud S, Lapostolle F, Dubien PY, Cristofini P, et al. Impact of Time to Treatment on Mortality After Prehospital Fibrinolysis or Primary Angioplasty: Data From the CAPTIM Randomized Clinical Trial. Circulation. 2003;108(23):2851-6.
8. Van De Werf F, Ristić AD, Averkov OV, Arias-Mendoza A, Lambert Y, Kerr Saraiva JF, et al. STREAM-2: Half-Dose Tenecteplase or Primary Percutaneous Coronary Intervention in Older Patients With ST-Segment–Elevation Myocardial Infarction: A Randomized, Open-Label Trial. Circulation. 2023;148(9):753-64.
9. Keeley EC, Boura JA, Grines CL. Primary angioplasty versus intravenous thrombolytic therapy for acute myocardial infarction: a quantitative review of 23 randomised trials. Lancet. 2003;361(9351):13-20.
10. Jollis JG, Granger CB, Zègre-Hemsey JK, Henry TD, Goyal A, Tamis-Holland JE, et al. Treatment Time and In-Hospital Mortality Among Patients With ST-Segment Elevation Myocardial Infarction, 2018-2021. JAMA. 2022;328(20):2033.
11. Cannon CP. Relationship of Symptom-Onset-to-Balloon Time and Door-to-Balloon Time With Mortality in Patients Undergoing Angioplasty for Acute Myocardial Infarction. JAMA. 2000;283(22):2941.
12. Rathore SS, Curtis JP, Chen J, Wang Y, Nallamothu BK, Epstein AJ, et al. Association of door-to-balloon time and mortality in patients admitted to hospital with ST elevation myocardial infarction: national cohort study. BMJ. 2009;338(may19 1):b1807.

13. De Luca G, Suryapranata H, Ottervanger JP, Antman EM. Time Delay to Treatment and Mortality in Primary Angioplasty for Acute Myocardial Infarction: Every Minute of Delay Counts. Circulation. 2004;109(10):1223-5.
14. Ibanez B, James S, Agewall S, Antunes MJ, Bucciarelli-Ducci C, Bueno H, et al. 2017 ESC Guidelines for the management of acute myocardial infarction in patients presenting with ST-segment elevation. Eur Heart J. 2018;39(2):119-77.
15. Dharma S, Andriantoro H, Dakota I, Sukmawan R, Firdaus I, Danny SS, et al. Hospital outcomes in STEMI patients after the introduction of a regional STEMI network in the metropolitan area of a developing country. AsiaIntervention. 2018;4(2):92-7.
16. O'Gara PT, Kushner FG, Ascheim DD, Casey DE Jr, Chung MK, de Lemos JA, et al. 2013 ACCF/AHA guideline for the management of ST-elevation myocardial infarction: a report of the American College of Cardiology Foundation/American Heart Association Task Force on Practice Guidelines. Circulation. 2013;127(4):e362-425. Erratum in: Circulation. 2013;128(25):e481.
17. Mohanan PP, Mathew R, Harikrishnan S, Krishnan MN, Zachariah G, Joseph J, et al. Presentation, management, and outcomes of 25 748 acute coronary syndrome admissions in Kerala, India: results from the Kerala ACS Registry. Eur Heart J. 2013;34(2):121-9.
18. Karthikeyan G, Mantoo MR, Bhargava B. Choosing the right model for STEMI care in India– Focus should remain on providing timely fibrinolytic therapy, for now. Indian J Med Res. 2022;156(1):17-20.
19. Alexander T, Mullasari AS, Joseph G, Kannan K, Veerasekar G, Victor SM, et al. A System of Care for Patients With ST-Segment Elevation Myocardial Infarction in India: The Tamil Nadu– ST-Segment Elevation Myocardial Infarction Program. JAMA Cardiol. 2017;2(5):498.
20. Chauhan V, Negi PC, Raina S, Raina S, Bhatnagar M, Guleri R, et al. Smartphone-based tele-electrocardiography support for primary care physicians reduces the pain-to-treatment time in acute coronary syndrome. J Telemed Telecare. 2018;24(8):540-6.
21. Rao SV, O'Donoghue ML, Ruel M, Rab T, Tamis-Holland JE, Alexander JH, et al. 2025 ACC/AHA/ACEP/NAEMSP/SCAI Guideline for the Management of Patients With Acute Coronary Syndromes: A Report of the American College of Cardiology/American Heart Association Joint Committee on Clinical Practice Guidelines. Circulation. 2025;151(13):e771-e862. Erratum in: Circulation. 2025;151(13):e865. Erratum in: Circulation. 2025;151(25):e1098.

SECTION 2

Critical Care

SECTION
2

INTRODUCTION

Critical Care

CHAPTER 8

Current Sepsis Guidelines: A Comprehensive Review

AR Balamurugan

INTRODUCTION

Sepsis is a complex and life-threatening clinical syndrome that continues to be one of the leading causes of mortality in hospitals worldwide. It is characterized by life-threatening organ dysfunction resulting from a dysregulated host response to infection. The condition can progress rapidly, leading to septic shock, multiorgan failure, and death if not promptly recognized and treated.

The Surviving Sepsis Campaign (SSC) was initiated in 2002 as an international collaboration between the European Society of Intensive Care Medicine (ESICM), the Society of Critical Care Medicine (SCCM), and the International Sepsis Forum (ISF). The campaign sought to reduce mortality from sepsis and septic shock by 25% within 5 years. Since its inception, SSC has produced a series of international guidelines that have become the foundation for evidence-based sepsis management across the globe.

The latest update, published in 2021, builds upon the previous versions and integrates advances in clinical evidence, diagnostic strategies, treatment protocols, and supportive care. This chapter provides a detailed review of the current sepsis guidelines, their evolution, diagnostic strategies, therapeutic bundles, hemodynamic and ventilatory support, adjunctive treatments, long-term outcomes, and recent advances.

EVOLUTION OF THE SURVIVING SEPSIS CAMPAIGN

The SSC has evolved considerably over the past two decades. The timeline of the campaign is important for understanding how sepsis care has shifted in response to emerging evidence:
- *2002:* SSC initiated with the Barcelona Declaration
- *2004:* First adult guidelines published, introducing the concept of early recognition and bundled care
- *2008:* SSC guidelines updated; industry independence emphasized; ISF partnership ended

- *2012:* Further refinement of bundles and incorporation of data from 30,000 patients in the SSC database demonstrated a 25% reduction in the relative risk of death.
- *2016:* Incorporation of sepsis-3 definitions; greater emphasis on individualized treatment
- *2018:* Identification of sepsis research priorities
- *2020:* Publication of SSC COVID-19 guidelines to address the unique challenges of sepsis during the pandemic
- *2021:* Latest comprehensive update to adult guidelines

NEW DEFINITION OF SEPSIS AND SEPTIC SHOCK

One of the most significant shifts in sepsis management came with the *sepsis-3 definitions*.
- *Sepsis*: It is defined as "life-threatening organ dysfunction caused by a dysregulated host response to infection." Operationally, it is an infection plus an increase in Sequential Organ Failure Assessment (SOFA) score of 2 or more points above baseline. This definition underscores that not all infections are sepsis; rather, sepsis requires evidence of organ dysfunction.
- *Septic shock*: It is defined as "a subset of sepsis in which underlying circulatory, cellular, and metabolic abnormalities are profound enough to substantially increase mortality." Clinically, septic shock is identified by infection plus hypotension requiring vasopressors to maintain mean arterial pressure (MAP) > 65 mm Hg, along with a lactate > 2 mmol/L despite adequate fluid resuscitation.

This refined definition places greater emphasis on organ dysfunction and hemodynamic instability rather than systemic inflammatory response alone.

SCREENING AND EARLY IDENTIFICATION

Timely recognition of sepsis is essential for initiating early treatment **(Fig. 1)**. The guidelines recommend two main tools:
1. *qSOFA (quick SOFA) score:* It is a simple bedside tool used outside the intensive care unit (ICU). Parameters include systolic blood pressure ≤ 100 mm Hg,

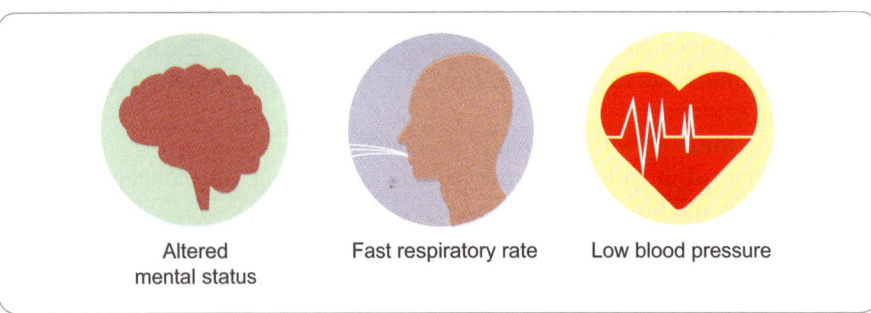

FIG. 1: Sepsis screening and early identification.

respiratory rate ≥ 22 breaths/min, and altered mental status. A score of 2 or more suggests a high risk of poor outcome and warrants further evaluation.
2. *SOFA score:* It is more comprehensive, covering six organ systems [respiratory, coagulation, liver, cardiovascular, central nervous system (CNS), and renal]. It quantifies severity and predicts outcomes. An initial SOFA < 9 predicts mortality below 33%, whereas a SOFA > 11 predicts mortality exceeding 95%.

By integrating screening tools with clinical judgment, clinicians can more rapidly identify at-risk patients and activate the sepsis bundle.

DIAGNOSTIC ALGORITHM

When sepsis is suspected, a structured diagnostic approach is essential.
- *Cultures:* Blood cultures should be obtained before starting antimicrobial therapy, provided this does not delay antibiotics by >45 minutes. Additional samples [urine, sputum, wound swabs, and cerebrospinal fluid (CSF)] should be obtained based on the suspected infection site.
- *Imaging:* Chest X-ray, computed tomography (CT), or ultrasound to identify infectious sources
- *Biomarkers:*
  - *Procalcitonin (PCT):* Helps guide discontinuation of antibiotics but not initiation
  - *C-reactive protein (CRP):* Nonspecific but useful for monitoring trends
  - *Lactate:* Elevated lactate is associated with higher mortality. Lactate clearance can be used as a resuscitation target.
- *Clinical evaluation:* Remains the cornerstone of diagnosis. Biomarkers are adjuncts, not replacements.

EARLY TREATMENT AND THE HOUR-1 BUNDLE

The SSC 2021 emphasizes the *hour-1 bundle,* reflecting the urgency of immediate intervention. The five steps are as follows:
1. Measure lactate and repeat if >2 mmol/L.
2. Obtain blood cultures before antibiotics.
3. Administer broad-spectrum antibiotics.
4. Deliver 30 mL/kg crystalloid for hypotension or lactate ≥ 4 mmol/L.
5. Apply vasopressors if hypotension persists to maintain MAP ≥ 65 mm Hg.

The goal is to initiate these interventions within the first hour of recognizing sepsis. Delays in antibiotic therapy are strongly associated with increased mortality **(Fig. 2)**.

INFECTION AND SOURCE CONTROL

Management of infection has two components: (1) Antimicrobial therapy and (2) source control.
1. *Antimicrobials*:
   - Should be administered within 1 hour of diagnosis
   - Broad-spectrum coverage is initiated and then narrowed based on culture results.

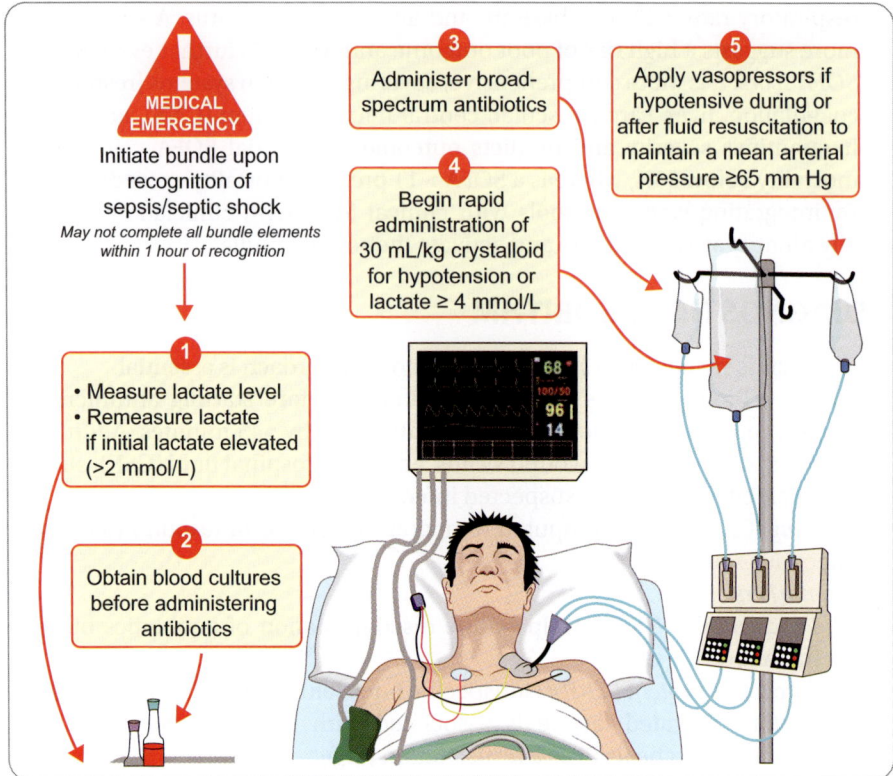

FIG. 2: Sepsis: Early treatment and the hour-1 bundle.

- Duration: 7–10 days for most cases
- Procalcitonin may support shortening or discontinuing therapy but should not be used to start antibiotics.
2. *Source control*:
    - Drainage of abscesses
    - Debridement of necrotic tissue
    - Removal of infected intravascular devices
    - Surgical intervention where indicated
    Failure of timely source control is a major cause of mortality in sepsis.

HEMODYNAMIC MANAGEMENT

Resuscitation strategies include fluids and vasopressors (**Fig. 3**).
- *Fluids*:
    - First-line: Crystalloids, with preference for balanced solutions like Ringer's lactate or PlasmaLyte
    - Normal saline is associated with hyperchloremic metabolic acidosis.
    - Albumin may be considered in patients needing large fluid volumes.
    - Hypotonic solutions and starch-based colloids [hydroxyethyl starch (HES), dextrans] are not recommended.

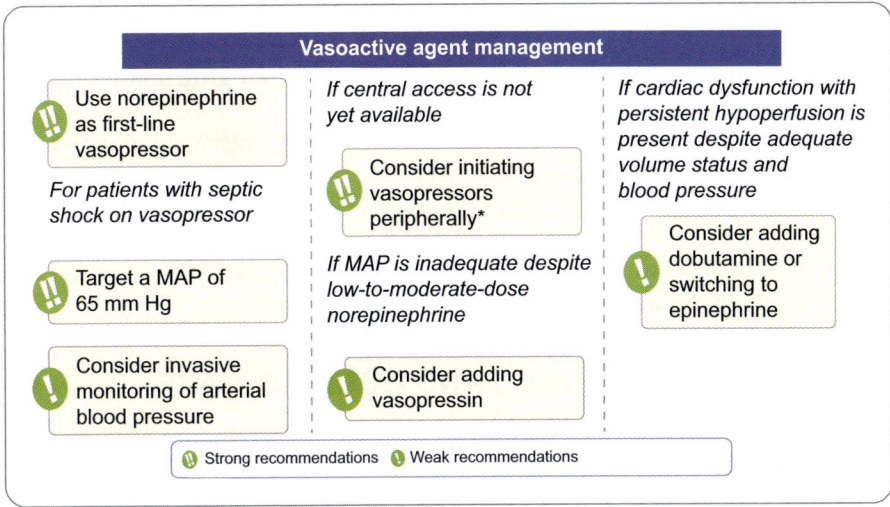

*When using vasopressors peripherally, they should be administered only for a short period of time and in a vein proximal to the antecubital fossa.

FIG. 3: Vasoactive agent management.
(MAP: mean arterial pressure)

- *Vasopressors*:
    - Norepinephrine is first-line.
    - Vasopressin or epinephrine may be added if norepinephrine is insufficient.
    - Dopamine is discouraged due to the increased risk of arrhythmias.
- *Targets*:
    - Maintain MAP ≥ 65 mm Hg.
    - Normalize lactate levels.
    - Use dynamic measures (e.g., passive leg raise) to assess fluid responsiveness.

VENTILATION IN SEPSIS-INDUCED ACUTE RESPIRATORY DISTRESS SYNDROME

Respiratory failure is common in sepsis and often manifests as acute respiratory distress syndrome (ARDS).
- *Mechanical ventilation*:
    - Use low tidal volume ventilation (6 mL/kg predicted body weight)
    - Plateau pressure ≤ 30 cmH$_2$O
    - Apply adequate positive end-expiratory pressure (PEEP) to prevent alveolar collapse.
    - Consider prone positioning (≥16 h/day) in moderate-to-severe ARDS.
- *Noninvasive ventilation (NIV)*:
    - May be attempted in selected cases but carries risks of gastric insufflation, aspiration, and discomfort
    - Most severe cases progress to invasive ventilation.

ADDITIONAL THERAPIES

- *Transfusion:* Restrictive strategy. Transfuse only if Hb < 7 g/dL unless ongoing bleeding or ischemia.
- *Corticosteroids:* Hydrocortisone 200 mg/day in patients with septic shock unresponsive to fluids and vasopressors
- *Renal replacement therapy (RRT):* Initiated for standard indications (e.g., hyperkalemia, acidosis, and uremia). Not sepsis-specific
- *Other therapies:* Immunoglobulin and extracorporeal blood purification are not routinely recommended due to low-quality evidence.

LONG-TERM OUTCOMES AND GOALS OF CARE

Survivorship after sepsis is increasingly recognized as a continuum. Patients who survive the acute illness often face:
- Persistent physical weakness
- Cognitive impairment
- Psychological sequelae [depression, anxiety, and post-traumatic stress disorder (PTSD)]
- Increased risk of recurrent infections

This constellation is termed *postsepsis syndrome.* Management includes early mobilization, nutritional rehabilitation, mental health support, and long-term follow-up.

Goals of care discussions are vital, particularly for elderly patients and those with comorbidities. Decisions about escalation or limitation of care should involve patients and families early in the course of illness.

RECENT ADVANCES

- *Procalcitonin:* Supports safe discontinuation of antibiotics, reducing unnecessary exposure
- *Presepsin:* Emerging biomarker with promise in early diagnosis and prognostication
- *Cell-free deoxyribonucleic acid (DNA):* Correlates with sepsis severity and mortality
- *Lactate clearance:* Now widely used as a resuscitation endpoint
- *Artificial intelligence:* Machine learning algorithms are being developed to predict sepsis onset and improve risk stratification.

These developments represent steps toward precision medicine in sepsis care.

CONCLUSION

Sepsis remains one of the most formidable challenges in critical care medicine. The SSC 2021 guidelines emphasize early recognition, prompt initiation of antimicrobials, rapid fluid resuscitation, appropriate vasopressor therapy, lung-protective ventilation strategies, and comprehensive follow-up for survivors.

The modern approach to sepsis balances evidence-based bundles with individualized patient care. As biomarker research and artificial intelligence mature, clinicians may gain powerful tools to predict, diagnose, and manage sepsis more effectively. Ultimately, the integration of timely intervention, multidisciplinary care, and long-term support offers the best opportunity to reduce mortality and improve the quality of life for sepsis survivors.

FURTHER READINGS

1. Evans L, Rhodes A, Alhazzani W, Antonelli M, Coopersmith CM, French C, et al. Surviving Sepsis Campaign: International Guidelines for Management of Sepsis and Septic Shock 2021. Intensive Care Med. 2021;47(11):1181-247.
2. Singer M, Deutschman CS, Seymour CW, Shankar-Hari M, Annane D, Bauer M, et al. The Third International Consensus Definitions for Sepsis and Septic Shock (Sepsis-3). JAMA. 2016;315(8):801-10.
3. Levy MM, Evans LE, Rhodes A. The Surviving Sepsis Campaign Bundle: 2018 update. Crit Care Med. 2018;46(6):997-1000.
4. Rhodes A, Evans LE, Alhazzani W, Antonelli M, Coopersmith CM, French C, et al. Surviving Sepsis Campaign: International Guidelines for Management of Sepsis and Septic Shock 2016. Intensive Care Med. 2017;43(3):304-77.
5. Shankar-Hari M, Phillips GS, Levy ML, Seymour CW, Liu VX, Deutschman CS, et al. Developing a new definition and assessing new clinical criteria for septic shock: for the Third International Consensus Definitions for Sepsis and Septic Shock (Sepsis-3). JAMA. 2016;315(8):775-87.

CHAPTER 9

Vasopressors and Inotropes in the Management of Shock

T Saravanan

INTRODUCTION

With an estimated 48.9 million cases recorded globally and over 11.0 million deaths from sepsis-related causes between 1990 and 2017, sepsis continues to be a major global health concern. This is currently the sixth most common reason for hospital stays in the United States. The high illness burden emphasizes how crucial it is to detect sepsis early and treat it well. Our knowledge and approach to treating severe sepsis and septic shock have greatly improved since the first formal definition of sepsis was established in 1991, thanks to a number of seminal investigations and clinical trials.

SEPSIS

Sepsis is defined formally as a complicated pathophysiological process in which an initial excessive inflammatory-immune response is triggered by a pathogen. Numerous biochemical pathways are either activated or suppressed as a result of this elevated reaction, which eventually leads to metabolic and circulatory dysfunction. Infection and at least two of the four systemic inflammatory response syndrome (SIRS) criteria are commonly used to identify sepsis clinically. Severe sepsis is defined as sepsis that results in organ dysfunction. Hemodynamic instability despite resuscitation, which is finally categorized as "septic shock" and is marked by severe circulatory collapse and decreased tissue oxygenation, is a result of this ongoing dysregulated reaction.

INTRAVENOUS FLUIDS

Intravenous fluid treatment during the acute period of septic shock is a topic of continuous discussion in the field of sepsis management. Although this is a minimal recommendation, the Surviving Sepsis Campaign (SSC) recommendations state that patients in septic shock or exhibiting symptoms of hypoperfusion should receive at least 30 mL/kg of intravenous crystalloid within the first 3 hours of resuscitation. A balanced crystalloid is currently the ideal fluid, and lactated Ringer's is chosen over regular saline because of the possibility of further acidosis as a result of hyperchloremia.

The Early Restrictive or Liberal Fluid Management for Sepsis-Induced Hypotension (CLOVERS) trial compared conventional fluid resuscitation to early vasopressor use and intravenous fluid restriction, finding that the conventional group received about 3.8 L of fluid while the restriction group received 1.8 L. The trial concluded that after 90 days, mortality and adverse events were similar between the two groups, regardless of the amount of fluid administered. Importantly, the American College of Emergency Physicians (ACEP) clinical policy does not recommend a standard fluid bolus but emphasizes the need for individualized fluid resuscitation based on the patient's specific condition. Furthermore, patients who exhibit symptoms of volume overload or who have a known low ejection fraction should have their fluid volume recommendations modified by the SSC. In conclusion, within the first 3 hours of resuscitation, 30 mL/kg of crystalloid (lactated Ringer's preferred over regular saline) should be administered. Alternatively, based on the CLOVERS trial, early vasopressor use may be considered if the patient is unresponsive to initial crystalloid therapy, all while using clinical judgment to avoid fluid overload.

■ VASOPRESSORS

The SSC recommendations advise starting vasopressor therapy gradually after sufficient volume resuscitation. Norepinephrine is the first-line treatment; if a mean arterial pressure (MAP) of >65 mm Hg cannot be reached, vasopressin is the second and epinephrine is the third. Dobutamine can be combined with norepinephrine or taken alone in cases of cardiac dysfunction. Notably, the CLOVERS and early use of norepinephrine in Septic Shock Resuscitation (CENSER) trials contrasted the early use of norepinephrine with traditional sepsis therapy, which involves intravenous fluids followed by vasopressors. While the CLOVERS trial revealed no difference in mortality or adverse events between the two regimens, the CENSER trial found that early norepinephrine usage improved shock management within 6 hours as compared to standard therapy. Instead of increasing norepinephrine doses, the guidelines advise adding vasopressin to adults with septic shock on norepinephrine who do not reach acceptable MAP (<65 mm Hg). To put it briefly, the algorithm for using vasopressors in severe sepsis and septic shock is as follows: A 30 mL/kg crystalloid fluid bolus (SSC guidelines) or early vasopressor use based on CLOVERS and CENSER trials is used first, followed by norepinephrine, vasopressin, and then epinephrine if no underlying cardiac dysfunction is suspected (think dobutamine).

■ PHARMACOLOGY OF VASOPRESSORS AND INOTROPES

Inotropes (levosimendan, milrinone, and dobutamine): Increase myocardial contractility. Vasopressors (norepinephrine, epinephrine, dopamine, phenylephrine, vasopressin, and angiotensin II): Increase vascular tone and MAP. Mechanism: Affect dopaminergic, angiotensin, calcium-sensitizing, and adrenergic (α, β) receptors. The aim is restoration of the perfusion pressure while reducing myocardial O_2 demand and side effects.

STEROIDS

The use of corticosteroids, especially in patients who need vasopressor support, is another contentious issue in the treatment of sepsis. In patients who still need vasopressor medication after receiving adequate fluid resuscitation, the SSC's current policy encourages the use of intravenous corticosteroids. The goal of this intervention is to enhance hemodynamic stability and lessen the length of time that vasopressor reliance lasts. Hydrocortisone is one often utilized regimen; a typical dose is 200 mg/day, given either continuously or as 50 mg every 6 hours.

This treatment plan is typically saved for patients who still require vasopressors even after receiving sufficient volume resuscitation. Interestingly, a number of studies have questioned the role of corticosteroids in sepsis management. Hydrocortisone, for instance, did not significantly lower the risk of progressing to septic shock within 14 days when compared to a placebo, according to the HYPRESS (Hydrocortisone for Prevention of Septic Shock) trial, which specifically looked at the early use of hydrocortisone in patients with severe sepsis who had not yet developed septic shock. The effectiveness of early corticosteroid therapy in sepsis, especially before shock has occurred, was called into question by this experiment.

Although the SSC recommends the use of corticosteroids for patients who continue to experience shock in spite of vasopressors, the evidence is still conflicting, and physicians must consider the advantages and disadvantages of each treatment individually. To summarize, in order to promote hemodynamic stability in sepsis with vasopressor reliance, the SSC advises using corticosteroids. Nevertheless, there is no discernible advantage to the HYPRESS study in preventing septic shock in patients who have not been shocked.

MANAGEMENT SPECIFIC TO SHOCK

Revascularization is the final treatment for cardiogenic shock, which is caused by left ventricular failure following an acute myocardial infarction. The medications include dobutamine, milrinone, levosimendan (limited), dopamine (less favored), and norepinephrine (preferred).
- *Hemorrhagic hypovolemic shock:* The first is to control bleeding and fluids; too much fluid can make things worse. Vasopressors are contentious; dobutamine/epinephrine is utilized for myocardial dysfunction; and norepinephrine is administered if fluids are insufficient.
- *Septic shock:* Get fluids and vasopressors early; aim for MAP ≥ 65 mm Hg. First-line treatment is norepinephrine; adjuncts include epinephrine, vasopressin for resistant patients, and dobutamine for cardiac dysfunction.
- *Anaphylactic shock:* The first line of treatment is epinephrine (IM), which stops bronchospasm, vasodilation, and airway edema.
- *Neurogenic shock:* Bradycardia and hypotension following spinal cord damage. Steer clear of dobutamine, norepinephrine/dopamine (high injuries), and phenylephrine (lower injuries).

DEVELOPMENTS AND PROSPECTS

Clinical: Vasopressin for refractory patients; levosimendan modest effect; norepinephrine safer than dopamine/epinephrine

Experimental: Norepinephrine enhances perfusion with fewer fluids, but vasopressin shows promise in hemorrhagic shock models.

Istaroxime, omecamtiv mecarbil, nitroxyl donors, and gene therapy (Ca^{2+} pump) are examples of novel agents.

CONCLUSION

Early diagnosis with fluids and vasoactive medications equals shock therapy. Vasopressin and epinephrine are adjuncts; dopamine is rarely utilized; norepinephrine is the cornerstone; and dobutamine is the key for poor output. Use the lowest effective doses because the evidence is still limited. In future, gene treatments and new inotropes could lead to better results.

FURTHER READINGS

1. Rudd KE, Johnson SC, Agesa KM, Shackelford KA, Tsoi D, Kiev Ian DR, et al. Global, regional, and national sepsis incidence and mortality, 1990–2017: analysis for the Global Burden of Disease Study. Lancet. 2020;18(395):200-11.
2. Arina P, Singer M. Pathophysiology of sepsis. Curr Opin Anaesthesiol. 2021;34(2):77-84.
3. King J, Chenoweth CE, England PC, Heiler A, Kenes MT, Raghavendran K, et al. Early recognition and initial management of sepsis in adult patients. Ann Arbor (MI): Michigan Medicine University of Michigan; 2023. [online] Available from https://www.ncbi.nlm.nih.gov/books/NBK598311/ [Last accessed October, 2025].
4. Evans L, Rhodes A, Alhazzani W, Antonelli M, Coopersmith C, French C, et al. Surviving sepsis campaign: international guide lines for management of sepsis and septic shock 2021. Intensive Care Med. 2021;47(11):1181-247.
5. Shapiro NI, Douglas IS, Brower RG, Brown SM, Exline MC, Ginde AA, et al. Early restrictive or liberal fluid management for sepsis-induced hypotension (CLOVERS). N Engl J Med. 2023;388(6):499-510.
6. Permpikul C, Tongyoo S, Viarasilpa T, Trainarongsakul T, Chakorn T, Udompanturak S. Early use of norepinephrine in septic shock resuscitation (CENSER). A randomized trial. Am J Respir Crit Care Med. 2019;199(9):1097-105.
7. Keh D, Trips E, Marx G, Wirtz SP, Abduljawwad E, Bercker S, et al. Effect of hydrocortisone on development of shock among patients with severe sepsis: the HYPRESS randomized clinical trial. JAMA. 2016;316(17):1775-85.

SECTION 3

Dermatology

SECTION 3

Dermatoses

CHAPTER 10

Dermatological Manifestations of Diabetes: When Glucose Marks the Skin

Satrajit Roy

■ INTRODUCTION

Diabetes mellitus (DM) is a chronic metabolic disorder characterized by hyperglycemia, resulting from defects in insulin secretion, insulin action, or both. Skin, being the largest organ, often reflects underlying systemic disorders including diabetes. Dermatological manifestations may appear before the diagnosis of diabetes or during its course, acting as a valuable clinical indicator of glycemic control. Approximately 30–70% of diabetic patients develop cutaneous manifestations during their lifetime.

■ PATHOPHYSIOLOGY

Chronic hyperglycemia contributes to nonenzymatic glycation of proteins, microangiopathy, neuropathy, and immune dysfunction, leading to skin barrier impairment and poor wound healing. Microangiopathy results in reduced perfusion, while neuropathy causes anhidrosis and altered sweating, predisposing to xerosis and fissuring. Advanced glycation end-products (AGEs) contribute to collagen cross-linking, loss of elasticity, and thickened skin seen in diabetic dermopathy and scleredema diabeticorum.

■ CLINICAL MANIFESTATIONS

Table 1 shows the classification of skin manifestations in diabetes.

TABLE 1: Common dermatological manifestations in diabetes.	
Category	Examples
Cutaneous markers of diabetes	Acanthosis nigricans and skin tags
Microangiopathic changes	Diabetic dermopathy and necrobiosis lipoidica
Neuropathic/Ischemic lesions	Foot ulcers and gangrene
Infectious conditions	Candidiasis and bacterial folliculitis
Drug-induced reactions	Insulin-induced lipoatrophy or lipohypertrophy and rash from oral hypoglycemics

Diagnosis

Diagnosis is primarily clinical, supported by laboratory confirmation of diabetes and exclusion of other dermatoses. Skin biopsy may be indicated in necrobiosis lipoidica or bullosis diabeticorum. Glycemic indices (HbA1c, fasting glucose) correlate with severity of some manifestations. Dermoscopy can aid in identifying microangiopathic changes.

■ MANAGEMENT

Management of dermatological manifestations in diabetes involves optimal glycemic control, skin care, and treatment of specific lesions. Regular emollient use alleviates xerosis. Topical and systemic antibiotics are used for bacterial infections, while antifungal agents treat candidiasis. Necrobiosis lipoidica may require topical corticosteroids or immunomodulators. Preventive care, including foot inspection and appropriate footwear, is crucial to avoid ulceration and gangrene.

■ OUTCOMES AND PROGNOSIS

Early recognition and management of cutaneous signs can prevent complications. Many lesions improve with glycemic control, while chronic ulcerations may lead to morbidity and even amputation. Patient education and multidisciplinary care are essential for favorable outcomes.

Key Points
- Skin manifestations may precede diabetes diagnosis.
- Chronic hyperglycemia alters skin structure and function.
- Diabetic dermopathy and infections are most common.
- Early detection improves prognosis and prevents complications.
- Multidisciplinary management enhances patient outcomes.

■ CONCLUSION

Cutaneous manifestations of diabetes are common, affecting up to 70% of patients, and often serve as vital diagnostic clues. Chronic hyperglycemia drives these changes through AGEs, microangiopathy, and neuropathy, leading to poor wound healing, infections, and specific dermatoses like diabetic dermopathy. Early recognition, meticulous glycemic control, and a multidisciplinary care approach are crucial for preventing complications such as chronic ulceration and amputation, thus improving patient prognosis.

FURTHER READINGS

1. Yosipovitch G, Hodak E, Vardi P, Shraga I, Karp M, Sprecher E, et al. The prevalence of cutaneous manifestations in IDDM patients and their association with diabetes risk factors and microvascular complications. Diabetes Care. 1998;21(8):1316-9.
2. Duff M, Demidova O, Blackburn S, Shubrook J. Cutaneous manifestations of diabetes mellitus. Clin Diabetes. 2015;33(1):40-8.
3. Kannan S, Ali A, Choudhary M. Advanced glycation end products in diabetes and its dermatological implications. Indian J Dermatol. 2019;64(2):110-6.
4. Bhat YJ, Gupta V, Kudyar RP. Cutaneous manifestations of diabetes mellitus. Int J Diabetes Dev Ctries. 2006;26(4):152-5.
5. Manjula VD, Shashikala K, Noronha TM, Shenoy N. Spectrum of cutaneous manifestations of diabetes mellitus and its correlation with HbA1c levels. J Evol Med Dent Sci. 2014;3(8):1966-74.

SECTION 4

Emergency Medicine

CHAPTER 11

Controversies in Snakebite Management: An Indian Perspective

Debasis Chakrabarti, Sayantani Bhadury

INTRODUCTION

Snakebite envenomation (SBE) was recognized by the World Health Organization (WHO) as a neglected tropical disease (NTD) in the year 2009 due to its high global burden and disproportionate impact on rural, impoverished populations. India alone contributes nearly half of global snakebite deaths, with recent studies estimating about 58,000 deaths per year.

A huge gap exists between the number of snakebite deaths reported from direct surveys and official data. Only 7.23% snakebite deaths were officially reported. Even today, only 22.19% of the snakebite victims attended the hospitals, rest approached traditional healers for treatment. States reporting a high incidence of snakebite include West Bengal, Tamil Nadu, Maharashtra, Uttar Pradesh, and Kerala.

Despite being preventable and treatable, snakebite management in India remains a significant challenge. Moreover, limited community awareness and dependence on traditional healers often delay definitive care.

TYPES OF POISONOUS SNAKES IN DIFFERENT REGIONS OF INDIA

India is home to over 300 snake species, of which >60 are venomous. The *"Big Four"* snakes—

Indian Cobra (Naja naja), Common Krait (Bungarus caeruleus), Russell's Viper (Daboia russelii), and Saw-scaled Viper (Echis carinatus)—are responsible for the majority of medically significant envenomations across the subcontinent.

The seasonal peak of snakebite is noted during the summer and rainy seasons. An increase in agricultural activity or heavy rain, leading to flooding of the natural habitat of snakes, increases the chance of snake-human contact. Flooding can lead to epidemics of snakebite **(Flowchart 1)**.

However, regional variations are significant. In *Northern India, Cobra* and *Russell's viper* predominate, while *Southern India* reports frequent envenomation from *Kraits, Saw-scaled vipers,* and the *Hump-nosed pit viper (Hypnale hypnale).* Mountain Pit Viper (*Ovophis monticola*) is found in the Darjeeling Hills of West

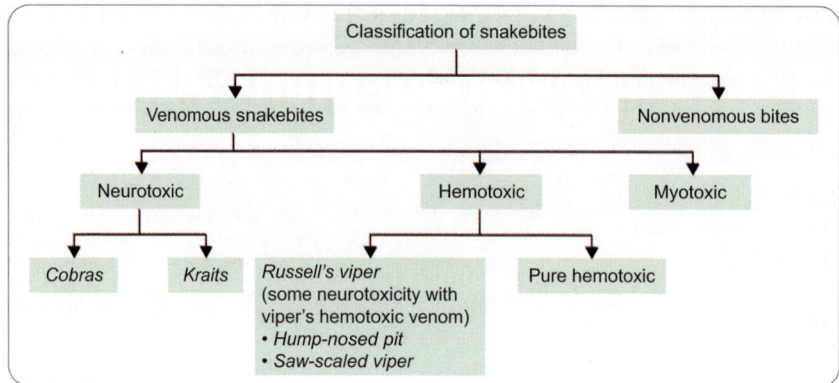

FLOWCHART 1: The classification of snakebites into venomous and nonvenomous categories.

Bengal. *Eastern India* sees *Cobra, Krait*, and *Green pit viper* bites, whereas *Western India*, particularly arid regions, reports high numbers of *Saw-scaled viper* cases. In the *Northeastern states*, the ecological diversity includes species such as *Trimeresurus* species, *King Cobra (Ophiophagus hannah)*, and *Naja kaouthia*, which are not covered by the currently available polyvalent antivenom.

This regional variation has major clinical implications since the efficacy of antivenom depends on the venom composition, which can vary significantly within the same species.

CLINICAL FEATURES

The clinical manifestations of snakebite depend on the species, venom type, and amount injected. Indian snakes produce three major clinical syndromes:
1. *Neurotoxic envenomation* (*Cobra and Krait*): It presents with ptosis, ophthalmoplegia, dysphagia, dysarthria, and descending paralysis, leading to respiratory failure. Krait bites often occur during sleep and may initially appear painless, leading to delayed recognition. Early morning "pain abdomen" is the most common presentation of Krait bite.
2. *Vasculotoxic (hemotoxic) envenomation* (*Viperidae*): It is characterized by local swelling, pain, ecchymosis, bleeding from puncture sites, spontaneous systemic bleeding, and coagulopathy. Acute kidney injury (AKI) due to hypotension, hemolysis, or disseminated intravascular coagulation (DIC) is a common complication.
3. *Myotoxic envenomation* (*sea snakes and some vipers*): It causes generalized myalgia, muscle tenderness, and dark urine due to myoglobinuria.

Local tissue necrosis, blistering, and gangrene are common in viper bites, often resulting in chronic disability. SBE is thus a multisystem emergency requiring rapid recognition and species-based management.

INVESTIGATIONS

The *20-minute whole blood clotting test (20 WBCT)* remains the cornerstone of bedside assessment for viper envenomation. Inability of the blood to clot within 20 minutes in a glass test tube indicates venom-induced consumption coagulopathy. If a neurotoxic bite is not surely proved and the first blood test is "clotted," the test should be carried out every hour for four times. If incoagulable blood is discovered thereafter, then 6-hourly cycles are adopted to test for the requirement for repeat doses of antisnake venom (ASV).

Other investigations include:
- *Hematology:* Complete blood count and peripheral smear for evidence of hemolysis
- *Coagulation profile:* Prothrombin time (PT)/international normalized ratio (INR), fibrinogen levels, and D-dimer, to monitor coagulopathy
- *Biochemistry:* Serum creatinine, electrolytes, and liver enzymes for systemic involvement
- *Urinalysis:* For hematuria or myoglobinuria
- *Imaging:* Ultrasound or Doppler when compartment syndrome or deep tissue injury is suspected

Emerging diagnostic tools, such as *enzyme-linked immunosorbent assays (ELISA)* for venom antigen detection and species-specific immunoassays, hold promise for identifying the offending species and quantifying venom load. However, these remain limited to research settings in India.

MANAGEMENT

First Aid and Prehospital Care

The WHO recommends immobilizing the bitten limb and reassuring the patient. The use of tourniquets, incision, suction, or application of traditional remedies is contraindicated, as they can worsen local tissue injury. The *pressure immobilization technique*, effective in neurotoxic bites, remains controversial in India due to a lack of standardization and risk of ischemic complications in viper bites. Bite marks to determine whether the biting species is venomous or nonvenomous are of no use.

In India, the first aid recommended is based around the mnemonic: *"Do it RIGHT."* It consists of:
- *R: Reassure.* Most crucial. Only 30% of bites by venomous species envenomate the patient.
- *I: Immobilize.* Immobilize the bitten limb in the same way as a fractured limb using bandages or cloth to hold the splints, not to occlude the blood supply or apply pressure.
- *GH: Go to the hospital immediately.* There is no alternative. Traditional remedies have no benefit in treating snakebite.
- *T: Tell the doctor* of progressive/new symptoms such as ptosis that manifest on the way to the hospital.

Hospital Management

The mainstay of definitive treatment is *ASV*, a polyvalent equine-derived immunoglobulin effective against the "Big Four". The recommended initial dose in India is *8–10 vials*, administered intravenously over 1 hour, though this may vary based on severity and species. Repeat doses are given if systemic signs persist or 20 WBCT remains abnormal after 6 hours. If a clotting defect is present, there will be active abnormal bleeding after 1 hour of first dose. Then repeat the second dose of 10 vials immediately. In viper bites, maximum of 30 vials of AVS may be needed.

Management of Neurotoxicity

In case of neurotoxic bites, once the first dose of AVS has been administered and a neostigmine test has been given, the victim is closely monitored. A neostigmine test is administered using 1.5 mg of neostigmine IM.

Injection atropine 0.6 mg intravenously (IV) must be given before neostigmine. Injection myopyrolate (neostigmine + glycopyrrolate) is an easily available alternative; one shot of injection is to be given @ 1 mL IV for 10 kg of body weight.

After 30 minutes, any improvement should be visible by an improvement in ptosis. Positive response to *"AN" trial* is measured as 50% or more recovery of the ptosis in 1 hour. The first sign of improvement is the ability to open the eyes (ptosis improves). If the response *(AN trial) is positive*, repeat dose of neostigmine 0.5 mg IM every 30 minutes for 5 doses with 0.6 mg of atropine IV over 8 hours by continuous infusion.

Supportive Therapy

- *Airway management and ventilatory support* are critical in neurotoxic envenomation.
- *Fluids and renal support* for shock and AKI
- *Tetanus prophylaxis* and *analgesia* as required
- *Antibiotics* are indicated for necrotic wounds or suspected infection.
- *Blood products* [fresh-frozen plasma (FFP) and cryoprecipitate] may be required for coagulopathy unresponsive to ASV.

Management of Antisnake Venom Reactions

Adverse reactions occur in 20–80% of cases due to heterologous protein content. The use of *low-dose intramuscular adrenaline (0.25–0.5 mg)* as premedication has been shown to significantly reduce severe reactions, though not all guidelines endorse routine prophylaxis.

Controversies in Snakebite Management

- *Timing and dosage of ASV:* There is no national consensus on the initial ASV dose or timing of repeat doses. Some clinicians advocate early aggressive dosing to neutralize circulating venom, while others favor titrated regimens to minimize adverse reactions.
- *Polyvalent versus monovalent ASV:* India relies on a single polyvalent ASV covering the "Big Four," leaving bites from region-specific species such as *Hypnale hypnale* and *Trimeresurus* species without effective therapy.

The debate continues whether *region-specific monovalent ASVs* should be developed, balancing the cost, logistics, and epidemiological needs.
- *Refractory coagulopathy:* Persistent incoagulable blood despite adequate ASV poses a therapeutic dilemma. Whether to continue ASV or switch to blood products such as FFP remains debatable due to a lack of standardized criteria.
- *Prehospital practices:* Use of traditional remedies, incision, suction, or herbal treatments remains common in rural India, delaying hospital presentation. The utility of *pressure immobilization* in neurotoxic bites versus its risks in vasculotoxic bites remains controversial.
- *Adjunctive therapies:* The use of *neostigmine* as an adjunct in *Cobra* or *Krait* bites has shown variable results. Similarly, *heparin, corticosteroids, and antibiotics* have limited evidence supporting their routine use.
- *Emerging therapeutics:* Recombinant antibodies, metal chelators, and small-molecule venom inhibitors are being explored as safer, more effective alternatives to conventional ASV. However, these remain experimental and inaccessible in endemic regions.

CONCLUSION

Snakebite management in India remains fraught with diagnostic uncertainty, therapeutic limitations, and public health challenges. Despite being one of the oldest medical emergencies known to mankind, it continues to cause preventable morbidity and mortality due to inconsistent practices and unresolved controversies.

Key areas demanding attention include the development of *region-specific ASVs*, improved *surveillance and reporting, standardized treatment protocols,* and *training of rural healthcare providers.* Strengthening research on venom composition, improving diagnostic capability, and ensuring equitable ASV access are essential to reduce the burden of this NTD.

A multidisciplinary, evidence-based approach—bridging clinical medicine, toxicology, and public health—is necessary to resolve these controversies and translate knowledge into effective, lifesaving care.

FURTHER READINGS

1. World Health Organization. Guidelines for the management of snake-bites, 2nd edition. WHO Regional Office for South-East Asia; 2016.
2. Suraweera W, Warrell DA, Whitaker R, Menon G, Rodrigues R, Fu SH, et al. Trends in snakebite deaths in India from 2000 to 2019 in a nationally representative mortality study. eLife. 2020;9:e54076.
3. Mohapatra B, Warrell DA, Suraweera W, Bhatia P, Dhingra N, Jotkar RM, et al. Snakebite mortality in India: a nationally representative mortality survey. PLoS Negl Trop Dis. 2011;5(4):e1018.
4. Warrell DA. Clinical toxicology of snakebite in Asia. In: Meier J, White J (Eds). Handbook of Clinical Toxicology of Animal Venoms and Poisons. CRC Press; 1995.
5. Government of India. National Snakebite Management Protocol, 2017. Directorate General of Health Services, Ministry of Health & Family Welfare.

SECTION 5

Endocrinology

CHAPTER 12

Male Osteoporosis: An Under-recognized and Growing Health Concern

Pankaj Singhania, Ayush Agarwal

INTRODUCTION

Osteoporosis is defined as a systemic skeletal disorder characterized by reduced bone mass and microarchitectural deterioration of bone tissue, which increases bone fragility and susceptibility to fractures. Although traditionally perceived as a disease predominantly affecting postmenopausal women, osteoporosis in men is a significant and growing health concern. Approximately one in five men over the age of 50 years will experience an osteoporotic fracture during their lifetime. Notably, men exhibit a higher risk of mortality following osteoporotic fractures than women, particularly in the case of hip fractures, where 1-year postfracture mortality can reach up to 37.5% in men. The underdiagnosis and undertreatment of osteoporosis in men contribute to this disparity, necessitating increased awareness, early detection, and effective management strategies tailored to the male population.

EPIDEMIOLOGY AND BURDEN OF DISEASE

Osteoporosis in men is an under-recognized public health issue with substantial personal and societal costs. Although the condition is less prevalent in men than in women, it is not uncommon. Approximately 20–30% of all osteoporotic fractures occur in men. In 2000 alone, 3.5 million fractures occurred in men worldwide. The burden of osteoporotic fractures in men is expected to rise dramatically due to global population aging, with projections indicating a 310% increase in fractures between 1990 and 2050. Mortality following a hip fracture is significantly higher in men than in women, ranging from 25 to 37% within the first year. Contributing factors include older age at the time of fracture, greater comorbidity burden, and increased risk of postoperative complications such as infections and cardiovascular events.

PATHOPHYSIOLOGY AND HORMONAL INFLUENCES

Bone metabolism in men is regulated by a complex interplay of hormones, including testosterone and estrogen. While androgens are essential for bone size and cortical bone mass through stimulation of periosteal apposition, estrogens play a critical role in maintaining trabecular bone mass and regulating bone turnover. Clinical cases of men with mutations in the aromatase gene or estrogen receptor have shown that even in the presence of normal or elevated testosterone levels, deficiency in estrogen signaling leads to severe osteoporosis, underlining its importance. With advancing age, men experience a gradual decline in testosterone and vitamin D levels, along with a rise in parathyroid hormone (PTH), all of which contribute to increased bone resorption and decreased bone formation. Unlike women, who undergo an abrupt loss of estrogen at menopause, men experience a more gradual decline in bone mineral density (BMD), typically starting around the age of 40 years and progressing at a rate of 0.5–1.0% annually.

RISK FACTORS

Risk factors for osteoporosis in men are multifactorial and include age-related bone loss, lifestyle factors, chronic diseases, medication use, and genetic predisposition. Key risk factors identified in systematic reviews include:
- Age ≥ 70 years
- History of low-trauma fracture after the age of 50 years
- Hypogonadism, including idiopathic or secondary causes (e.g., pituitary or testicular dysfunction)
- Chronic use of glucocorticoids (≥7.5 mg/day prednisone equivalent)
- Excessive alcohol intake (≥3 units/day) and active smoking
- Chronic diseases such as chronic obstructive pulmonary disease (COPD), rheumatoid arthritis, celiac disease, and diabetes mellitus
- Low body weight [body mass index (BMI) < 20 kg/m^2] and physical inactivity
- Family history of osteoporosis or hip fracture

The FRAX tool integrates many of these risk factors to estimate the 10-year probability of hip and major osteoporotic fractures.

DIAGNOSIS AND EVALUATION

Evaluation of osteoporosis in men includes assessment of clinical risk factors, BMD, and laboratory testing. BMD is measured using dual-energy X-ray absorptiometry (DXA), targeting the lumbar spine and hip. Despite anatomical differences, diagnosis in men is based on the same T-score threshold (≤–2.5) using the National Health and Nutrition Examination Survey (NHANES) female reference database. Forearm DXA (one-third radius) is recommended when hip or spine sites are not interpretable or in patients with hyperparathyroidism or on androgen deprivation therapy (ADT).

The FRAX tool calculates 10-year probabilities of major osteoporotic and hip fractures based on clinical risk factors with or without BMD. Recent enhancements, such as FRAXplus, include modifications for recent fracture, glucocorticoid dose, and trabecular bone score.

Laboratory testing is essential to identify secondary causes and includes serum calcium, phosphate, creatinine, alkaline phosphatase, liver enzymes, 25-hydroxyvitamin D, testosterone, complete blood count, and urinary calcium.

Additional tests like serum protein electrophoresis, thyroid function, and celiac screening may be performed based on clinical context. Vertebral fracture assessment (VFA) or lateral spine radiographs are recommended in men with unexplained height loss or back pain.

TREATMENT AND MANAGEMENT

Management of male osteoporosis involves a combination of lifestyle modifications and pharmacotherapy.

Lifestyle:
- Ensure calcium intake of 1,000–1,200 mg/day, preferably from dietary sources. Supplement if needed.
- Maintain serum 25(OH)D levels ≥ 30 ng/mL through sun exposure or supplementation.
- Engage in weight-bearing/resistance exercises for 30–40 minutes, three to four times/week.
- Avoid smoking and limit alcohol intake to <3 units/day.

Pharmacologic therapy:
- Oral bisphosphonates (e.g., alendronate and risedronate) are first-line due to efficacy and cost-effectiveness.
- Zoledronate [intravenous (IV)] is suitable for those intolerant to oral agents or with recent hip fractures.
- Denosumab is effective in increasing BMD and is particularly useful in ADT-induced bone loss.
- Teriparatide or abaloparatide (anabolic agents) is reserved for severe osteoporosis or multiple vertebral fractures.
- Testosterone therapy is considered for hypogonadal men with testosterone < 200 ng/dL and symptoms, but should not replace bone-specific drugs in high-risk individuals.

MONITORING AND FOLLOW-UP

Monitoring involves periodic reassessment of BMD, typically every 1–2 years. A plateau in BMD may warrant reduced frequency of scans. Bone turnover markers (e.g., serum CTX and P1NP) can be measured 3–6 months after initiating therapy to assess adherence and biochemical response. Monitoring serum testosterone is also recommended in men receiving hormone therapy.

SPECIAL POPULATION

Men receiving ADT for prostate cancer are at increased risk for osteoporosis. Guidelines recommend baseline and periodic DXA, vitamin D, and calcium supplementation, and pharmacologic therapy if BMD is low or fracture risk is high. Men with recent fragility fractures, especially vertebral or hip fractures, represent another high-priority group for initiation of treatment.

CHRONIC DISEASES ASSOCIATED WITH SECONDARY OSTEOPOROSIS

Several chronic diseases are associated with secondary osteoporosis in men, including:
- COPD—chronic inflammation and corticosteroid use
- Hypogonadism—reduced bone formation due to low testosterone
- Celiac disease—malabsorption of calcium and vitamin D
- Glucocorticoid therapy—direct suppression of osteoblast function
- Diabetes mellitus—altered bone quality and increased fracture risk

FUTURE DIRECTIONS AND RESEARCH GAPS

Despite increasing recognition, male osteoporosis remains under-researched. Few trials assess fracture endpoints in men. Most data are extrapolated from studies in women. There is a need for:
- Randomized controlled trials (RCTs) with fracture outcomes in male cohorts
- Long-term data on sequential therapy
- Evaluation of newer agents (e.g., romosozumab) in men
- Health-economic analyses tailored to men
- Improved awareness and education to enhance diagnosis and treatment adherence

CONCLUSION

Osteoporosis in men is associated with significant morbidity and mortality but remains underdiagnosed and undertreated. Effective management requires early identification, risk stratification using BMD and FRAX, correction of modifiable risk factors, and timely initiation of pharmacological therapy. Clinicians must be vigilant in recognizing at-risk individuals, especially those with hypogonadism, chronic illness, or prior fractures. Greater awareness and implementation of evidence-based guidelines will improve outcomes for men with osteoporosis.

FURTHER READINGS

1. Orwoll E, Ettinger M, Weiss S, Miller P, Kendler D, Graham J, et al. Alendronate for the treatment of osteoporosis in men. N Engl J Med. 2000;343(9):604-10.
2. Fuggle NR, Beaudart C, Bruyère O, Abrahamsen B, Al-Daghri N, Burlet N, et al. Evidence-based guideline for the management of osteoporosis in men. Nat Rev Rheumatol. 2024;20(4):241-51.
3. Watts NB, Adler RA, Bilezikian JP, Drake MT, Eastell R, Orwoll ES, et al. Osteoporosis in men: an Endocrine Society clinical practice guideline. J Clin Endocrinol Metab. 2012;97(6):1802-22.
4. Björnsdottir S, Clarke BL, Mannstadt M, Langdahl BL. Male osteoporosis—what are the causes, diagnostic challenges, and management. Best Pract Res Clin Rheumatol. 2022;36(3):101766.
5. Föger-Samwald U, Dovjak P, Azizi-Semrad U, Kerschan-Schindl K, Pietschmann P. Osteoporosis: pathophysiology and therapeutic options. EXCLI J. 2020;19:1017-37.

CHAPTER 13

Testosterone: Facts and Myths

Ranjodh Gill

■ INTRODUCTION

Testosterone is primarily produced in the testes with an insignificant contribution from the adrenal cortex. While testosterone levels naturally decline with age, particularly after the age of 30 years, many patients and healthcare providers associate this decline with a variety of nonspecific symptoms such as fatigue, reduced libido, and muscle weakness. The growing trend of TRT for aging men, however, has given rise to numerous misconceptions and debates surrounding its safety, efficacy, and long-term consequences.

■ TESTOSTERONE PHYSIOLOGY: FACTS

- *Definition:* Diagnosis of hypogonadism requires both the presence of symptoms and signs consistent with testosterone (T) deficiency and unequivocally and consistently low serum T concentrations on at least two separate occasions.
- *Diagnostic criteria:* The diagnosis of testosterone deficiency is based on clinical symptoms in conjunction with blood tests that measure total testosterone levels, typically in the morning when levels are highest. Levels below 300 ng/dL are considered low, though individual patient symptoms and preferences should guide treatment decisions.
- *Production and regulation*: The production of testosterone from Leydig cells in testes is regulated by the hypothalamic–pituitary–gonadal (HPG) axis, which exhibits a circadian rhythm with peak levels typically occurring in the morning, with a second small peak in early evening.
- *Testosterone's role in the body:* Testosterone is responsible for a wide array of physiological processes, namely:
  - *Sexual function:* It is crucial for the development of secondary sexual characteristics such as increased muscle mass, facial hair, and deepening of the voice in males. It also plays a key role in maintaining libido and erectile function.
  - *Bone health:* Testosterone is essential for the maintenance of bone density. Low levels are associated with an increased risk of bone loss. Testosterone

replacement certainly increases bone mass, but it is not known whether there is reduction in fracture risk.
  - *Mood and cognition:* Testosterone has a significant impact on mood regulation, cognition, and mental clarity. Low testosterone levels have been linked with depression, irritability, and cognitive decline.
  - *Metabolism:* Testosterone contributes to the regulation of fat distribution and muscle mass. It has anabolic effects, promoting muscle growth and strength.
  - *Testosterone replacement:* Before starting testosterone, the benefits and risks of such an intervention should be discussed with the patient, with a clear plan for efficacy and safety monitoring. It is generally safer to use a topical agent that achieves a more steady and sustained testosterone level, avoiding peaks and troughs and mitigating some of the side effects associated with superphysiologic testosterone levels.
- *Testosterone levels and aging:* Testosterone levels naturally decline with age, with a decrease of about 1% per year after the age of 30 years. This gradual decline is sometimes referred to as "andropause" or "male menopause." This is a very gradual process due to pathophysiological changes occurring at the gonadal, pituitary, and hypothalamic levels. It is thought to be adaptive, and most men either do not recognize symptoms or get accustomed to them. Moreover, we do not have age-adjusted normative testosterone values. Symptoms such as reduced libido, fatigue, and decreased muscle mass are commonly associated with low testosterone levels in aging men, but many of these symptoms overlap with other age-related conditions and are multifactorial in etiology, making diagnosis challenging.

TESTOSTERONE MYTHS

- *Testosterone therapy causes prostate cancer:* It is true that testosterone increases prostate volume by causing its hyperplasia and may lead to lower urinary tract symptoms. While it may also promote the growth of existing prostate cancer cells, there is no conclusive evidence to suggest that TRT causes prostate cancer in healthy men. However, men with a history of prostate cancer should avoid TRT.
- *Testosterone therapy leads to heart disease:* Early studies suggested a potential link between TRT and increased heart attack risk, but more recent research, including large cohort studies, has not found a clear causal relationship between testosterone therapy and heart disease. In fact, some studies suggest that testosterone may have a protective effect on the cardiovascular system by improving lipid profiles, reducing visceral fat, and promoting better endothelial function.
- *Testosterone and fertility:* It is true that exogenous testosterone can suppress sperm production by inhibiting the HPG axis. A fair number of young men of reproductive age are erroneously started on testosterone without proper counseling and endanger becoming infertile. This occurs due to suppression of luteinizing hormone (LH), leading to low endogenous gonadal testosterone, which is needed for sperm production and maturity. Additionally, testosterone

also leads to suppression of follicle-stimulating hormone (FSH), which directly suppresses spermatogenesis through the seminiferous tubules. They can recover fertility after stopping testosterone or with appropriate interventions, such as the use of human chorionic gonadotropin (HCG) or selective estrogen receptor modulators (SERMs). However, there is a long latency period in recovery of the HPG axis after stopping testosterone, which can last several months. Therefore, men seeking fertility preservation should avoid starting testosterone until after fathering children and discuss their options with their provider or a fertility specialist before beginning TRT.
- *Higher testosterone means greater masculinity or better performance:* A prevalent myth is that higher levels of testosterone automatically lead to better athletic performance, enhanced muscle growth, or improved masculinity. However, the relationship between testosterone and athletic performance is complex and depends on several factors, including genetics, diet, exercise, and overall health. Additionally, excessively high levels of testosterone, whether through supplementation or abuse, can lead to negative side effects such as aggression, venous thromboembolism, and adverse cardiovascular outcomes.

CONCLUSION

Testosterone is a critical hormone with wide-ranging effects on health and well-being. Despite the growing use of TRT therapy, many myths and misconceptions persist. For physicians, understanding the nuanced clinical data surrounding testosterone is essential for providing effective care. By debunking myths and focusing on evidence-based facts, clinicians can ensure that testosterone therapy is used safely and appropriately for patients, whether for hypogonadism or age-related testosterone decline. The ongoing research into the long-term effects of testosterone therapy, particularly in older men, will continue to shape best practices in the years to come.

Key takeaways for physicians:
- Be aware of the physiological role of testosterone, particularly in aging and hypogonadism.
- Diagnose testosterone deficiency with appropriate testing and clinical evaluation.
- Dispel myths around the risks of testosterone therapy, particularly in relation to prostate cancer, cardiovascular disease, and infertility.
- Approach testosterone therapy in aging men with caution, balancing the benefits with potential risks.

FURTHER READINGS

1. Bhasin S, Ozimek N. Optimizing diagnostic accuracy and treatment decisions in men with testosterone deficiency. Endocr Pract. 2021;27(12):1252-9.
2. Bhasin S, Brito JP, Cunningham GR, Hayes FJ, Hodis HN, Matsumoto AM, et al. Testosterone therapy in men with hypogonadism: an Endocrine Society Clinical practice guideline. J Clin Endocrinol Metab. 2018;103:1715.

3. Bhasin S, Snyder PJ. Testosterone treatment in middle-aged and older Men with hypogonadism. N Engl J Med. 2025;393(6):581-91.
4. Qaseem A, Horwitch CA, Vijan S, Etxeandia-Ikobaltzeta I, Kansagara D, Forciea MA, et al.; Clinical Guidelines Committee of the American College of Physicians. Testosterone treatment in adult men with age-related low testosterone: a clinical guideline from the American College of Physicians. Ann Intern Med. 2020;172(2):126-33.
5. Yeap BB, Wu FCW. Clinical practice update on testosterone therapy for male hypogonadism: contrasting perspectives to optimize care. Clin Endocrinol. 2019;90(1):56-65.

CHAPTER 14

Sugar in the Shadows: Rare Tales from the Diabetic Spectrum

Ram Babu, Raghavi Abhilesh Bembey

■ INTRODUCTION

The most severe acute metabolic decompensations in individuals with diabetes mellitus are diabetic ketoacidosis (DKA) and hyperglycemic hyperosmolar state (HHS). Many patients, particularly those with undiagnosed diabetes or poorly controlled existing diabetes, may manifest as unusual or organ-specific symptoms that may not immediately suggest an underlying glycemic disorder. These rare presentations pose diagnostic challenges, leading to delays in appropriate management and potentially increasing morbidity and mortality.

■ CENTRAL NERVOUS SYSTEM

Variants and Severe Forms of Diabetic Amyotrophy (Bruns–Garland Syndrome)

Classic diabetic amyotrophy involves acute, asymmetric, painful proximal weakness and wasting in the lower limbs, often with autonomic dysfunction and weight loss. It involves the upper limbs more, can be bilateral and asymmetric, or present with a more fulminant course of weakness and muscle atrophy. Sensory symptoms are less prominent than pain and motor weakness. It is an ischemic-inflammatory process affecting the lumbosacral plexus or multiple nerve roots (immune-mediated microvasculitis). Magnetic resonance imaging (MRI) of the spine/plexus may show nerve root enhancement.

Diabetic Striatopathy (Nonketotic Hyperglycemic Hemichorea; Chorea Hyperglycemia Basal Ganglia Syndrome)

Diabetic striatopathy, nonketotic hyperglycemic hemichorea (NHH) or chorea hyperglycemia basal ganglia (C-H-BG) syndrome, is a rare but distinctive neurological complication primarily associated with nonketotic hyperglycemia in patients with poorly controlled diabetes mellitus.

Clinical presentation: It is common in elderly individuals, typically with a mean age in their 70s, with female predominance. It can be the initial presenting manifestation of previously undiagnosed diabetes. The clinical hallmark is the acute or subacute onset of involuntary hyperkinetic movements, most commonly hemichorea (affecting one side of the body) or hemiballismus (more proximal, large-amplitude flinging movements of a limb). These movements are typically continuous during wakefulness, nonrhythmic, irregular and can involve both proximal and distal muscles of the affected limbs. The movements are characteristically contralateral to the affected basal ganglia (striatum) seen on neuroimaging. A key feature is that these involuntary movements usually cease during sleep and may be exacerbated by stress or voluntary actions. While limb involvement is prominent, facial sparing can occur.

Characteristic neuroimaging [computed tomography (CT)/MRI]: Brain MRI is the imaging modality of choice for evaluating suspected diabetic striatopathy. The most consistent and characteristic finding is hyperintensity in the affected striatum (putamen and/or caudate nucleus), contralateral to the clinical symptoms. The signal intensity on T2-weighted imaging (T2WI) and fluid attenuated inversion recovery (FLAIR) sequences is variable. The cornerstone of management for diabetic striatopathy is the prompt detection of hyperglycemia and its effective control with correction of the nonketotic hyperosmolar state, which involves intravenous fluid administration to correct dehydration and hyperosmolarity with insulin therapy. With successful glycemic control, the involuntary movements often improve significantly or resolve completely over days to weeks. If choreiform movements are severe, disabling, or persist despite adequate glycemic control, adjunctive symptomatic pharmacological therapy may be necessary like typical antipsychotics (dopamine D2 receptor antagonists)—haloperidol in low doses (e.g., 0.5–2 mg daily); atypical antipsychotics—risperidone or olanzapine is effective and potentially better tolerated; dopamine-depleting agents [vesicular monoamine transporter type 2 (VMAT2) inhibitors]—tetrabenazine or reserpine can be considered, particularly if antipsychotics are ineffective or poorly tolerated; benzodiazepines: clonazepam or diazepam may provide some symptomatic relief, possibly due to their gamma aminobutyric acid (GABA)-enhancing effects or sedative properties; anticonvulsants—sodium valproate or topiramate has been used anecdotally. The prognosis is generally favorable, with most patients experiencing complete or near-complete resolution of choreiform movements and neuroimaging abnormalities once hyperglycemia is controlled.

Nonketotic Hyperglycemic Seizures

Seizures are a recognized neurological complication of hyperglycemic crises and can range between focal (including epilepsia partialis continua) and generalized seizures, due to severe complications such as cerebral edema, profound electrolyte disturbances. Primary management is the gradual correction of hyperglycemia, hyperosmolality, dehydration, and any significant electrolyte imbalances.

Focal Neurological Deficits in Hyperglycemia

Hyperglycemia can manifest as focal neurological deficits. Diagnostic clues to differentiate it from stroke include presence of marked hyperglycemia (often >600 mg/dL) and calculated or measured hyperosmolality, clinical signs of severe dehydration, fluctuating nature of neurological symptoms, improvement with initial hydration and glucose-lowering measures, or absence of clear evidence of large vessel occlusion on acute stroke imaging protocols. HHS can be the first presentation of diabetes, so a lack of prior diabetes diagnosis should not exclude it. Neuroimaging (CT/MRI)—in hyperglycemia-induced focal deficits, brain CT or MRI is normal.

Meningeal Syndrome and Aseptic Meningitis in Diabetic Ketoacidosis

Characterized by signs of meningeal irritation, presents with altered mental status (disorientation, agitation, and confusion), headache, neck stiffness, and positive Kernig's and/or Brudzinski's signs, alongside the typical metabolic features of DKA. The primary diagnostic challenge is to differentiate this DKA-associated meningeal syndrome from acute bacterial or viral meningitis, done by performing a lumbar puncture (LP) and cerebrospinal fluid (CSF) analysis. The primary management is the standard treatment for DKA; if infectious meningitis cannot be confidently excluded, empirical antimicrobial therapy is to be initiated promptly after LP and blood cultures are obtained. The symptoms of meningism in DKA typically resolve rapidly (e.g., within 24 hours).

Craniofacial Hyperkinesias (Hemifacial Spasm, Blepharospasm, Oromandibular Dystonia)

Hyperglycemic state can present with unusual craniofacial hyperkinetic movement disorders. These can occur singly or multiple types of movement disorders may manifest in a single patient.
- *Hemifacial spasm (HFS)*: Involuntary, paroxysmal, or persistent twitching of the muscles innervated by the facial nerve on one side of the face. HFS can be an initial manifestation of uncontrolled diabetes mellitus, while pathophysiology is not established. Proposed mechanisms include transient ischemia or metabolic insult to the facial nerve due to hyperosmolarity, or a direct neurotoxic effect of hyperglycemia on the nerve or its central pathways. A crucial clinical feature is that these episodes resolve rapidly and completely following the correction of hyperglycemia and metabolic stabilization. Brain MRI is normal.
- *Blepharospasm*: Characterized by involuntary, forceful contractions of the eyelid muscles (orbicularis oculi), leading to episodic eye closure. When associated with HHS, improve with metabolic correction.
- *Oromandibular dystonia (OMD)*: This involves involuntary spasms and movements of the muscles of the jaw, mouth, and tongue, leading to difficulties with speaking, chewing, or causing abnormal facial grimacing, impaired oral intake.

These hyperglycaemia induced craniofacial hyperkinesias are refractory to standard treatments for movement disorders, such as antiepileptic drugs or neuroleptics, but show a dramatic response to insulin therapy and the normalization of the metabolic state. The diverse array of these rare movement disorders reported in HHS, often resolving with metabolic correction, suggests a profound but frequently reversible functional derangement of complex brainstem and basal ganglia circuits due to hyperosmolar stress, rather than indicative of permanent structural damage. This implies a high degree of metabolic sensitivity within these specific neural pathways.

Myoclonus and opsoclonus: Myoclonus is characterized by sudden, brief, shock-like involuntary muscle jerks, can affect various body parts, including the head, neck, or limbs, and may sometimes be reflexive (stimulus-sensitive). Opsoclonus is a disorder of eye movements characterized by rapid, involuntary, multivectorial (horizontal, vertical, and torsional), conjugate saccadic intrusions, often described as "dancing eyes", occurs due to significant metabolic dysfunction of neurons within critical brainstem or cerebellar areas that control and coordinate eye movements. Both typically resolves with the correction of the underlying metabolic abnormalities.

CARDIOVASCULAR SYSTEM

While atherosclerotic cardiovascular disease is a pervasive chronic complication of diabetes, acute and severe hyperglycemic states can precipitate or unmask distinct, less common cardiac syndromes.

Myocardial Injury and Electrocardiogram Changes Mimicking Acute Coronary Syndrome

The electrocardiogram (ECG) changes in DKA/HHS that mimic acute coronary syndrome (ACS), particularly ST-segment elevation myocardial infarction (STEMI), can be differentiated as discussed in **Table 1**.

TABLE 1: Differentiating pseudoinfarction from true acute coronary syndrome (ACS).

Differentiating factor	Pseudoinfarction (in DKA/HHS)	True acute coronary syndrome (ACS)
ECG response to metabolic correction	Hallmark is the resolution or significant improvement of ECG abnormalities (e.g., ST elevation) as metabolic derangements are corrected	ECG abnormalities (e.g., ST elevation) persist despite metabolic correction and require coronary intervention
Cardiac biomarkers (troponins)	Can be mildly elevated	Typically shows markedly elevated and rapidly rising troponin levels
Echocardiography and angiography	May show global hypokinesis or nonspecific wall motion abnormalities, with normal vessels	Regional wall motion abnormalities and block correspond to the territory of the occluded coronary artery

(DKA: diabetic ketoacidosis; ECG: electrocardiogram; HHS: hyperglycemic hyperosmolar state)

Arrhythmias (Atrial Fibrillation, Ventricular Tachycardia, and Atrioventricular Blocks)

Hyperglycemic crises are frequently complicated by cardiac arrhythmias, which can range from relatively benign supraventricular tachycardias to life-threatening ventricular arrhythmias and conduction disturbances. These are often driven by profound metabolic and electrolyte disturbances **(Tables 2 and 3)**.

TABLE 2: Unusual hematological findings in hyperglycemia.

Finding	Pathophysiology and mechanisms	Diagnosis
Hyperviscosity syndrome (HVS)	Caused by a clinically significant increase in blood viscosity due to: *Extreme hyperglycemia* (>1,000–1,500 mg/dL) leading to osmotic diuresis, severe dehydration, and hemoconcentration. *Reduced RBC deformability* due to the effects of high glucose • *Severe hypertriglyceridemia* (chylomicronemia syndrome)	*Definitive test*: Measurement of *plasma viscosity* (symptoms typically occur >3.0–4.0 cP)

(RBC: red blood cell)

TABLE 3: Rare gastroenterological presentations of hyperglycemia.

System/Condition	Pathophysiology and key presentations	Diagnostic approach	Management and prognosis
Gastrointestinal emergencies			

Severe gastroparesis precipitating crises/intestinal obstruction	• *Pathophysiology*: Autonomic neuropathy delays gastric emptying, leading to a vicious cycle of food/insulin mismatch
	• *Presentation*: Recurrent DKA/HHS with intractable nausea, vomiting of old food, and glycemic lability
		Gastric emptying study: Gold standard to confirm delayed emptying after excluding mechanical obstruction	• *Acute*: Standard DKA/HHS management
			• *Chronic*:
			  ○ *Diet*: Small, low-fat/low-fiber meals
			  ○ *Meds*: Prokinetics, antiemetics
			  ○ *Insulin*: Pump therapy may offer flexibility

Acute colonic pseudo-obstruction (Ogilvie's)	• *Pathophysiology*: Acute, massive colonic dilation without mechanical blockage, due to autonomic imbalance • *Presentation*: Progressive, massive abdominal distension. High risk of cecal perforation if the diameter is >12 cm	*CT scan*: Confirms massive colonic dilation and rules out a mechanical cause	• *Medical*: Conservative care (NPO, NG tube) • *Neostigmine* IV under cardiac monitoring can induce decompression • *Interventional*: Colonoscopic decompression if medical therapy fails

(CT: computed tomography; DKA: diabetic ketoacidosis; HHS: hyperglycemic hyperosmolar state; IV: intravenous; NPO: nil per os; NG: nasogastric)

HEMATOLOGICAL PRESENTATION

Hematological findings in hyperglycemia are given in **Table 2**.

MISCELLANEOUS SYSTEM

Rare gastroenterological presentations of hyperglycemia are given in **Table 3**.

MUSCULOSKELETAL SYSTEM

- Rhabdomyolysis
- Acute Charcot arthropathy

CONCLUSION

Hyperglycemia, far from being a simple biochemical abnormality with a narrow set of classic symptoms and chronic complications, reveals itself as a potent systemic disruptor capable of precipitating a wide and often bewildering array of rare and atypical clinical manifestations. As detailed throughout this chapter, these uncommon presentations can span every organ system, masquerading as primary disorders of the affected organ system, leading to potential delays in recognizing the pivotal role of dysglycemia. Therefore, a cornerstone of effective clinical practice must be the cultivation of a high index of suspicion for underlying or coexisting hyperglycemia when faced with acute, unexplained, or atypical illness, particularly in vulnerable populations such as the elderly or those with known risk factors for diabetes.

FURTHER READINGS

1. Desai R, Singh S, Syed MH, Dave H, Hasnain M, Zahid D, et al. Temporal trends in the prevalence of diabetes decompensation (diabetic ketoacidosis and hyperosmolar hyperglycemic state) among adult patients hospitalized with diabetes mellitus: a nationwide analysis stratified by age, gender, and race. Cureus. 2019;11:e4353.
2. Guisado R, Arieff AI. Neurological manifestations of diabetic comas: correlation with biochemical alterations in the brain. Metabolism. 1975;24:665-79.
3. Blonde L, Umpierrez GE, Reddy SS, McGill JB, Berga SL, Bush M, et al. American Association of Clinical Endocrinology clinical practice guideline: developing a diabetes mellitus comprehensive care plan-2022 update. Endocr Pract. 2022;28(10):923-1049.

CHAPTER 15

A Missed Diagnosis: Why Primary Aldosteronism Deserves More Attention?

Bimal K Agrawal

■ INTRODUCTION

Aldosterone production is physiologically governed by the renin–angiotensin–aldosterone system (RAAS). In *primary aldosteronism (PA)*, the adrenal glands autonomously secrete aldosterone, independent of renin. Hypertension is one of the most prevalent chronic diseases worldwide, driving cardiovascular morbidity and mortality. While often categorized as "essential hypertension," a substantial proportion arises from secondary causes. Among them, PA stands out as both common and treatable. Yet, it remains underdiagnosed, leading to missed opportunities for targeted therapy and risk reduction. If systematically screened, 10–25% of patients labeled as primary hypertension could actually be reclassified as PA. This chapter highlights why PA remains overlooked and why it deserves greater clinical attention.

■ EPIDEMIOLOGY: MORE COMMON THAN BELIEVED

Once thought rare, PA is now recognized as the most frequent cause of secondary hypertension. It accounts for 5–10% of all hypertensives and up to 20% of those with resistant hypertension. Despite this, real-world detection remains low due to inconsistent screening and misconceptions about its rarity. Clinicians are often deterred by the perceived complexity of the diagnostic algorithm, resulting in underdiagnosis.

■ PATHOPHYSIOLOGY: MORE THAN BLOOD PRESSURE

Primary aldosteronism is marked by autonomous aldosterone secretion from the zona glomerulosa. Excess aldosterone drives sodium retention, potassium loss, and plasma volume expansion, producing sustained hypertension. Importantly, aldosterone has *direct profibrotic and proinflammatory effects* on the heart, vessels, and kidneys. This leads to cardiac fibrosis, nephrosclerosis, and vascular remodeling.

Consequences extend beyond hypertension: Patients with PA have higher risks of *stroke, atrial fibrillation, left ventricular hypertrophy, heart failure, and chronic kidney disease*. Higher glomerular filtration rate (GFR) and albuminuria predispose to renal decline. PA is also linked to *metabolic syndrome, diabetes, and obstructive sleep apnea*, likely due to insulin resistance. Hypercalciuria contributes to osteoporosis and fractures.

CLINICAL CLUES AND MISSED OPPORTUNITIES

The classic presentation of hypertension with hypokalemia is uncommon. Most patients present with normokalemia and hypertension, indistinguishable from essential hypertension. Consequently, PA prevalence is underestimated.

Screening with *aldosterone–renin ratio (ARR)* is underutilized. Confirmatory testing (e.g., aldosterone suppression with saline loading) is often avoided because of logistical challenges or contraindications in patients with renal/cardiac disease. The absence of standardized confirmatory pathways further discourages clinicians. As a result, many patients are misclassified as having essential hypertension and treated nonspecifically rather than with targeted therapy.

COMORBIDITIES ASSOCIATED WITH PRIMARY ALDOSTERONISM

Large studies consistently show that PA confers *greater cardiovascular and renal risk than essential hypertension* at similar blood pressure levels. For example:
- A two- to threefold higher risk of atrial fibrillation and stroke. In one study, 42.5% of hypertensives with atrial fibrillation had PA.
- Increased rates of left ventricular hypertrophy (concentric and eccentric), dilated cardiomyopathy, and heart failure
- Accelerated renal function decline
- Lower reported quality of life

Notably, nearly 20% of patients with *diabetes and hypertension* may also have PA. These data emphasize that PA is not merely "another hypertension subtype," but a condition with unique systemic consequences.

TREATMENT: CURE OR CONTROL

Timely diagnosis is crucial because treatment is highly effective.
- *Unilateral disease (adrenal adenoma or hyperplasia)*: Patients willing for surgery should be imaged with computed tomography (CT), followed by adrenal venous sampling to confirm laterality. Surgery (unilateral adrenalectomy) can normalize blood pressure or reduce medication needs. Patients declining surgery will benefit from medical therapy.
- *Bilateral disease*: Managed with *mineralocorticoid receptor antagonists (MRAs)* such as spironolactone or eplerenone. These reduce blood pressure and counteract aldosterone's vascular and cardiac toxicity. Spironolactone is

initiated at 12.5–25 mg/day and titrated up to 200 mg/day. Eplerenone (25–50 mg twice daily, maximum 200 mg twice a day) is preferred if spironolactone causes endocrine side effects like gynecomastia, erectile dysfunction in males, and menstrual irregularity in females. If MRAs are contraindicated, epithelial sodium channel (*ENaC*) *inhibitors* (amiloride and triamterene) may be used.
- *Lifestyle*: All patients should follow a *low-salt diet (<5 g/day)*. Interestingly, PA patients have a higher salt taste threshold, but after adrenalectomy or MRA therapy, this normalizes, improving compliance with restriction.

Thus, identifying PA enables precision therapy—curative in some, disease-modifying in others.

MOVING FORWARD: PRACTICAL APPROACH

Despite robust evidence, PA screening is rarely performed, usually reserved for patients with resistant hypertension or established complications. The recent *European Society of Cardiology (ESC) 2024 guidelines* recommend screening all hypertensives. Early testing avoids the dilemma of medication withdrawal in advanced hypertension, which complicates ARR interpretation.

Screening should focus on *high-risk groups*: Resistant hypertension, early onset hypertension, hypokalemia (spontaneous or diuretic-induced), atrial fibrillation, obstructive sleep apnea, diabetes with hypertension, and family history of PA.

The *Endocrine Society guidelines (2025)* recommend ARR measurement in all hypertensives. Ideally, sampling occurs in the morning with the patient seated and not salt-restricted. Antihypertensives do not need to be stopped initially If ARR is inconclusive but suspicion remains, repeat testing after adjusting interfering medications is advised. Hypokalemia should be corrected prior to screening.

Notably, *spironolactone has been shown to be superior to bisoprolol and doxazosin* in resistant hypertension. Broader adoption of ARR testing and standardized algorithms could convert many cases of "treated" hypertension into "cured" or better-controlled hypertension.

CONCLUSION

Primary aldosteronism remains a frequently missed diagnosis with serious consequences. Despite being the leading treatable cause of secondary hypertension, it is still overshadowed by the broad label of "essential hypertension." Recognizing PA goes beyond controlling blood pressure—it prevents long-term cardiovascular and renal disease, improves quality of life, and offers cure in selected cases. Systematic awareness, early screening, and guideline-directed management are crucial to bridging the gap between *hypertension control* and *hypertension cure*.

KEY POINTS

- Primary aldosteronism is a *common secondary cause of hypertension*, present in up to 20% of resistant cases.

- *Cardiovascular and renal risks* are disproportionately higher than in essential hypertension [atrial fibrillation, stroke, left ventricular hypertrophy (LVH), chronic kidney disease (CKD), obstructive sleep apnea (OSA), and diabetes].
- *High-risk groups* include patients with resistant hypertension, hypokalemia, atrial fibrillation, young-onset hypertension, OSA, diabetes, or early stroke.
- ARR screening is simple and should not be withheld due to concerns about confirmatory testing.
- Abnormal ARR warrants treatment with MRAs; selected patients benefit from adrenalectomy.
- Only a minority of PA patients are surgical candidates, but all benefit from tailored therapy and salt restriction.

FURTHER READINGS

1. Funder JW, Carey RM, Mantero F, Murad MH, Reincke M, Shibata H, et al. The management of primary aldosteronism: case detection, diagnosis, and treatment: an Endocrine Society Clinical Practice guideline. J Clin Endocrinol Metab. 2016;101(5):1889-916.
2. Monticone S, Burrello J, Tizzani D, Bertello C, Viola A, Buffolo F, et al. Prevalence and clinical manifestations of primary aldosteronism encountered in primary care practice. J Am Coll Cardiol. 2017;69(14):1811-20.
3. Mulatero P, Monticone S, Deinum J, Amar L, Prejbisz A, Zennaro MC, et al. Genetics, prevalence, screening, and confirmation of primary aldosteronism: a position statement and consensus of the Working Group on Endocrine Hypertension of the European Society of Hypertension. J Hypertens. 2020;38(10):1919-28.
4. Rossi GP, Bernini G, Caliumi C, Desideri G, Fabris B, Ferri C, et al. A prospective study of the prevalence of primary aldosteronism in 1,125 hypertensive patients. J Am Coll Cardiol. 2006;48(11):2293-300.
5. Hundemer GL, Curhan GC, Yozamp N, Wang M, Vaidya A. Cardiometabolic outcomes and mortality in medically treated primary aldosteronism: a retrospective cohort study. Lancet Diabetes Endocrinol. 2018;6(1):51-9.

CHAPTER 16

Beyond Blood Glucose: The Multisystem Magic of SGLT-2 Inhibitors

Vijay Kumar

INTRODUCTION

Sodium-glucose cotransporter-2 inhibitors (SGLT-2 inhibitors) represent one of the most transformative classes of drugs in modern medicine. Initially developed as glucose-lowering agents for type 2 diabetes mellitus (T2DM), they act by blocking glucose and sodium reabsorption in the proximal renal tubule, resulting in glycosuria, natriuresis, and osmotic diuresis. This leads to modest reductions in glycated hemoglobin (HbA1c, ~0.5–0.8%), body weight, and blood pressure.

Unexpectedly, large randomized controlled trials (RCTs) demonstrated that SGLT-2 inhibitors reduces hospitalization for heart failure (HF), slow chronic kidney disease (CKD) progression, and improve survival, even in nondiabetic patients. These findings prompted a paradigm shift: SGLT-2 inhibitors are now incorporated into both cardiovascular (CV) and renal guidelines. The American Heart Association/American College of Cardiology/Heart Failure Society of America (AHA/ACC/HFSA) 2022 guideline positions them as foundational therapy for HF, while the Kidney Disease: Improving Global Outcomes (KDIGO) 2022 and 2024 guidelines recommend them in diabetic and nondiabetic CKD with estimated glomerular filtration rate (eGFR) $\geq$ 20 mL/min/1.73 m^2.

This review synthesizes the proven benefits, discusses potential roles under active investigation, and highlights adverse effects, with emphasis on mechanistic pathways linking renal, cardiac, and systemic protection.

PROVEN BENEFITS

Heart Failure

Heart Failure with Reduced Ejection Fraction (Ejection Fraction $\leq$ 40%)

The strongest early evidence for SGLT-2 inhibitor in HF emerged from patients with reduced ejection fraction. Multiple large randomized trials and meta-analysis have shown proven benefit including *DAPA-HF* where 4,744 patients with heart failure with reduced ejection fraction (HFrEF), both diabetic and nondiabetic were enrolled. In this trial, dapagliflozin reduced CV death or worsening HF by 26% [hazard ratio (HR) 0.74; 95% confidence interval (CI) 0.65–0.85]. The absolute risk reduction (ARR) was 4.9% over 18 months [number needed to treat (NNT) = 21]. Similarly in *EMPEROR-reduced* trial with 3,730 patients with HFrEF, empagliflozin reduced CV death or HF hospitalization by 25% (HR 0.75; 95% CI 0.65–0.86) and slowed annual eGFR decline by 1.73 mL/min/1.73 m².

Heart Failure with Mid-range Ejection Fraction and Heart Failure with Preserved Ejection Fraction

For decades, no therapy consistently improved outcomes in HFpEF. SGLT-2 inhibitor changed this landscape as shown in multiple trials like in *EMPEROR-preserved* enrolled 5,988 patients with EF > 40%. Empagliflozin reduced CV death or HF hospitalization by 21% (HR 0.79; 95% CI 0.69–0.90), mainly through fewer HF hospitalizations. In *DELIVER*, 6,263 patients with EF > 40% were studied. Analysis revealed that dapagliflozin reduced CV death or worsening HF by 18% (HR 0.82; 95% CI 0.73–0.92), ARR 3.1% over 2.3 years.

Similarly in acute heart failure, EMPULSE trial, 530 hospitalized patients with acute HF were studied. Analysis showed that empagliflozin improved a composite of death, HF events, and quality of life (win ratio 1.36, $p = 0.005$).

In post-myocardial infarction (MI) HF prevention: DAPA-MI enrolled 4,017 post-MI patients without diabetes or HF. In this trial, dapagliflozin reduced new-onset diabetes (33% lower risk) and body weight but did not reduce CV death or recurrent MI. *Similarly in EMPACT-MI* trial with 6,522 post-MI patients, empagliflozin did not reduce all-cause death or first HF hospitalization (HR 0.90), but reduced recurrent HF admissions (rate ratio 0.77).

Mechanistic Basis in Heart Failure

Sodium-glucose cotransporter-2 inhibitors improve outcomes through multiple converging mechanisms such as:
- *Hemodynamic unloading*: Natriuresis and osmotic diuresis reduce preload and afterload.
- *Energetics*: Enhanced ketone oxidation increases myocardial adenosine triphosphate (ATP) efficiency.
- *Cellular ion handling*: Na^+/H^+ exchanger inhibition reduces intracellular sodium and calcium overload.
- *Antifibrotic effects*: Suppression of transforming growth factor-β (TGF-β) and proinflammatory cytokines mitigates myocardial fibrosis.
- *Cardiorenal synergy*: Slower CKD progression reduces the cardiorenal feedback loop.

AHA/ACC/HFSA 2022: SGLT-2 INHIBITORS ARE CLASS I IN HFrEF AND CLASS IIA IN HFmrEF/HFpEF

Chronic Kidney Disease and Proteinuria

In DAPA-CKD trial, 4,304 patients with CKD, including 32% without diabetes were enrolled. Trial showed that dapagliflozin reduced kidney failure, sustained

≥50% eGFR decline, or renal/CV death by 39% (HR 0.61; 95% CI 0.51–0.72). ARR 5.3%, NNT = 19. All-cause mortality fell by 31% (HR 0.69).

EMPA-KIDNEY enrolled 6,609 CKD patients, 54% without diabetes. Empagliflozin reduced kidney disease progression or CV death by 28% (HR 0.72; 95% CI 0.64–0.82). Benefits extended to patients with low or absent albuminuria.

Both trials demonstrated substantial proteinuria reduction, with ~29% fall in urine albumin-creatinine ratio (UACR) observed in DAPA-CKD.

Proposed mechanisms to these benefits include lowering intraglomerular pressure by tubuloglomerular feedback restoration, albuminuria reduction by decreasing tubular protein load and toxicity. It acts on antifibrotic pathways to reduce inflammation and fibrosis. It also causes erythropoietin stimulation which leads to better renal oxygenation and hematopoiesis.

Due to consistent benefits in clinical trials KDIGO 2022 has recommended SGLT-2 inhibitor in T2DM + CKD with eGFR ≥ 20 (grade 1A).

KDIGO 2024 further extended this to include nondiabetic CKD:
- *1A*: CKD with eGFR ≥ 20 and UACR ≥ 200 mg/g, or any HF irrespective of albuminuria.
- *2B*: CKD with eGFR 20–45 and UACR < 200 mg/g.

Blood Pressure

Sodium-glucose cotransporter-2 inhibitors consistently lower blood pressure by modest but durable amounts. Meta-analyses show average systolic BP reduction of 3–5 mm Hg and diastolic reduction of ~2 mm Hg, independent of background antihypertensive therapy. These effects are mediated by natriuresis, plasma volume contraction, reduced arterial stiffness, and suppression of sympathetic activity. Endothelial function improvements have also been documented in mechanistic studies. While not a replacement for traditional antihypertensives, this effect is additive and particularly valuable in CKD and HF populations. Ongoing research is evaluating their role in resistant hypertension.

Weight

Weight reduction with SGLT-2 inhibitor is modest but clinically relevant, averaging 2–3 kg sustained over years. The primary driver is caloric loss through glycosuria (~200–300 kcal/day), but imaging studies confirm preferential reductions in visceral and hepatic fat. This contributes to improved insulin sensitivity, smaller waist circumference, and favorable metabolic risk profiles. Importantly, weight reduction occurs even when combined with glucagon-like peptide-1 (GLP-1) receptor agonists, making SGLT-2 inhibitor attractive as part of multidrug regimens. Research is ongoing into their role in nonalcoholic fatty liver disease (NAFLD) and weight regain prevention post-bariatric surgery.

Uric Acid and Gout

Sodium-glucose cotransporter-2 inhibitors lower serum uric acid by 0.6–1.0 mg/dL, mediated by uricosuria through GLUT9 and URAT1 transporters. This translates to a 30–40% reduction in incident gout in pooled analyses. Lower uric acid may also contribute to renoprotection by reducing crystal deposition and oxidative stress. Current studies are evaluating their potential role as adjuncts in gout management and hyperuricemia-related CKD progression.

MORTALITY AND ATHEROSCLEROTIC CARDIOVASCULAR DISEASE OUTCOMES

- *EMPA-REG outcome*: Empagliflozin reduced CV death by 38% (HR 0.62) and all-cause mortality by 32% in T2DM with atherosclerotic cardiovascular disease (ASCVD).
- *CANVAS*: Canagliflozin reduced major adverse cardiovascular event (MACE) (HR 0.86) but raised amputation concerns.
- *DECLARE–TIMI 58*: Dapagliflozin was neutral for MACE but reduced HF hospitalization (HR 0.73).

POTENTIAL BENEFITS AND ONGOING RESEARCH

Post-myocardial Infarction

Sodium-glucose cotransporter-2 inhibitors may attenuate adverse ventricular remodeling after MI through hemodynamic unloading, improved myocardial energetics, and anti-inflammatory effects. DAPA-MI and EMPACT-MI confirmed metabolic benefits and fewer recurrent HF admissions, though mortality benefit remains unproven. Ongoing mechanistic studies are exploring whether early initiation post-MI can improve infarct healing, fibrosis suppression, and long-term LV remodeling.

Erectile Dysfunction

Erectile dysfunction (ED) is highly prevalent in diabetes and CV disease due to endothelial dysfunction and oxidative stress. Pilot studies show improved erectile scores with dapagliflozin, possibly via nitric oxide restoration and oxidative stress reduction. Larger randomized trials are needed, with ongoing research investigating synergistic effects with phosphodiesterase type 5 (PDE-5) inhibitors.

Respiratory Disease

Patients with diabetes on SGLT-2 inhibitor appear to have lower rates of COPD exacerbations and pneumonia hospitalizations in real-world data. Proposed mechanisms include reduced pulmonary congestion from natriuresis and systemic anti-inflammatory effects. Dedicated prospective studies are underway to confirm respiratory benefits, particularly in patients with comorbid HF and COPD.

Migraine

Animal studies demonstrate reduced cortical spreading depolarizations with SGLT-2 inhibitor, suggesting antimigraine potential. Improved mitochondrial function and reduced oxidative stress are proposed mediators. Human studies are still lacking, but early phase clinical trials are exploring whether SGLT-2 inhibitor can reduce migraine frequency in metabolic syndrome populations.

Depression

Large cohort studies report a 15–20% lower incidence of depression among SGLT-2 inhibitor users versus dipeptidyl peptidase 4 inhibitor (DPP-4i) or sulfonylureas. Potential mechanisms include reduction of systemic inflammation, improved cerebral perfusion, and neurohormonal modulation. Trials are ongoing to test whether SGLT-2 inhibitor can directly improve mood or adjunctively treat depression in diabetes.

Cognitive Decline

Animal studies indicate SGLT-2 inhibitor may reduce amyloid-β deposition, enhance hippocampal mitochondrial function, and suppress neuroinflammation. This has led to pilot trials examining cognitive outcomes in elderly patients with diabetes or CKD. Larger ongoing studies (e.g., NCT04503104) are evaluating whether these agents can slow progression of mild cognitive impairment or Alzheimer's disease.

Hematology

Sodium-glucose cotransporter-2 inhibitors raise hematocrit by ~2–3% through erythropoietin stimulation, improving oxygen delivery. This may enhance exercise tolerance in HF. Ongoing studies are investigating whether this effect directly contributes to outcome benefits.

Liver Disease

Sodium-glucose cotransporter-2 inhibitors reduce hepatic steatosis and alanine transaminase (ALT) levels in small NAFLD trials. Ongoing phase 2/3 studies are assessing histological endpoints in nonalcoholic steatohepatitis (NASH).

Inflammation and Oncology

Sodium-glucose cotransporter-2 inhibitors inhibit the NLRP3 inflammasome in preclinical models, reducing systemic inflammation. Experimental oncology studies suggest they may impair tumor growth by limiting glucose availability, though no clinical data yet exist.

ADVERSE EFFECTS

Sodium-glucose cotransporter-2 inhibitors are well tolerated overall.
- *Common*: Genital mycotic infections, mild dehydration, and transient eGFR dip.
- *Rare but serious*: Euglycemic diabetic ketoacidosis (DKA), Fournier's gangrene, and canagliflozin-associated amputation risk.

- *Contraindications*: Type 1 diabetes, active DKA, pregnancy/lactation, severe hypotension, initiation if eGFR <20.

CONCLUSION

Sodium-glucose cotransporter-2 inhibitors have moved from glucose-lowering agents to cornerstones of cardiorenal-metabolic therapy. They reduce HF hospitalization and mortality, slow CKD progression in diabetic and nondiabetic proteinuria, and improve metabolic parameters such as blood pressure, weight, and uric acid.

Guidelines have embraced these findings—AHA/ACC/HFSA 2022 gives them class I in HFrEF and IIa in HFmrEF/HFpEF; KDIGO 2022/2024 recommends them for CKD with eGFR ≥ 20.

Emerging data suggest possible benefits in post-MI care, ED, respiratory disease, neurological disorders, liver disease, and even oncology. While these remain exploratory, the mechanistic rationale is compelling.

With strong efficacy, broad applicability, and manageable safety, SGLT-2 inhibitors now stand as true multisystem protective therapies.

FURTHER READINGS

1. DeFronzo RA, Ferrannini E, Chen R, Mehta AE. SGLT2 inhibitors and diabetes management. Diabetes Care. 2015;38(11);2110-9.
2. Heidenreich PA, Bozkurt B, Aguilar D, Allen LA, Byku AS, Chang PP, et al. 2022 AHA/ACC/HFSA Guideline for the Management of Heart Failure: A Report of the American College of Cardiology/American Heart Association Joint Committee on Clinical Practice Guidelines. Circulation. 2022;145(18);e895-e1032.
3. Kidney Disease: Improving Global Outcomes (KDIGO) Diabetes Work Group. KDIGO 2022 Clinical Practice Guideline for Diabetes Management in Chronic Kidney Disease. Kidney Int. 2022;102(5S):S1-S127.
4. Kidney Disease: Improving Global Outcomes (KDIGO) CKD Work Group. KDIGO 2024 Clinical Practice Guideline for the Evaluation and Management of Chronic Kidney Disease. Kidney Int. 2024;105(4S):S117-S314.
5. McMurray JJV, Solomon SD, Inzucchi SE, Køber L, Kosiborod MN, Martinez FA, et al. Dapagliflozin in Patients with Heart Failure and Reduced Ejection Fraction. N Engl J Med. 2019:21;381(21):1995-2008.

CHAPTER 17

Circadian Rhythm Disruption in Endocrinology

Gagan Priya

INTRODUCTION

In recent years, circadian disruption has become a growing public-health concern. Artificial lighting, shift work, excessive screen exposure, and erratic meal timing have collectively distanced human life from natural light-dark cycles. This misalignment between our internal clocks and the external environment is now recognized as a key contributor to obesity, diabetes, sleep disorders, mood changes, reproductive dysfunction, and even cancer. Understanding the science of circadian biology therefore holds direct clinical relevance. By recognizing how timing affects physiology, physicians can better guide patients toward healthier behaviors and treatment outcomes.

In this chapter, we discuss the physiology of circadian rhythms (CRs), explore how their disruption contributes to endocrine and metabolic disorders, and highlight key clinical evidence and practical strategies for restoring rhythm alignment and improving health outcomes.

RHYTHMS IN NATURE

Rhythms lie at the core of nature, from sunrise to sunset, and from tides to hormones. Same rhythmic patterns, called biological rhythms, regulate nearly every physiological process in living organisms. Depending on their periodicity, they are classified as circadian (around 24 hours), ultradian (<20 hours), infradian (>28 hours), or circannual (~1 year). Among them, the circadian rhythm is the most influential, synchronizing our body's internal clocks with the 24-hour light–dark cycle.

Every living organism, from single-celled algae to humans, exhibits such rhythmicity. In humans, these rhythms control sleep-wake cycles, hormonal secretion, metabolism, body temperature, and immune regulation. The recurring oscillation of physiological variables, described in terms of amplitude, period, mesor (mean level), and phase **(Fig. 1)**, is not merely a pattern but a fundamental property of life.

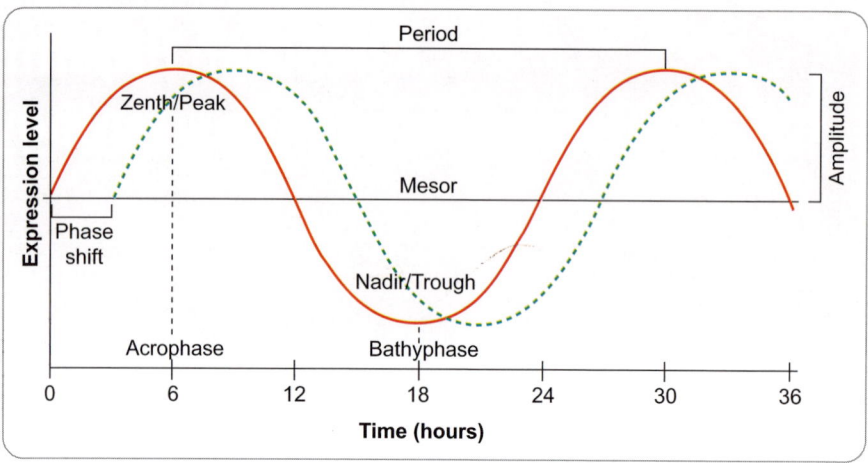

FIG. 1: A typical circadian rhythm represents a cosine wave. Period refers to the duration of a complete cycle (24 hours for circadian rhythm). Phase is an instantaneous value of a variable at the predetermined time—phase shift could mean the cycle is either delayed or early. Mesor (or medium) is the mean value of any rhythmic variable. Amplitude is the maximum deviation from the mesor. Zenith/Peak is the highest level while nadir or trough is the lowest level from the mesor.

EVOLUTION OF CIRCADIAN RHYTHMS

Life evolved under predictable environmental cycles of light/dark (day/night) and temperature. Organisms developed internal time-keeping systems to anticipate such changes rather than merely react to them. Two broad systems regulate homeostasis:

1. Circadian timing system (CTS) enables anticipatory and rhythmic responses to predictable daily changes.
2. Stress response system provides reactive and on-demand responses to unpredictable challenges.

Through millions of years, this capacity to allocate energy and functions across day/night cycles improved survival and performance. The CTS is a hierarchical network comprising a central clock and multiple peripheral clocks distributed across tissues **(Fig. 2)**:

- *Central clock (master clock):* The suprachiasmatic nucleus (SCN) in the hypothalamus, consisting of about 20,000 neurons, acts as the master pacemaker. It receives light signals via the retinohypothalamic tract, interpreting day/night information and coordinating body rhythms accordingly.
- *Peripheral clocks:* Nearly every organ—liver, pancreas, heart, muscle, adipose tissue, and even gut microbiota—contains its own molecular clock. These peripheral clocks regulate tissue-specific gene expression, ensuring that metabolic, hormonal, and behavioral functions occur at the right time of day.

Communication between central and peripheral clocks occurs through neural pathways, autonomic signals, and hormonal cues such as cortisol (peaking in the morning) and melatonin (rising at night).

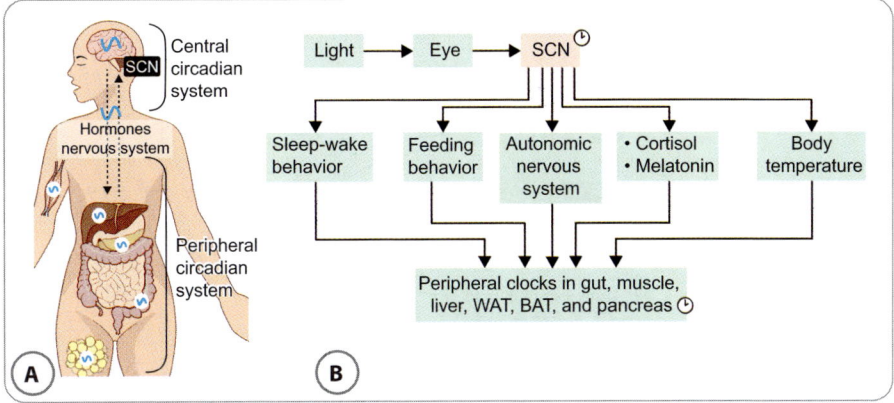

FIGS. 2A AND B: Components of the circadian timing system (SCN). (A) Central clock in suprachiasmatic nucleus (SCN) in hypothalamus via neuroendocrine pathways. (B) The SCN projects information to peripheral clocks in metabolically active tissues such as liver, gut, muscle, white adipose tissue (WAT), brown adipose tissue (BAT), and pancreas to synchronize their functioning via an intricate network. This communication is mediated via regulation of sleep-wake and feeding behaviors, autonomic nervous system, hormones including cortisol and melatonin, and body temperature.

MOLECULAR BASIS OF CIRCADIAN RHYTHMS

At the molecular level, circadian rhythms arise from transcription–translation feedback loops (TTFLs) **(Fig. 3)** driven by *core clock genes*, *CLOCK* and *BMAL1* that activate transcription of *PER* (period) and *CRY* (cryptochrome) genes. *PER* and *CRY* proteins accumulate and inhibit their own transcription, creating a roughly 24-hour oscillation. A secondary loop involving *REV-ERB* and *ROR* genes stabilizes *BMAL1* expression and maintains rhythm robustness. These self-sustained oscillations generate rhythmic expression of thousands of *clock-output genes* that affect up to 25% of the human genome, influencing nearly every biological system.

ZEITGEBERS: THE TIMEKEEPERS

Circadian rhythms remain synchronized with the environment through external cues called zeitgebers (time-givers or timekeepers). The primary zeitgeber for the central clock is light. Peripheral clocks are strongly influenced by food intake, metabolic signals, body temperature, and hormones. The central clock acts as the master-clock which orchestrates and coordinates the functioning of peripheral clocks, and both of these take cues from the external and internal environment. When all clocks remain in harmony and synchronization, central with peripheral, and body with environment, the system functions as a finely tuned orchestra. Desynchrony, on the other hand, leads to physiological "noise" and disease.

Figure 4 illustrates the intricate network of the circadian timing system and role of zeitgebers.

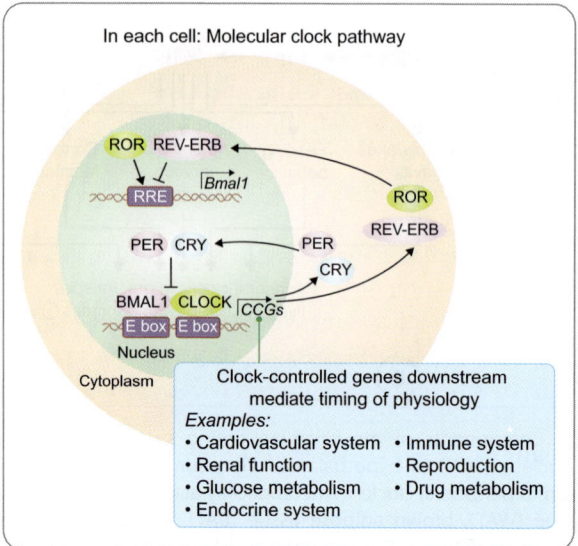

FIG. 3: Molecular mechanisms underlying circadian rhythms. There are core clock genes (CCG) and clock output genes (COG). At dawn, *CLOCK:BMAL1* stimulates expression of *PER* and *CRY* repressor genes. These also lead to expression of thousands of downstream genes or COGs. *PER* and *CRY* form a dimer in cytoplasm which is transported to nucleus and inhibits further transcriptional activity by interacting with *CLOCK/BMAL1*. *PER* and *CRY* proteins are destructed by *CK1* releasing *CLOCK:BMAL1* and a new cycle recurs every 24 hours. *CLOCK:BMAL1* controls transcription of *ROR* and *REV-ER*: *ROR* is a positive regulator while *REV-ERB* is a negative regulator of *BMAL1* transcription. Core loop (*CLOCK/BMAL1* and *PER/CRY*) is responsible for generating molecular rhythms while *REV-ERB* and *ROR* regulate *BMAL1* expression to confer rhythm stability and robustness.

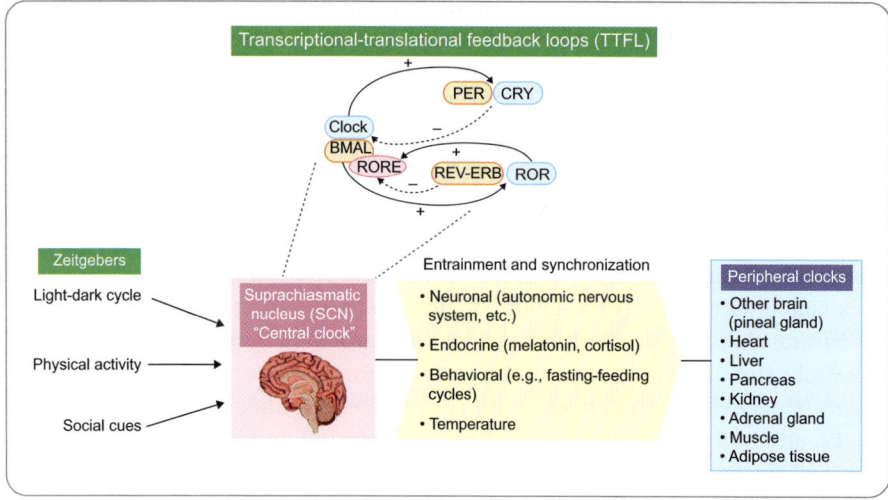

FIG. 4: The complex network of the circadian timing system. The central clock receives external cues and entrains the peripheral clocks, keeping the biological systems in synchronization.

Most hormone axes exhibit well-defined daily oscillations depending on their physiological role, e.g., cortisol peaks in the early morning, growth hormone rises during sleep, and thyroid-stimulating hormone (TSH) increases in the late evening. These rhythmic secretions ensure optimal timing of energy utilization, repair, and recovery. Similarly, metabolic processes, including glucose regulation, also show clear circadian variation. Clamp studies demonstrate that insulin secretion and glucagon-like polypeptide-1 (GLP-)1 responses are stronger in the morning than at night. Similarly, insulin sensitivity and glucose uptake in muscle and adipose tissue are maximal in early hours while hepatic glucose production decreases after feeding and follows meal timing. The gut microbiota also exhibits rhythmic changes, influencing the release of short-chain fatty acids, bile acids, and cytokines that modulate host metabolism. Consequently, glucose tolerance and energy expenditure are best in the morning, aligning with the body's evolutionary design.

CIRCADIAN DISRUPTION AND ITS IMPACT ON ENDOCRINE AND METABOLIC HEALTH

Modern society challenges these natural rhythms. Artificial light exposure, erratic sleep schedules, late-night eating, and shift work all cause a misalignment between internal and external time cues, called circadian disruption. In the US, nearly 15% of workers perform night shifts, while 70% of adults experience chronic "social jet lag" living by a schedule that conflicts with their biological clock. When the body's clocks go out of phase, efficiency drops. Circadian disruption has been associated with:

- Obesity and metabolic syndrome
- Insulin resistance and type 2 diabetes
- Hypertension and cardiovascular disease
- Polycystic ovary syndrome (PCOS) and infertility
- Cancers, mood disorders, and neurodegeneration

Multiple lines of evidence **(Table 1)** confirm the causal role of circadian dysregulation in metabolic disease. Sleep quantity and quality also matter. Both short and prolonged sleep durations correlate with increased risk of diabetes, with the lowest risk seen at 7–8 hours per night.

Beyond glucose metabolism, circadian disruption affects multiple endocrine axes.

- *Reproductive system:* Irregular sleep, light exposure at night, and shift work can disturb gonadotropin and steroid hormone rhythms, contributing to menstrual irregularities and infertility.
- *Thyroid axis:* TSH and thyroid hormone levels fluctuate diurnally; with evening elevations often blunted in night-shift workers.
- *Endocrine tumors:* Clock genes regulate cell-cycle control, DNA repair, and tumor microenvironment. Dysregulation of these genes is implicated in endocrine malignancies including adrenal, thyroid, and pituitary tumors.

TABLE 1: Evidence linking circadian disruption and risk of obesity and other metabolic disorders.

Line of evidence	Findings and clinical implications
Animal models	• Deletion of key clock genes in mice (e.g., *BMAL1*) results in increased appetite, obesity, hyperglycemia, and premature aging • Surgical removal of suprachiasmatic nucleus resulted in altered microbiota, tumors, and immune dysfunction
Human data	• Specific single nucleotide polymorphisms (SNPs) in *BMAL1*, *CRY2*, and *PER2* have been linked to glucose intolerance and metabolic risk • Shift workers display higher rates of obesity, insulin resistance, and diabetes • Social jet lag—the mismatch between biological and social time—is associated with impaired glucose metabolism • Chronotype studies show that individuals with "evening preference" (late chronotype) have higher glycated hemoglobin (HbA1c), lower activity, and greater cardiometabolic risk

CLINICAL IMPLICATIONS AND LIFESTYLE INTERVENTIONS

From a physician's perspective, understanding circadian biology offers new levers for prevention and treatment.

- *Lifestyle modification:* Large cohort data including the Nurses Health Study (I and II) demonstrate that the combination of shift work and unhealthy lifestyle increases diabetes risk almost three-fold. However, much of this excess risk is modifiable through diet, exercise, and sleep hygiene. Therefore, physicians should encourage healthier lifestyle practices which honor circadian biology, as enlisted in **Box 1**.
- *Chrononutrition:* "Chrononutrition" emphasizes when we eat, not just what we eat. Early eating windows (e.g., 10-hour eating between 8 AM and 6 PM) improve insulin sensitivity, fasting glucose, and gut microbiota composition. Late eating or irregular meal patterns disrupt clock gene expression and glucose metabolism. Time-restricted eating (TRE) studies show greater metabolic benefit when meals are concentrated in the earlier part of the day.
- *Chronotherapy:* The timing of certain medications may influence efficacy and safety. For example, glucocorticoids are timed in morning to align with physiological cortisol peaks, reducing hypothalamic–pituitary–adrenal (HPA) suppression and metabolic side effects. Short-acting statins (e.g., simvastatin) are more effective when taken at night due to nocturnal hydroxymethylglutaryl-coenzyme A (HMG-CoA) reductase activity. Growth hormone (GH) injections are administered at night to mimic the nocturnal GH secretion.
- *Emerging therapeutic approaches:* Pharmacological modulation of the CTS to improve metabolism is an interesting area of development. Melatonin, when taken in the early evening, can resynchronize the sleep–wake cycle, though results in diabetes remain mixed. Berberine, a botanical compound and REV-ERB agonist, has shown metabolic benefits including improved insulin

> **BOX 1: Lifestyle behaviors that honor circadian rhythm and reduce circadian disruption.**
> - Regular sleep schedules, with 7–8 hours of nightly sleep
> - Appropriate sleep hygiene—dark, comfortable room, keep devices on silent
> - Consistent meal timing
> - Avoiding late-night eating
> - Early-morning natural light exposure
> - Reducing screen time in night
> - Minimizing rotating or night-shift frequency whenever possible

sensitivity. Nobiletin, a citrus-derived RORα agonist, enhances circadian amplitude and reduces adiposity in preclinical studies. Further, novel REV-ERB agonists and CRY stabilizers are under investigation for obesity, metabolic syndrome, and sleep disorders.

CONCLUSION

The science of circadian rhythms is no longer a niche field—it is foundational to understanding human health. Physicians, regardless of specialty, must appreciate the temporal dimension of disease and therapy. By integrating circadian principles into patient care, be it counseling shift workers, optimizing drug timing, or advocating early-day meals, we can enhance metabolic health and overall well-being.

Just as the Earth turns predictably each day, our bodies too thrive when their internal clocks stay in synchronized with nature's rhythm.

FURTHER READINGS

1. Potter GD, Skene DJ, Arendt J, Cade JE, Grant PJ, Hardie LJ. Circadian Rhythm and Sleep Disruption: Causes, Metabolic Consequences, and Countermeasures. Endocr Rev. 2016;37(6): 584-608.
2. Reinke H, Asher G. Crosstalk between metabolism and circadian clocks. Nat Rev Mol Cell Biol. 2019;20(4):227-41.
3. Longo VD, Panda S. Fasting, Circadian Rhythms, and Time-Restricted Feeding in Healthy Lifespan. Cell Metab. 2016;23(6):1048-59.
4. Stenvers DJ, Scheer FAJL, Schrauwen P, la Fleur SE, Kalsbeek A. Circadian clocks and insulin resistance. Nat Rev Endocrinol. 2019;15(2):75-89.
5. Tahara Y, Shibata S. Chrono-nutrition and metabolic health. J Pharmacol Sci. 2018;137(2): 97-103.

SECTION 6

Gastroenterology

CHAPTER 18

Gut Microbiota and Its Role in Immunity

Princi Jain, Srinivasa Murthy, SS Dariya

INTRODUCTION

The gut microbiota is composed of trillions of microorganisms residing in the human gastrointestinal (GI) tract and has emerged as an essential contributor to host immunity. Once considered a passive presence, this complex microbial ecosystem plays a pivotal role in the development, modulation, and function of both innate and adaptive immune responses. Dysbiosis or alteration in gut microbial balance has been linked to a broad spectrum of immune-mediated diseases, spanning from autoimmune disorders to chronic inflammatory conditions and susceptibility to infections. This chapter spotlights the intricate interactions between gut microbiota and the host immune system.

COMPOSITION AND DYNAMICS OF THE GUT MICROBIOTA

The human gut harbors approximately 100 trillion microbes, including bacteria, archaea, viruses, and fungi. The major bacterial phyla are Firmicutes, Bacteroidetes, Actinobacteria, Proteobacteria, Fusobacteria, and Verrucomicrobia, with Firmicutes and Bacteroidetes dominating in healthy adults. The gut microbiota exhibits high interindividual variability, shaped by factors such as age, genetics, diet, medications, environmental exposures, and anatomical location along the GI tract **(Fig. 1)**.

ESTABLISHMENT OF GUT MICROBIOTA AND IMMUNE SYSTEM MATURATION

- *Early life colonization and immune development*: Initial gut colonization is shaped by birth method (vaginal vs. C-section), maternal microbiota, and feeding type (breastmilk vs. formula), with vaginal delivery transferring maternal vaginal/enteric bacteria while C-section favoring skin microbes. This early microbial exposure drives gut-associated lymphoid tissue (GALT) development, mucosal immunity maturation, and commensal tolerance.

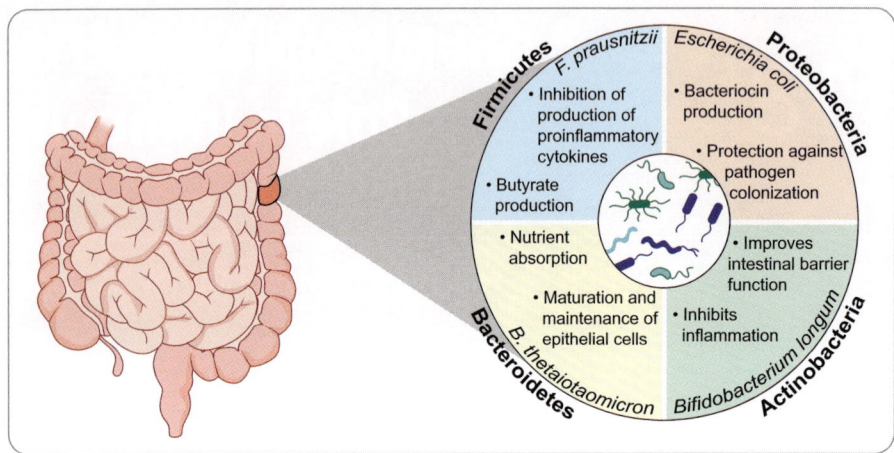

FIG. 1: Main phyla and functions associated with the intestinal microbiota.

Breastmilk further supports immune education via secretory immunoglobulin A (sIgA) and immunomodulatory factors during immune system priming.
- *Mechanisms linking gut microbiota to innate immunity*: The gut microbiota profoundly influences innate immunity through multiple mechanisms. Microbial-associated molecular patterns (MAMPs), like lipopolysaccharide (LPS), peptidoglycan, and flagellin, are detected by host pattern recognition receptors [PRRs; toll-like receptors (TLRs), and nucleotide-binding oligomerization domain (NOD)-like receptors (NLRs)] on epithelial and immune cells. This triggers signaling cascades that regulate mucosal homeostasis or inflammation. Commensals strengthen the epithelial barrier by stimulating antimicrobial peptide (AMP) production (defensins and RegIIIγ), enhancing mucus secretion, and reinforcing tight junctions. They also shape sIgA responses, promoting immune exclusion of pathogens while maintaining tolerance to beneficial microbes. Germ-free studies reveal the microbiota's essential role in immune development—its absence leads to underdeveloped GALT, reduced Tregs, and impaired sIgA production, defects reversible upon microbial colonization. These interactions demonstrate how microbiota-innate immunity crosstalk maintains barrier function while balancing tolerance and defense **(Fig. 2)**.
- *Gut microbiota and adaptive immunity*: The gut microbiota critically shapes adaptive immunity through T- and B-cell regulation. Short-chain fatty acids (SCFAs) like butyrate and propionate promote regulatory T-cell (Treg) differentiation, maintaining immune tolerance, while segmented filamentous bacteria (SFB) drive Th17 cell development—essential for mucosal defense but potentially proinflammatory if dysregulated. Microbial signals also guide B-cell maturation and IgA secretion, which neutralizes luminal pathogens and maintains microbial homeostasis. Dendritic cells sample gut bacteria, presenting antigens in mesenteric lymph nodes to coordinate T-/B-cell responses. This delicate balance between proinflammatory and regulatory mechanisms ensures effective pathogen defense without excessive inflammation.

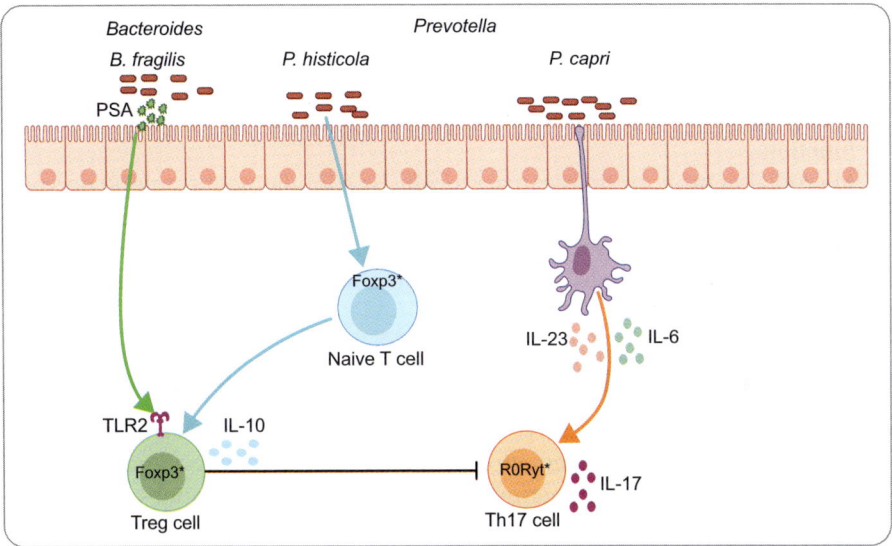

FIG. 2: *Bacteroides fragilis* promotes anti-inflammatory responses by inducing Tregs [via TLR2/PSA signaling] that secrete interleukin (IL)-10, suppressing Th17. *Prevotella copri* enhances Th17 via dendritic cell-derived IL-6/IL-23, while *Prevotella histicola* reduces proinflammatory cytokines [IL-2, IL-17, and tumor necrosis factor alpha (TNF-α)] by boosting Tregs. These interactions modulate gut immunity and influence systemic inflammation.

(IL: interleukin; PSA: polysaccharide A; TLR2: toll-like receptor 2)

NEUROHORMONES AND THEIR ROLE IN MICROBIAL EFFECT

The gut microbiota is now recognized as a dynamic endocrine organ, profoundly influencing host neuroendocrine function by generating and modulating neurohormones, bioactive molecules that impact both local and systemic physiology.

Microbial Synthesis of Neurohormones

Specific gut bacterial strains have the enzymatic machinery to produce neuroactive compounds, including:

- *Gamma-aminobutyric acid (GABA):* Certain *Lactobacillus* and *Bifidobacterium* species decarboxylate glutamate to generate GABA, a major inhibitory neurotransmitter with effects on gut motility and visceral pain perception. Microbial GABA can modulate enteric neural circuits and even influence central stress responses.
- *Serotonin [5-hydroxytryptamine (5-HT)]:* While over 90% of peripheral serotonin is produced by enterochromaffin cells, gut microbiota such as *Bifidobacterium* and *Lactobacillus* regulate tryptophan metabolism and stimulate host serotonin biosynthesis, altering GI transit, behavior, and immune responses.
- *Dopamine and catecholamines: Enterococcus* and *Escherichia* species are capable of producing dopamine, noradrenaline, and adrenaline, which

influence GI secretions, local immune tone, and potentially distal neural signaling.
- *Histamine and other bioamines:* Microbial decarboxylation of amino acids yields histamine and tyramine, affecting mucosal immunity and gut sensory function.

Microbial neurohormones can act locally by stimulating the enteric nervous system or systemically via vagal afferents, sometimes crossing the intestinal barrier to enter circulation. Conversely, host neurohormones (e.g., stress hormones cortisol and catecholamines) modulate microbial growth and virulence gene expression **(Fig. 3)**.

Key Microbial Metabolites and Hormonal Pathways (Fig. 4)

- *Short-chain fatty acids:* SCFAs—primarily acetate, propionate, and butyrate—result from microbial fermentation of dietary fibers and play critical roles in:
  - Stimulating enteroendocrine cells to release gut hormones [glucagon-like peptide 1 (GLP-1) and peptide YY (PYY)], thereby regulating insulin secretion, appetite, and energy expenditure

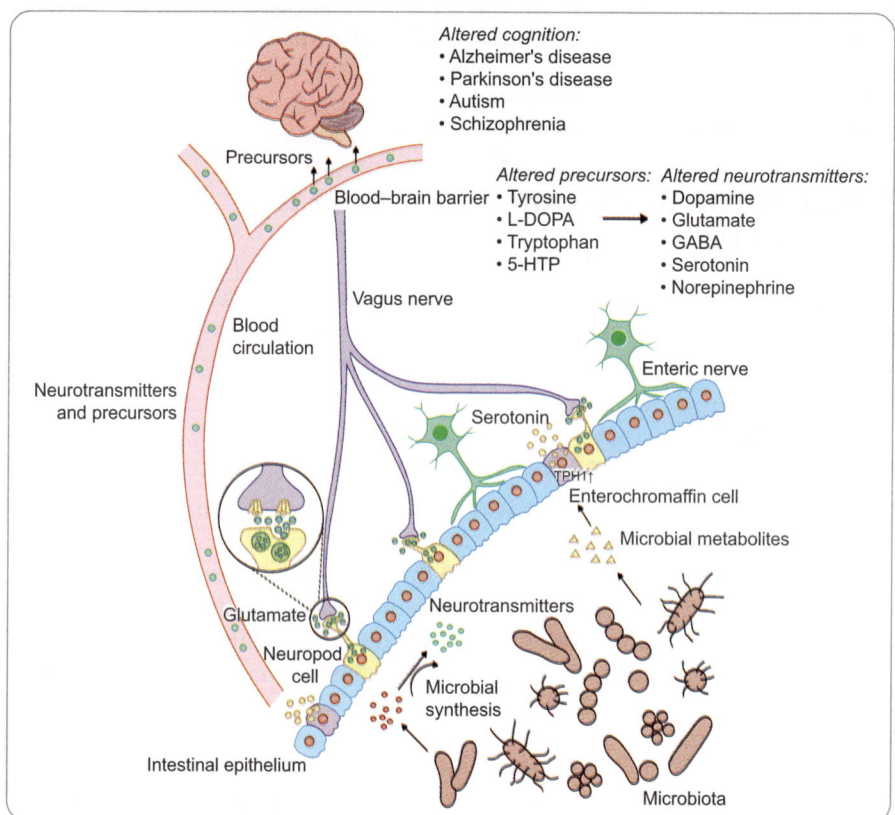

FIG. 3: Gut microbiota influences cognition by producing neurotransmitters or their precursors (e.g., serotonin via TPH1 in enterochromaffin cells) or stimulating enteroendocrine cells.
(5-HTP: 5-hydroxytryptophan; GABA: gamma-aminobutyric acid; TPH1: tryptophan hydroxylase 1)

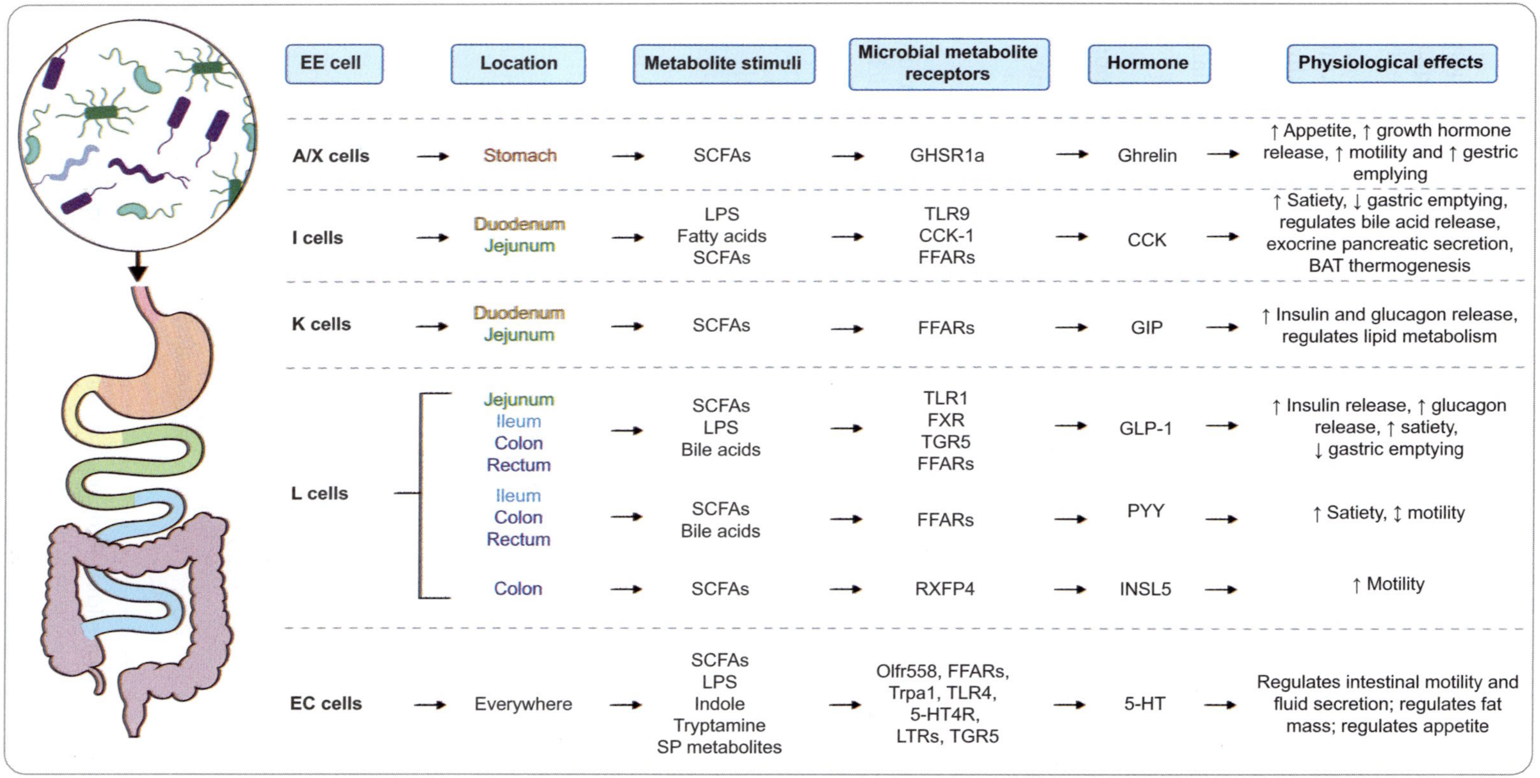

EE cell	Location	Metabolite stimuli	Microbial metabolite receptors	Hormone	Physiological effects
A/X cells	Stomach	SCFAs	GHSR1a	Ghrelin	↑ Appetite, ↑ growth hormone release, ↑ motility and ↑ gastric emptying
I cells	Duodenum, Jejunum	LPS, Fatty acids, SCFAs	TLR9, CCK-1, FFARs	CCK	↑ Satiety, ↓ gastric emptying, regulates bile acid release, exocrine pancreatic secretion, BAT thermogenesis
K cells	Duodenum, Jejunum	SCFAs	FFARs	GIP	↑ Insulin and glucagon release, regulates lipid metabolism
L cells	Jejunum, Ileum, Colon, Rectum	SCFAs, LPS, Bile acids	TLR1, FXR, TGR5, FFARs	GLP-1	↑ Insulin release, ↑ glucagon release, ↑ satiety, ↓ gastric emptying
L cells	Ileum, Colon, Rectum	SCFAs, Bile acids	FFARs	PYY	↑ Satiety, ↓ motility
L cells	Colon	SCFAs	RXFP4	INSL5	↑ Motility
EC cells	Everywhere	SCFAs, LPS, Indole, Tryptamine, SP metabolites	Olfr558, FFARs, Trpa1, TLR4, 5-HT4R, LTRs, TGR5	5-HT	Regulates intestinal motility and fluid secretion; regulates fat mass; regulates appetite

FIG. 4: Gut microbiota metabolites (SCFAs, bile acids, and indole) bind receptors on enteroendocrine cells (EECs), triggering hormone release that regulates appetite, gut motility, insulin, thermogenesis, and lipid metabolism across the GI tract.

[CCK: cholecystokinin; EC cell: enterochromaffin cell; EE cell: enteroendocrine cell; FFARs: free fatty acid receptors; FXR: farnesoid X receptor; GHSR1: growth hormone secretagogue receptor 1; GI: gastrointestinal; GLP-1: glucagon-like peptide 1; INSL5: insulin-like peptide 5; LPS: lipopolysaccharide; LTRs: long terminal repeats; PYY: peptide YY; RXFP4: relaxin family peptide receptor 4; SCFAs: short-chain fatty acids; 5-HT: 5-hydroxytryptamine (serotonin); 5-HT4R: 5-hydroxytryptamine receptor 4; TLR: toll-like receptor]

        ○ Enhancing intestinal barrier function, reducing systemic inflammation, and modulating the hypothalamic–pituitary–adrenal (HPA) axis
- *Bile acid derivatives:* Microbiota-driven deconjugation and transformation of bile acids impact farnesoid X receptor (FXR) and TGR5 signaling, influencing lipid metabolism, glucose homeostasis, and hormonal feedback on the liver and pancreas.
- *Tryptophan metabolites:* Metabolic pathways governed by gut flora determine the fate of tryptophan, affecting serotonin levels and kynurenine pathway intermediates that modulate behavioral and immune responses.
- Certain bacterial proteins mimic host peptide hormones, such as ClpB (caseinolytic protease B), which exhibits alpha-melanocyte-stimulating hormone-like activity, thus influencing satiety signaling and potentially appetite disorders.
- The gut microbiota regulates hormonal axes by modulating appetite hormones (GLP-1, PYY, and ghrelin), insulin sensitivity via SCFAs, and reproductive function through microbial β-glucuronidases that shape the estrobolome.

GUT MICROBIOME AND DISEASES

Emerging research underscores the gut microbiome's profound impact on a broad array of human diseases, extending well beyond the GI tract to include metabolic, inflammatory, and immune-mediated disorders **(Fig. 5)**.

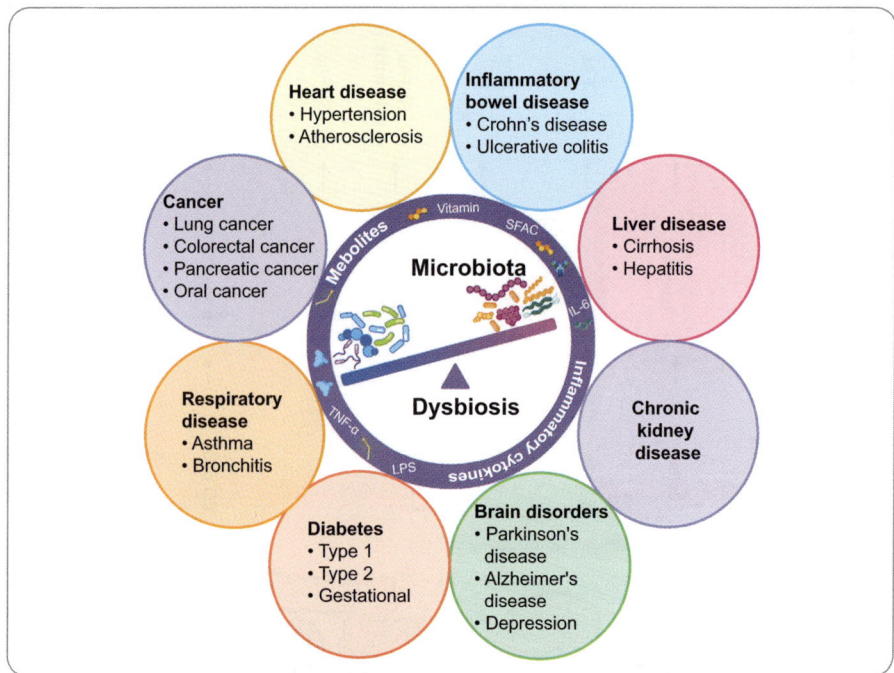

FIG. 5: Human microbiota dysbiosis contributes to various diseases.

(IL: interleukin; LPS: lipopolysaccharide; SCFAs: short-chain fatty acids; TNF-α: tumor necrosis factor-alpha)

Gut Dysbiosis and Inflammatory Bowel Disease

Inflammatory bowel disease (IBD), comprehending Crohn's disease (CD) and ulcerative colitis (UC), arises from chronic GI inflammation driven by genetic susceptibility, immune dysregulation, and gut microbial dysbiosis. A healthy gut microbiota, dominated by Firmicutes and Bacteroidetes, maintains immune tolerance, produces anti-inflammatory SCFAs, and reinforces the mucosal barrier. In IBD, this balance is disrupted, marked by reduced microbial diversity, depletion of beneficial SCFA producers (e.g., *Faecalibacterium prausnitzii*), and expansion of proinflammatory *Proteobacteria* (e.g., adherent-invasive *Escherichia coli*).

Dysbiosis exacerbates IBD through multiple mechanisms: Immune dysregulation—loss of commensals impairs Treg-mediated tolerance, while pathobionts activate dendritic cells, promoting Th17-driven inflammation. Barrier dysfunction—thinned mucus layers and disrupted tight junctions permit bacterial translocation, sustaining immune activation. Genetic-microbial crosstalk—mutations in PRRs (e.g., NOD2 and TLRs) impair microbial sensing, triggering maladaptive immune responses in susceptible hosts. Environmental factors (diet, stress, and medications) further shape dysbiosis, amplifying disease.

Clinically, IBD patients exhibit reduced alpha diversity, Firmicutes/Bacteroidetes depletion, and Proteobacteria overgrowth. Animal studies confirm that IBD-derived microbiota transfers induce colitis, highlighting microbial causality. Emerging therapies like probiotics and fecal microbiota transplantation (FMT) aim to restore microbial equilibrium, offering potential remission. These findings underscore dysbiosis as a central player in IBD pathogenesis.

Gut Microbiota and Mechanism of Carcinogenesis

The gut microbiota plays a dual role in cancer development by acting as both a protector and a perpetrator, particularly in GI malignancies such as colorectal and pancreatic cancer. Several mechanisms underlie this involvement:

- *Genotoxic metabolites*—certain bacteria produce deoxyribonucleic acid (DNA)-damaging metabolites (e.g., secondary bile acids, reactive oxygen species, and biogenic amines), driving genomic instability and mutations, a hallmark of cancer.
- *Chronic inflammation*—dysbiosis promotes low-grade, persistent inflammation, a known precursor to tumorigenesis in the colon, pancreas, and stomach.
- *Immune modulation*—microbes alter immune surveillance by inducing immunosuppressive regulatory T-cell responses or impairing cytotoxic lymphocyte activity, facilitating tumor immune escape.
- *Metabolic reprogramming*—shifts in microbial fermentative activity, including changes in SCFA producers, influence colonocyte metabolism and tumor microenvironments.

Key bacterial players include *Fusobacterium nucleatum* and *Bacteroides fragilis*, which are enriched in tumors and promote inflammation and carcinogenic signaling, while *Roseburia intestinalis* and *F. prausnitzii*, butyrate-producing, anti-inflammatory species, are often depleted during carcinogenesis.

Gut Microbiome in Obesity

The gut microbiota plays a key role in obesity through multiple mechanisms. First, certain microbes enhance energy harvest by breaking down indigestible polysaccharides, increasing caloric absorption. Second, SCFA imbalances disrupt appetite-regulating hormones (GLP-1, PYY), gut barrier integrity, and systemic inflammation. Microbial composition shifts also matter—elevated Firmicutes/Bacteroidetes ratios correlate with higher body mass index (BMI), whereas *Akkermansia muciniphila* is associated with leanness.

Additionally, microbes influence bile acid metabolism, altering lipid absorption and metabolic regulation. Finally, dysbiosis-induced endotoxemia triggers adipose tissue inflammation and insulin resistance, thus exacerbating metabolic dysfunction. These interactions highlight the microbiota's central role in obesity's complex pathogenesis.

Gut Microbiome and Diabetes Mellitus

Gut microbial dysbiosis significantly impacts glucose metabolism and insulin sensitivity through multiple pathways. Impaired intestinal barrier function permits endotoxin translocation, promoting inflammation and insulin resistance. The loss of butyrate-producing bacteria weakens the gut barrier and disrupts immunoregulation. Additionally, altered microbial metabolites, including SCFAs and bile acids, influence incretin secretion and hepatic glucose processing. In type 2 diabetes mellitus (T2DM), reduced microbial diversity is a hallmark, accompanied by taxonomic shifts—increased *Bacteroides* and *Clostridium*, alongside decreased *Lactobacillus*, *Bifidobacterium*, and *Faecalibacterium*. These microbial alterations collectively contribute to metabolic dysfunction, highlighting the gut microbiome's critical role in glucose regulation.

Gut Microbiome in Chronic Inflammation and Autoimmunity

The gut microbiome plays a pivotal role in chronic inflammatory and autoimmune diseases through immune dysregulation and barrier dysfunction. Dysbiosis disrupts the Th17/Treg balance, promoting systemic autoimmunity, while impaired barrier integrity allows bacterial translocation, triggering inflammation. In rheumatoid arthritis (RA), reduced *Bifidobacteria* and *B. fragilis* alongside proinflammatory overgrowth exacerbate disease. Systemic lupus erythematosus (SLE) exhibits altered *Lachnospiraceae* and *Ruminococcaceae*, with bacterial products stimulating type I interferon responses. Mechanisms include molecular mimicry, where microbial antigens cross-react with host proteins, and metabolite-mediated immune modulation. Similarly, in allergies and asthma, early-life dysbiosis skews immunity toward Th2 responses, while reduced SCFAs and depleted *Bifidobacterium* and *F. prausnitzii* correlate with atopy. These findings underscore the microbiome's systemic influence on immune-mediated diseases.

Other Diseases Associated with Gut Microbial Dysbiosis

The gut–brain axis represents a critical bidirectional communication system where gut microbiota significantly influence mental health. Dysbiosis contributes to psychiatric disorders by producing neuroactive metabolites (e.g., serotonin and GABA), triggering inflammation via microbial translocation (e.g., LPS), and disrupting the HPA axis, thereby affecting stress responses. Impaired gut barrier function further exacerbates mood disorders through systemic endotoxemia. These mechanisms collectively link microbial imbalance to anxiety, depression, and stress-related conditions, thus highlighting the role of microbiota in psychological well-being.

Altered gut microbiota increases production of proatherogenic metabolites such as trimethylamine N-oxide (TMAO), implicating the microbiome in vascular inflammation and cardiovascular risk.

Microbiota-driven changes in gut permeability and immune signaling are crucial factors in the pathogenesis of nonalcoholic fatty liver and steatohepatitis.

CLINICAL IMPLICATIONS: DIAGNOSTIC AND THERAPEUTIC OPPORTUNITIES

- *Biomarkers:* Specific microbial signatures are being explored as disease biomarkers, particularly in cancer and metabolic disorders.
- *Dietary interventions:* Manipulating diet alters microbial profiles, offering non-invasive disease modulation.
- *Probiotics/Prebiotics:* Clinical trials demonstrate some benefit in restoring microbial balance, though efficacy depends on disease context and microbial strain.
- *Fecal microbiota transplantation:* It shows efficacy in recurrent *Clostridioides difficile* infection and is under investigation for chronic inflammatory and metabolic diseases.

CONCLUSION

The gut microbiome serves as a key regulator of health, influencing cancer, metabolic disorders, and immune-mediated diseases through metabolic, immune, and neural networks. It shapes immune development, barrier function, and systemic homeostasis. Advances in microbiome science are revealing novel diagnostic and therapeutic strategies, from precision microbial engineering to targeted interventions, offering transformative potential for chronic disease prevention and treatment by restoring host–microbe symbiosis.

FURTHER READINGS

1. Hou K, Wu ZX, Chen XY, Wang JQ, Zhang D, Xiao C, et al. Microbiota in health and diseases. Signal Transduct Target Ther. 2022;7(1):135.
2. Maciel-Fiuza MF, Muller GC, Campos DMS, do Socorro Silva Costa P, Peruzzo J, Bonamigo RR, et al. Role of gut microbiota in infectious and inflammatory diseases. Front Microbiol. 2023;14:1098386.
3. Maynard CL, Elson CO, Hatton RD, Weaver CT. Reciprocal interactions of the intestinal microbiota and immune system. Nature. 2012;489(7415):231-41.
4. Pires L, Gonzalez-Paramás AM, Heleno SA, Calhelha RC. Gut microbiota as an endocrine organ: unveiling its role in human physiology and health. Appl Sci. 2024;14(20):9383.
5. Chen Y, Xu J, Chen Y. Regulation of neurotransmitters by the gut microbiota and effects on cognition in neurological disorders. Nutrients. 2021;13(6):2099.

SECTION 7

General Medicine

CHAPTER 19

Artificial Intelligence in Healthcare: Revolutionizing Medicine and Paving the Way for Future

Amandeep Kaur

INTRODUCTION

Artificial intelligence (AI) is defined as the display of human intelligence by machines. It comprises deep learning and machine learning (ML). It benefits patients with accurate diagnosis, appropriate treatment, and prognosis.

TYPES OF ARTIFICIAL INTELLIGENCE IN HEALTHCARE

Artificial intelligence is a common term used for various forms of processes. These can be explained as follows:
- *ML:* Supervised or semisupervised by a programmer
- *Deep learning:* It is a type of ML with deeper levels. It is inspired by the structure and function of the brain. Deep learning allows a computer program to analyze the problem and come up with solutions on its own, something like what a human (or animal) brain does every second.
- *Natural language processing (NLP):* Helps understand the human language, both verbal and written, thus helping in the documentation of notes, as well can be used for research purposes
- *Robotic process automation (RPA):* Helps in the administrative work in the bigger organizations

ARTIFICIAL INTELLIGENCE APPLICATIONS IN HEALTHCARE

Use of Artificial Intelligence in Medicine and Healthcare

Artificial intelligence has been helping us in different subsections of medicine. These are described as in the following text.

AI in the Diagnosis of the Disease

Machine learning models are used for observing certain vital signs of patients and are helping us in predicting the risk factors for certain diseases. They have been accurately used to predict diseases as sepsis so that earlier treatments can be initiated.

AI in Imaging

The artificial neural network has been said to diagnose the radiological images accurately. It has also helped us to store several images.

Accelerated Drug Development

Artificial intelligence-assisted drug discovery technology is used to study the physicochemical and biological properties of the drugs, and this has helped us to develop newer drugs. AI has also helped us to develop newer drug combinations as per the patient's requirement. It has also lowered the cost and reduced the time taken for developing new drugs.

Error Reduction

Artificial intelligence-powered tools have made life easy for physicians and healthcare workers as they accurately make decisions and help in drug management.

AI in Data Provision

Artificial intelligence is helping several patients with management of their diet, planning exercises, and keeping record of their diseases and their management. Urgencies and emergencies can be alerted to the healthcare workers via mobile apps. It can accumulate much larger amounts of data compared to the previous methods.

Streamlining Tasks

Healthcare practices are changing everywhere. Artificial intelligence innovative tools are helping:
- Collect and maintain healthcare records
- Schedule appointments
- Track patients' clinical presentation
- Keep a review of the medical insurance claims

Time Management and Optimal Use of Resources

- AI has saved a lot of time, and this has helped to see an increased number of patients, leading to increased productivity.
- Low cost
- Reduced medication errors, increased efficiency in maintaining workflow, and decreased frauds in insurance claims

Research Assistance

- AI has given access to a large amount of data to researchers worldwide.
- Individualized software packages are being developed by different institutions for the storage of research data.

Reduction of the Physician's Stress
Excess workloads and long duration of working hours have made the physicians feel stressed. AI has helped to streamline the entire course of the patient data, and this has also saved time and hence reduced the workload and pressure.

Precision Treatment
Artificial intelligence has helped physicians provide personalized care to their patients.
- With AI-assisted tools, precision medicine can be provided for the treatment of diseases.
- It has helped individualize treatment plans and prognosis of patients.

Limitations of Artificial Intelligence in Medicine
Human Surveillance
Despite their efficacy, AI applications still require considerable human surveillance. All the medical professionals need to be trained in the use of AI, and it will take a considerable time. Being a machine, there is always a possibility of error.

Overlooking of Social Variables
Artificial intelligence does not consider the socioeconomic status of the patient as well as the personal preferences.

Leads to Unemployment
Artificial intelligence is suspected to lead to unemployment as it has reduced the time consumption and cost of care. This process may already be underway, resulting in a decrease in the number of employees across all sectors of society.

Possible Imprecisions
Artificial intelligence in medicine is based on the already existing information regarding any disease. For rare diseases, adequate information is not available, so this may hinder the appropriate diagnosis and management. Diseases may also vary as per the environmental factors, and this may also hinder the management.

Security Risks
Dependent on large data networks, AI systems are susceptible to security risks. AI itself has now become a reason for cyberattacks.

Artificial Intelligence in Detection, Prediction, Diagnosis, Grading, and Prognosis of Diseases
A few examples are cited in the following text.

Cancer
- AI has significantly improved early detection and accurate diagnosis of cancers, enhancing treatment outcomes.
- Lung cancer detection using convolutional neural networks (CNNs) achieved accuracy rates of 99% in distinguishing malignant from benign tumors.
- AI-assisted mammography has shown superior performance compared to radiologists in breast cancer detection.
- Deep learning models have improved cervical cancer screening, reducing unnecessary colposcopies with higher sensitivity and specificity.

Artificial intelligence applications in colorectal cancer have enhanced diagnostic accuracy and treatment optimization.

Cardiology
- Manual assessment by echocardiography is limited by expertise. AI has been used in echo to accurately diagnose different pathologies.
- Patients with ST-elevation myocardial infarction (STEMI) and atrial fibrillation can be easily diagnosed by AI through accurate echocardiogram (ECG) predictions.
- Early home recognition of cardiac arrest and timely activation of emergency services have helped save patients.

Diabetes
- Automatic retinal screening helps to interpret and diagnose diabetic retinopathy from fundus images without involving an ophthalmologist.
- AI has been used to play an important role in the administration of insulin via continuous glucose monitoring and self-monitoring blood glucose by sending appropriate information about insulin dosage without a diabetologist.
- Predict hypoglycemia
- Predict the risk factors of diabetes

Neurological Conditions
Artificial intelligence, such as machine learning, has helped in the diagnosis and assessment of neurological conditions as strokes, epilepsies, and concussions.
- Predict embolic stroke by assessing atrial fibrillation
- Predict epilepsy based on electroencephalogram (EEG)

Artificial Intelligence in Pharmaceutical Research and Development
- AI reduces time and costs in drug development, improving efficiency in drug discovery and screening processes.
- Algorithms like AlphaFold predict protein structures, aiding in drug target identification for diseases like COVID-19.

- AI-based drug screening has shown accuracy rates of 84–87% in predicting pharmacokinetic attributes and toxicity.
- Clinical trial design can be optimized using AI, improving patient selection and compliance with protocols.

Artificial Intelligence in Basic Science

- AI aids in understanding complex biological mechanisms and relationships, enhancing research in various scientific fields.
- Integrated models using ML can reveal causal relationships in biological signals and drug mechanisms.
- AI has potential applications in identifying genetic mutations and their roles in cancer development.

FUTURE CHALLENGES

- Data access and sharing remain significant barriers to AI implementation in medicine, particularly in remote areas.
- AI is vulnerable to transparency and bias issues.
- Continued research is needed to validate AI technologies and ensure their safe and equitable application in healthcare.

With further improvement in the AI models soon, AI will assist in improving the patient's experience of care, enhance the caregiver experience, and reduce the time and cost of healthcare.

FINAL QUESTIONS: STILL TO BE ANSWERED?

In an artificially managed healthcare system, who will have the final word after the machine delivers a decision, the human doctor or the AI doctor? And what if something goes wrong: With whom will the liability lie in such cases?

CONCLUSION

The integration of AI is fundamentally transforming healthcare, moving beyond traditional methods to enable accurate diagnosis, personalized treatment, and optimized operations. Technologies like deep learning, natural language processing, and robotic automation are driving advancements across various medical domains.

However, the realization of AI's full potential depends on successfully addressing crucial challenges, particularly around data privacy, ethical governance, and mitigating potential algorithmic bias. While AI is poised to enhance the patient and caregiver experience, the critical question remains regarding liability and accountability in an artificially-managed healthcare system. The future lies in robust validation, ethical guidelines, and ensuring AI serves to augment human expertise, leading to a safer, more equitable, and more efficient healthcare system for all.

FURTHER READINGS

1. The Royal Society. (2017). Machine Learning: The Power and Promise of Computers That Learn by Example. [online] Available from https://royalsociety.org/~/media/policy/projects/machine-learning/publications/machine-learning-report.pdf [Last accessed October, 2025].
2. Topol EJ. High-performance medicine: the convergence of human and artificial intelligence. Nat Med. 2019;25:44-56.
3. Kelly CJ, Karthikesalingam A, Suleyman M, Corrado G, King D. Key challenges for delivering clinical impact with artificial intelligence. BMC Med. 2019;17:195.
4. Davahli MR, Karwowski W, Fiok K, Wan T, Parsaei HR. Controlling safety of artificial intelligence-based systems in healthcare. Symmetry. 2021;13:102.
5. Nachev P, Herron D, McNally N, Rees G, Williams B. Redefining the research hospital. NPJ Digit Med. 2019;2:119.

SECTION 8

Hematology

CHAPTER 20

Hemophilia: Current Approach and Future Outlook

Sudhir Kumar Atri, Piyush Malik

INTRODUCTION

Hemophilia is an inherited bleeding disorder caused by a deficiency or dysfunction of clotting factor VIII (hemophilia A) or IX (hemophilia B).

EPIDEMIOLOGY

Globally, the estimated prevalence of hemophilia is approximately 1.1 million cases. The condition has no racial or ethnic predilection but is more often diagnosed in high-income countries due to better surveillance.
- *Hemophilia A:* Accounts for 80–85% of cases. The incidence is ~1 per 5,000 male births. Around 30% of new cases are due to spontaneous mutations in the *F8* gene, which encodes factor VIII.
- *Hemophilia B:* Occurs in ~1 per 25,000–30,000 male births and results from *F9* gene mutations. It accounts for 15–20% of cases. Like hemophilia A, ~30% of cases arise from new mutations.
- *Carrier detection and prenatal diagnosis:* Advances in molecular genetics allow identification of carriers and prenatal testing, which is essential for genetic counseling and family planning in affected families.

SEVERITY

Severity is defined by residual factor levels:
- *Severe (<1%):* Characterized by spontaneous bleeding, especially hemarthrosis and intramuscular hematomas, often without trauma
- *Moderate (1–5%):* Bleeding occurs after minor trauma or surgery, with occasional spontaneous episodes.
- *Mild (5–40%):* Patients usually present after surgery or major trauma, as spontaneous bleeds are uncommon.

The severity classification is crucial for treatment decisions and predicting long-term complications.

CLINICAL PRESENTATION

Hemophilia A and B are clinically indistinguishable. The bleeding phenotype depends on severity, frequency of exposure to trauma, and treatment access.
- *Frequency by site:* Joints (70–80%), muscles (10–20%), other sites such as viscera (5–10%), and central nervous system (CNS; <5%)
- *Common manifestations:*
    - *Hemarthroses:* The hallmark of severe disease. Hinge joints such as knees, elbows, and ankles are most affected. Recurrent bleeds cause synovial hypertrophy, cartilage destruction, and "target joints," leading to hemophilic arthropathy.
    - *Hematomas:* Bleeding into deep muscles (iliopsoas, quadriceps, and forearm) may cause compartment syndrome or nerve compression.
    - *Visceral bleeding:* Gastrointestinal (GI) hemorrhage may present as melena or hematemesis, while hematuria is frequent.
    - *Intracranial hemorrhage:* Though rare, it is the most fatal complication. It may follow trauma or occur spontaneously, requiring urgent replacement therapy.
    - *Mucosal bleeds:* Epistaxis, gingival bleeding, and hemoptysis are frequent in moderate disease.
    - *Postsurgical bleeding:* Dental extractions or surgical procedures often unmask undiagnosed mild cases.

Chronic complications include arthropathy, muscle contractures, reduced mobility, and psychosocial burden. Early initiation of prophylaxis prevents irreversible damage.

INHIBITORS

The most significant complication in treatment is the development of *inhibitors*, which are antibodies against infused factor concentrates.
- *Incidence:* Seen in 25–30% of severe hemophilia A and 3–5% of hemophilia B patients
- *Risk factors:* Severe disease, intensive exposure at young age, family history, large gene deletions, ethnicity, and type of factor concentrate used
- *Impact:* Inhibitors render factor replacement ineffective, leading to poor bleed control and rapid joint damage. In hemophilia B, inhibitors may trigger severe allergic reactions or nephrotic syndrome.

CLINICAL DIAGNOSIS

Laboratory diagnosis is based on coagulation testing:
- *Screening tests:* Normal platelet count and prothrombin time (PT); prolonged activated partial thromboplastin time (aPTT) that corrects with mixing studies unless inhibitors are present
- *Specific assays:* Factor VIII and IX activity assays confirm the deficiency. Both one-stage and chromogenic assays are used; the latter is more reliable for factor VIII.

- *Genetic testing:* Identifies causative mutations, useful for carrier detection and prenatal diagnosis.

TREATMENT

- *Replacement therapy:* The cornerstone of management is the replacement of missing clotting factor.
  - *Factor VIII and IX concentrates:* Both plasma-derived and recombinant products are available. Recombinant concentrates are preferred due to lower infection risk.
  - *Extended half-life (EHL) products:* Achieved by Fc fusion or PEGylation, allowing less frequent dosing. The EHL factor VIII extends half-life by 1.5-fold, while the EHL factor IX extends by three- to fivefold, enabling dosing once weekly or less.
  - *Prophylaxis:* Regular infusion of factor concentrates prevents recurrent joint bleeds and arthropathy. Primary prophylaxis started before the first joint bleed offers the best long-term outcomes.
- *Bypassing agents:* Used in patients with inhibitors—
  - *Activated prothrombin complex concentrate (aPCC/FEIBA).*
  - *Recombinant activated factor VII (rFVIIa).* These agents bypass the factor VIII/IX to generate thrombin. They are effective but short-acting, requiring repeated doses.
- *Immune tolerance induction (ITI):*
  - High-dose regular factor infusion aims to eradicate inhibitors by inducing immune tolerance.
  - Success rate ~70–80% in hemophilia A; less effective in hemophilia B
- *Nonfactor therapy:*
  - *Emicizumab:* A bispecific antibody that mimics FVIII by bridging FIXa and FX. Administered subcutaneously weekly or monthly, it dramatically reduces the annual bleed rate and is effective even with inhibitors.
  - *Fitusiran:* Small interfering RNA that reduces antithrombin, rebalancing hemostasis. Approved in 2025, it requires monitoring for thrombotic risk.
  - *Concizumab and marstacimab:* Anti-tissue factor pathway inhibitor (TFPI) antibodies under trial
- *Adjunctive therapy:*
  - *Desmopressin (DDAVP):* Stimulates the release of endogenous factor VIII; useful in mild hemophilia A
  - *Antifibrinolytics (tranexamic acid, epsilon aminocaproic acid):* Effective for mucosal bleeds and dental procedures but contraindicated in hematuria
  - *Supportive care:* Physiotherapy, orthopedic interventions, and pain management are integral to comprehensive care.

PREVENTIVE CARE

- *POLICE (Protection, Optimal Loading, Ice, Compression, Elevation) protocol:* Applied during acute bleeds to reduce damage

- *Rehabilitation:* Early physiotherapy restores joint function, prevents stiffness, and reduces long-term disability.
- *Multidisciplinary approach:* Regular follow-up with hematologists, orthopedists, physiotherapists, and psychosocial support teams ensures optimal care.

DOSING GUIDELINES

Recommended target factor levels vary with bleed type:
- *Joint/Muscle bleeds:* 40–60% for 1–3 days
- *Iliopsoas bleeds:* Initial 80–100% and then 30–60% for 3–5 days with physiotherapy
- *CNS/Neck bleeds:* Initial 80–100% and then ≥50% for 1–3 weeks
- *GI bleeds:* Initial 80–100% and then ≥50% for 1–2 weeks
- *Major surgery:* Preoperative 80–100% and then taper gradually for 1–2 weeks postoperative

FUTURE PROSPECTS

Gene Therapy

The most exciting advance in hemophilia management is *gene therapy*, aiming to provide long-term endogenous factor production.
- *Approved therapies:*
  - ROCTAVIAN (valoctocogene roxaparvovec): For hemophilia A, delivers FVIII transgene via AAV5 vector.
  - HEMGENIX (etranacogene dezaparvovec) and BEQVEZ (fidanacogene elaparvovec): For hemophilia B, sustaining FIX levels up to 30% 1 year after infusion
- *Durability:* Clinical trials show sustained factor expression for several years, though levels gradually decline.
- *Challenges:* High cost, limited durability, liver enzyme elevations, and restricted eligibility (e.g., pre-existing AAV antibodies)

GLOBAL GENE THERAPY REGISTRY

The *WFH Gene Therapy Registry (GTR)* was established in 2022 to track long-term outcomes, durability, and rare side effects globally. It ensures systematic postapproval surveillance and real-world data collection from multiple countries.

Emerging Nonfactor Therapies

- *Fitusiran:* Approved in 2025 for hemophilia A or B, with or without inhibitors. Monthly subcutaneous dosing offers a convenient alternative.
- *Marstacimab:* Anti-TFPI antibody in phase III trials demonstrated superiority over on-demand therapy.
- *NXT007:* A next-generation bispecific antibody with higher potency than emicizumab, currently in advanced trials.

CHALLENGES AND SETBACKS

Despite breakthroughs, several programs have been discontinued due to cost or safety concerns. Hematology organizations emphasize the need for renewed investment to maintain innovation and improve access.

CONCLUSION

Hemophilia management has evolved from factor replacement to innovative therapies like extended half-life products and nonfactor treatments such as emicizumab. Gene therapy offers the potential for long-term factor production. The focus remains on prophylaxis, inhibitor management, and a multidisciplinary approach to prevent long-term complications and improve the quality-of-life for patients.

FURTHER READINGS

1. Srivastava A, Brewer AK, Mauser-Bunschoten EP, Key NS, Kitchen S, Llinas A, et al. Guidelines for the management of hemophilia. Haemophilia. 2013;19(1):e1-47.
2. Iorio A, Stonebraker JS, Chambost H, Makris M, Coffin D, Herr C, et al. Establishing the prevalence and prevalence at birth of hemophilia in males: a meta-analytic approach using national registries. Ann Intern Med. 2019;171(8):540-6.
3. Hay CR, Baglin TP, Collins PW, Hill FG, Keeling DM. The diagnosis and management of factor VIII and IX inhibitors: a guideline from the UK Haemophilia Centre Doctors' Organization (UKHCDO). Br J Haematol. 2000;111(1):591-605.
4. Peyvandi F, Garagiola I, Young G. The past and future of haemophilia: diagnosis, treatments, and its complications. Lancet. 2016;388(10040):187-97.
5. Samelson-Jones BJ, Small JC, George LA. Roctavian gene therapy for hemophilia A. Blood Adv. 2024;8(19):5179-89.
6. Konkle BA, Peyvandi F, Coffin D, Naccache M, Youttananukorn T, Pierce GF; WFH Gene Therapy Registry Steering Committee. Landmark endorsement of a global registry: The European Medicines Agency (EMA) Committee for Medicinal Products for Human Use (CHMP) publicly endorses World Federation of Hemophilia Gene Therapy Registry as global standard. Haemophilia. 2024;30(1):232-52.

CHAPTER 21

Transfusion Practices in Clinical Medicine

Kanchan Bhardwaj, BL Bhardwaj, Harnoor Singh

INTRODUCTION

Clinical transfusion procedure comprises the appropriate use of blood/component, safe transfusion practices, and all clinical aspects of blood transfusion. It includes both the risks and benefits of transfusion. Patients should be transfused only when there is evidence for a potential benefit outweighing the risk.

MULTIPLE TRANSFUSIONS

Multiple transfusions are repeated transfusions over a long period of time. In these conditions, packed red blood cell (PRBC) transfusions are preferred. In cases where nonhemolytic transfusion reactions are reported, leukocyte-reduced PRBCs are preferred. Blood components used should be <10 days old. They develop long-term complications, namely transmission of blood-borne infections, alloimmunization, and iron overload.

THALASSEMIA

Thalassemia major patients are given PRBC (with hematocrit around 0.65) after assessing clinical parameters. Hemoglobin (Hb) level < 7 g/dL on two successive occasions separated by at least 2 weeks (patient on folic acid replacement, and there should be no other aggravating cause, i.e., infection, bleeding, etc.). Growth of the patient is hampered, marrow expansion leads to unnatural bony growth, and organ failure develops. If these clinical features are present in spite of the Hb levels being >7 and <10 g/dL, chronic transfusion therapy is needed. The aim of PRBC transfusion is to ensure an adequate Hb level so that oxygen delivery to the tissues is not hampered. This can be assessed by normal growth spurts and increased energy. Suppressed overactive erythropoiesis leading to normal bone without deformities.

The schedule of PRBC therapy should be at 2–5-week interval. The interval is based on the volume of PRBC so that pretransfusion Hb remains >9 g/dL, but post-transfusion Hb should not go > 12 g/dL. The amount of PRBCs to be transfused is calculated by the patient's pretransfusion Hb and weight. 3–4 mL/kg of PRBC will raise the Hb by 1 g/dL in the absence of hypersplenism. In a single transfusion, the target is to raise the Hb by 4 g/dL if the transfusion is done at 3–5-week interval. Serum ferritin (SF) should be done at 3-month interval after the transfusion of 10 units of PRBCs. Iron chelation therapy should be started and SF should be maintained between 300 and 1,000 ng/mL. Close relatives' blood should not be transfused.

SICKLE CELL DISEASE

During acute illness, PRBC transfusion plays an important role. It is lifesaving in severe complications. It is done when Hb < 1–2 g/dL, below the baseline, and the patient shows any sign of cardiovascular compromise. Indications for PRBC transfusion include acute exacerbation of the patient's baseline anemia (e.g., sequestration and aplastic crisis) that increases oxygen-carrying capacity, life-threatening vaso-occlusive episode, and preparation for surgical procedures. Slow correction of anemia, 4–5 mL/kg PRBC over 4 hours, often with frusemide or isovolumic partial exchange transfusion, may be needed to prevent precipitation of heart failure. PRBC transfusion at a dose of 10 mL/kg for Hb < 4–5 g/dL and signs of cardiovascular compromise should be done. Transfusion may be needed for Hb < 7–8 g/dL for patients with relatively high baseline Hb sickle cell levels. A post-transfusion Hb level of <8–9 g/dL is generally recommended to avoid the risk of hyperviscosity that may occur several days later when RBCs sequestered in the spleen may return to the circulation and increase the Hb 1–2 mg/dL above the post-transfusion levels. Partial exchange transfusion by erythrocytapheresis may be needed for life-threatening illness. Erythrocytapheresis to achieve Hb 10 g/dL and keep Hb Sickle (patient's RBC) <30%.

AUTOIMMUNE HEMOLYTIC ANEMIA

Autoimmune hemolytic anemia (AIHA) is an autoimmune-mediated destruction of a patient's RBC by autoantibodies bound to the RBC membrane and activated complement proteins. The autoantibodies are not identifiable in the majority of cases, as they are formed against various targets. RBC destruction can occur directly in the circulation or by the macrophages of the reticuloendothelial system. AIHA is classified as primary (idiopathic) and secondary due to infection, drugs, immune diseases, malignancy, transplantation, etc. Clinical presentation in AIHA is dependent on the mode of onset, type of antibody, and severity of anemia. Usually, the patient comes with acute severe symptoms of hemoglobinuria, dyspnea, abdominal pain, fever, malaise, and jaundice with a history of postinfectious and drug-induced AIHA, as well as paroxysmal cold hemoglobinuria (PCH). Patients with cold AIHA or cold agglutinin disease have a chronic indolent course with symptoms of cold-dependent acrocyanosis, acral numbness, or cold sensitivity. Anemia in these patients worsens after cold exposure. Warm AIHA may have a chronic course with symptoms mainly attributed to anemia, like malaise, dyspnea on exertion, etc. The presence of lymphadenopathy, splenomegaly, or any other organomegaly points toward secondary AIHA. On investigation, normocytic/

macrocytic anemia, reticulocytosis, low serum haptoglobin, elevated lactate dehydrogenase, increased unconjugated bilirubin, and a positive direct Coombs test point toward AIHA.

In AIHA, it may not be possible to find a compatible donor unit for PRBC transfusion. In critical cases, transfusion should not be avoided or delayed because of uncertainty in cross-matching, and incompatible ("least incompatible") units may have to be transfused. The possibility of alloantibody masked by autoantibody must be ruled out by clinical history (e.g., alloantibody is unlikely in previously nontransfused males) and laboratory testing. PRBC transfusion can be safely given if alloantibodies can be ruled out, although cross-matching in such cases is incompatible. ABO and Rh(D) matched blood must be transfused. In cold AIHA, PRBCs must be warmed ideally using in-line filters or at least prewarmed. The decision to transfuse should be individualized depending upon the age, symptoms, clinical signs, rate of development, and severity of anemia in the patient. The aim of hemotherapy is to alleviate acute symptoms due to the severity of anemia rather than achieve the target Hb. Complete remission of AIHA may not be possible in primary AIHA but can be achieved in secondary AIHA, although this is much delayed. This usually means Hb > 11 g/dL without signs of hemolysis, irrespective of direct Coombs test status. Remission (partial) is the absence of a blood transfusion requirement and a satisfactory clinical status with Hb > 9 g/dL. Treatment is customized individually to suit the patient's requirement.

PLATELET TRANSFUSION

Platelets are derived from the whole blood [platelet concentrate (PC)] or by using the apheresis technique [single donor platelet (SDP)]. Dosage: 1 unit of PC/10 kg in an adult, i.e., 4–6 units of PC or 1 unit of SDP, should raise the platelet count by 20,000–40,000/µL. In splenomegaly, disseminated intravascular coagulation (DIC), active bleeding, fever, or septicemia, the increment will be less. The World Health Organization (WHO) bleeding score is given in **Table 1**. Platelet transfusion is therapeutic to treat bleeding or prophylactic to prevent bleeding. For patients with a WHO bleeding score of ≤1, prophylactic transfusion is given, and with a bleeding score of ≥2, therapeutic transfusion is given **(Table 2)**.

TRANSFUSION IN ONCOLOGY

Bone marrow in oncology patients may be suppressed. Repeated RBC and platelets may lead to the need for human leukocyte antigen (HLA)-matched plateletpheresis components because of incompatibility problems. Platelet transfusion requirements may also necessitate a change from Rh-negative to Rh-positive products. RhIG may be given to women of childbearing potential to protect against immunization. One 300 µg dose of RhIG can neutralize the effect of up to 15 mL of Rh-positive cells (<0.5 mL of Rh-positive RBCs are present in one unit of SDP and 4 mL of RBCs are present in a pooled platelet unit). So one dose of RhIG can be used for 30 SDP or 4 platelet pools. Chronic lymphocytic leukemia and lymphoma are frequently complicated by AIHA, increased destruction of

Grade of bleeding	Type of bleeding
1	• Petechiae/purpura that is localized to 1/2 dependent sites or is sparse/nonconfluent • Oropharyngeal bleeding, epistaxis of < 30 mm duration
2	• Melaena, hematemesis, hemoptysis, fresh blood in stool, musculoskeletal/soft-tissue bleeding not requiring RBC transfusion within 24 hours of onset, and without hemodynamic instability • Profuse epistaxis or oropharyngeal bleeding > 30 mm • Symptomatic oral bleeding or the one causing major discomfort • Multiple bruises, each >2 cm or anyone >10 cm • Petechiae/purpura that is diffuse • Visible blood in the urine • Abnormal bleeding from procedure sites • Unexpected vaginal bleeding saturating more than 2 pads with blood in a 24-hour period • Bleeding in cavity fluids evident microscopically • Retinal hemorrhage without visual impairment
3	• Bleeding requiring RBC transfusion specifically for support of bleeding within 24 hours of onset and without hemodynamic instability • Bleeding in body cavity fluids grossly visible • Cerebral bleeding noted on CT without neurological signs ans symptoms
4	• Debilitating bleeding, including retinal bleeding and visual impairment • Nonfatal cerebral bleeding with neurological signs/symptoms • Bleeding associated with hemodynamic instability (hypotension > 30 mm Hg change in systolic/diastolic BP) • Fatal bleeding from any source

TABLE 1: World Health Organization (WHO) bleeding score.

RBCs, and pretransfusion testing problems. Hodgkin's disease and lymphoma are at an increased risk of transfusion-associated graft-versus-host disease because of chemotherapy drugs used for treatment. Therefore, these patients should receive irradiated cellular components.

COAGULATION FACTOR DEFICIENCIES

Hemophilia A is deficiency of factor VIII levels, although the clinical disease is apparent when the factor VIII level is <10% (normal is 50–150%). Individuals with a level <1% have severe and spontaneous bleeding into the muscles and joints. Factor VIII concentrates/recombinant factor VIII are used. *Hemophilia B* is deficiency of factor IX. It is treated with factor IX concentrates/recombinant factor IX or prothrombin complex concentrates.

Von Willebrand's disease has the deficiency of von Willebrand factor (vWF). Type I von Willebrand disease has a reduced amount of vWF multimers. Type IIA has a deficiency of high molecular weight multimers, whereas type IIB has

TABLE 2: Platelet transfusion trigger.

Indications	Transfusion trigger
Prophylactic transfusion	
WHO score 0–1 No clinically significant bleeding, no invasive procedures planned; cataract surgery, BM aspiration	≤10,000/μL
As above with additional risk factors for bleeding, e.g., venous central lines	≤20,000/μL
Lumbar puncture	≤40,000/μL
Insertion/Removal of epidural catheter	≤80,000/μL
Major surgery, percutaneous liver/renal biopsy	≤50,000/μL
Neurosurgery	≤100,000/μL
WHO bleeding score > 2	No trigger, manage individually
Therapeutic transfusion	
WHO bleeding score > 2, severe life-threatening bleeding	No trigger, manage individually, and maintain platelet count ≥ 50,000/μL
Multiple trauma, brain injury/spontaneous intracerebral hemorrhage	≤100,000/μL
Non-life-threatening bleed	≤30,000/μL
Transfusion in immune thrombocytopenia	
No bleeding	≤5,000/μL
Invasive procedure	1 adult/pediatric dose prior to intervention
Life-threatening bleeding	≥2 adult/pediatric dose of platelets and IVIG

(BM: bone marrow; IVIG: intravenous immunoglobulin; WHO: World Health Organization)

abnormal high molecular weight multimers that have increased avidity for binding to platelets. In type III, no vWF is produced. Desmopressin [also known as DDAVP (1-deamino-8-D-arginine vasopressin)], a synthetic vasopressin analog, can simulate the release of vWF from the vascular endothelium in type I. DDAVP is contraindicated in type IIB disease. Many factor VIII products are used in type I/IIA/III when DDAVP has failed.

All coagulation factors and many thrombolytic proteins are produced in the liver except vWF. In severe liver failure, multiple coagulation factor deficiencies occur. Plasma contains all these proteins, so it is used in these cases. *Vitamin K* aids in the activation of factors II, VII, IX, and X. In its absence or use of drugs that interfere with vitamin K metabolism, such as warfarin, the factors are not activated. Vitamin K administration rather than plasma transfusion is recommended to correct vitamin K deficiency or warfarin overdose. In cases of signs of hemorrhage or impending surgery, plasma transfusion may be given, as it takes several hours for vitamin K effectiveness.

Disseminated intravascular coagulation is uncontrolled activation and consumption of coagulation proteins, causing small thrombi within the vascular system throughout the body. Treatment is aimed at correcting the cause of DIC—sepsis, disseminated malignancy, certain acute leukemias, obstetric complications, or shock. In some cases, transfusion of plasma, platelets, and/or cryoprecipitate may be required. Monitoring the prothrombin time (PT), activated partial thromboplastin time (aPTT), platelet count, fibrinogen, Hb, and hematocrit levels helps direct the choice of the next component to be used.

Platelet functional disorders are caused by drugs, uremia, or congenital abnormalities. Platelet transfusions in these patients should be reserved for treating hemorrhage or the impending need for adequate hemostasis (surgical procedure) to decrease the development of platelet refractoriness. Drugs that interfere with platelet function, such as clopidogrel, are commonly used in cardiovascular disease and are irreversible for the life of the platelet. Therefore, discontinuing the drug for 5-7 days before surgery will minimize hemorrhage. In uremia, DDAVP releases fresh, functional vWF from endothelial cells. Dialysis removes by-products of protein metabolism that degrade vWF and coat platelets, making both nonfunctional.

CONCLUSION

Effective transfusion practice requires careful selection of appropriate blood components and adherence to safe procedures to maximize patient benefit while minimizing risk. For patients requiring multiple transfusions, managing alloimmunization and iron overload is crucial, demanding vigilance and long-term care tailored to the underlying condition like thalassemia.

FURTHER READINGS

1. Agnihotri N, Agnihotri A. Transfusion of blood components. In: Gupta S, Marwaha N, Chaudhary R, Rajan S, Gupta D, Kaur R (Eds). Transfusion Medicine Technical Manual. Director General of Health Services. Ministry of Health and Family Welfare. Government of India, 3rd edition. 2022. pp. 164-79.
2. Ghosh K, Colah R, Manglani M, Choudhry VP, Verma I, Madan N, et al. Guidelines for screening, diagnosis, and management of hemoglobinopathies. Indian J Hum Genet. 2014;20:101-19.
3. Kaufman RM, Shehata N. Hemotherapy decisions and their outcomes. In: Fug MK (Ed). Technical Manual, 19th edition. Bethesda, MD: AABB; 2017. pp. 505-26.
4. Estcourt LJ, Birchall J, Allard S, Bassey SJ, Hersey P, Kerr JP, et al. on behalf of the British Committee for Standards in Haematology. Guidelines for the use of platelet transfusions. Br J Hematol. 2017;176(3):365-94.
5. Kennedy MS, Harmening D, Rhees J. Transfusion therapy. In: Harmening DM (Ed). Modern Blood Banking and Transfusion Practices, 7th edition. Philadelphia, PA: FA Davis Company; 2019. pp. 355-72.

CHAPTER 22

Hemophagocytic Lymphohistiocytosis: An Overview

Rajesh Kumar, Shilpa Atwal

■ INTRODUCTION

Hemophagocytic lymphohistiocytosis (HLH) is an aggressive and life-threatening hyperinflammatory syndrome resulting from uncontrolled activation of immune cells—particularly natural killer (NK) cells, cytotoxic T cells, and macrophages—leading to cytokine storm, tissue damage, and multiorgan failure. It most often affects infants from birth to 18 months of age but may occur in adults of all ages.

Hemophagocytic lymphohistiocytosis can occur as a familial or sporadic disorder as a result of triggers by various events that disrupt immune homeostasis, such as infections, malignancies, rheumatologic disorders, and immune deficiencies.

Prompt and adequate treatment is critical for successful outcomes, but delayed diagnosis is a common barrier. Factors leading to delayed diagnosis include rare and variable clinical presentation and lack of specificity of clinical and laboratory findings, which may overlap with other disease conditions.

■ TERMINOLOGY

Consistent with the recommendations from the North American Consortium for Histiocytosis (NACHO), the terminologies used are as follows:

Hemophagocytic lymphohistiocytosis syndrome: A clinical condition of severe immune hyperactivation which may be associated with a gene defect of lymphocyte cytotoxicity, infection, cancer, rheumatological disease, or immunodeficiency

Hemophagocytic lymphohistiocytosis disease: An HLH syndrome resulting from distinctive immune activation

Macrophage activating syndrome (MAS): A form of HLH that occurs primarily in juvenile idiopathic arthritis (JIA) or other rheumatological conditions

Human leukocyte antigen (HLA) disease mimics: Diseases mimicking HLH syndrome

CLASSIFICATION

Hemophagocytic lymphohistiocytosis is categorized into the following:
- *Primary (familial) HLH (pHLH):* Driven by inherited genetic mutations affecting cytotoxic lymphocyte function, often presenting in infancy or childhood
- *Secondary (acquired) HLH (sHLH):* Arises in response to infections, malignancies, autoimmune/autoinflammatory diseases, or certain therapies such as chimeric antigen receptor (CAR) T-cell therapy or immune checkpoint inhibitor therapy.

PATHOPHYSIOLOGY AND GENETIC INSIGHTS

Primary Hemophagocytic Lymphohistiocytosis

Genetic Considerations
- Mutations in genes such as *PRF1* (encoding perforin), *UNC13D*, *STX11*, *STXBP2*, and others compromise cytotoxic killing—leading to hyperactivation of T cells and macrophages via unchecked interferon gamma (IFN-γ) release
- For instance, *FHL2* due to *PRF1* mutations accounts for approximately 20–50% of familial cases. Hypomorphic mutations may present later in life, while null mutations manifest in infancy.

A *study from North India (2025)* characterizes clinicopathologic and immunogenetic features of eight FHL2 cases, expanding insights into regional genetic variants and their presentations.

FHL2 and FHL3 are most prevalent in Indian pHLH cases, with significant mutational diversity and frequent novel variants.

Combining *flow cytometry functional tests* with genetic sequencing accelerates accurate classification and diagnosis **(Table 1)**.

Secondary Hemophagocytic Lymphohistiocytosis

Secondary HLH results from increased CD8+ T-cell responses against infections, malignancy, autoimmune disease, and other inflammatory states.

These stimuli result in the engulfment of normal hematopoietic cells in the bone marrow, liver, and spleen as a result of uncontrolled inflammation and macrophage activation.

Macrophage activating syndrome is a term used for HLH driven by a rheumatologic or autoimmune disorder, including systemic lupus erythematosus and systemic onset JIA.

Tropical infections—scrub typhus, dengue, enteric fever, leishmaniosis, hepatitis E virus (HEV), malaria, dengue—play a central role in Indian sHLH demographics.

There have also been cases of sHLH reported in the setting of vaccination.

TABLE 1: Genes implicated in familial (primary) HLH and associated immune dysregulation.

Disease/Syndrome	Cytogenetic location	Gene	Protein	Function	Clinical features
Familial HLH type 1	9q21.3-22	Unknown	Unknown	Unknown	–
Familial HLH type 2	10q21-22	PRF1	Perforin	Pore formation	–
Familial HLH type 3	17q25	UNC13D	Munc13-4	Granule priming	–
Familial HLH type 4	6q24	STX11	Syntaxin-11	Granule fusion	–
Familial HLH type 5	19p13.2	STXBP2	Munc18-2	Granule fusion	Colitis, sensorineural hearing loss
Chediak–Higashi syndrome	1q42-43	LYST	LYST	Granule trafficking	Oculocutaneous albinism, neurologic dysfunction, cytoplasmic granules
Griscelli syndrome	15q21	RAB27a	Rab27a	Granule docking	Hypopigmentation
Hermansky–Pudlak syndrome	5q14.1	AP3B1	AP3B1	Granule trafficking	Oculocutaneous albinism, granulomatous colitis, pulmonary fibrosis
X-linked lymphoproliferative disease	Xq24-25	SH2D1A	SAP	Signaling in T and NK cells	EBV lymphoproliferation
X-linked inhibitor of apoptosis deficiency	Xq25	BIRC4	XIAP	Signaling pathways involving NF-κB	Refractory colitis, EBV lymphoproliferation

(EBV: Epstein–Barr virus; HLH: hemophagocytic lymphohistiocytosis; NFNK: natural killer)

EPIDEMIOLOGY

Hemophagocytic lymphohistiocytosis primarily occurs in the pediatric age group but is reported in all age groups. Infants, mostly < 3 months old, are commonly affected. The male:female ratio is about 1:1 in infants, whereas in adults, a light male predisposition is seen. The median age of presentation of children is 8 months, whereas adults typically present with a median age of 49 years.

CLINICAL FEATURES

Fever is reported as the most common symptom, present in about 95% cases of HLH. Other presenting symptoms include organomegaly (e.g., lymphadenopathy, hepatomegaly, and splenomegaly), liver dysfunction, coagulopathy, and skin changes. Hepatomegaly is found more frequently in children (approximately 95%) than in adults (18–67%). Splenomegaly is observed in ~ 50–83% of adults.

Laboratory investigations usually demonstrate bicytopenia (92%)/pancytopenia, hypertriglyceridemia, hypofibrinogenemia (90%), hyperferritinemia (94%), elevated soluble CD25 [interleukin-2 (IL-2)] levels (97%), abnormal liver tests, low or absent NK cell activity (71%), and/or hemophagocytosis in the bone marrow (82%) or elsewhere.

NEUROLOGICAL INVOLVEMENT

- Central nervous system (CNS) involvement can be the first site of clinical presentation in HLH, and between 10 and 70% of adults with HLH have been cited to have neurological involvement.
- Clinically, this can present as seizures, ataxia, cranial nerve palsies, and/or encephalitis. Performing a lumbar puncture and measuring neopterin levels when suspecting CNS HLH should be pursued, as it can help delineate CNS involvement in the setting of HLH from similarly presenting conditions such as demyelinating syndromes, infections, malignancy, and CNS vasculitis. Neopterin can be elevated in the cerebrospinal fluid in those with HLH.

HEMOPHAGOCYTIC LYMPHOHISTIOCYTOSIS TRIGGERS

Immune Activation

Infections [Epstein–Barr virus (EBV), cytomegalovirus (CMV), parvovirus, HZV, herpes simplex virus (HSV), measles, human herpesvirus (HHV), H1N1 influenza, human immunodeficiency virus (HIV)], malignancies, and the treatment of rheumatological disorders are common triggers in both genetic and sporadic cases.

Immunodeficiencies: Inherited or acquired

Diagnostic Criteria and Consensus Guidelines

HLH 2024 Criteria

Diagnosis of HLH traditionally relies on: The *HLH-2024 criteria*, requiring require five of the eight criteria—
1. Persistent fever (>38.5°C)
2. Splenomegaly (>2 cm below the costal margin)
3. Cytopenias (≥2 lineages)
4. Hb < 90 g/L
5. Platelets < 100×10^9 L; neutrophils < 10^9 L
6. Hypertriglyceridemia and/or hyperfibrinogenemia
7. Fibrinogen < 1.5 g/L; Tg ≥ 3 mmol
8. Ferritin ≥ 500 ng/mL
9. Hemophagocytosis in bone marrow or other tissues
10. Elevated soluble CD25 (sIL-2 receptor) > 2,400 units/mL

In the revised HLH-2004 criteria, also known as the HLH-2024 diagnostic criteria, the Histiocyte Society has suggested utilizing genetic and lymphocyte cytotoxicity assays as two distinct diagnostic strategies, in addition to five of the seven original (NK-cell activity omitted) clinical criteria in the HLH-2004 trial.

An international panel of experts reported that HLH 2024 criteria were 99% accurate in differentiating HLH from infections or systemic JIA.

It is important to note that these criteria have never been fully validated in adults and serve as a guide and prediction tool rather than a complete, validated diagnostic tool.

■ PREDICTIVE MODELS

H Score

The H Score is used as a risk stratification model that generates a probability for the presence of sHLH. The H Score was published in 2014 by Fardet et al. and utilizes nine criteria to predict the probability of a patient having HLH.
The nine criteria included are:
1. Known underlying immunosuppression
2. Elevated temperature
3. Organomegaly (spleen and/or liver)
4. Number of cytopenias (one, two, or three cell lines)
5. Ferritin level
6. Triglyceride levels
7. Fibrinogen level
8. Alanine aminotransferase (ALT) level
9. Hemophagocytosis present in bone marrow aspirate

The scoring system ranges from 0 to 337, with a higher score corresponding to an increased probability of HLH. An H Score > 250 confers a 99% probability of HLH compared to an H Score < 90, which confers a <1% probability.

The H Score has been compared to the HLH-2004 criteria and was found to be more sensitive and specific than the HLH-2004 criteria on the initial presentation of the patient, but has similar diagnostic accuracy as the patient becomes more critically ill.

Optimized HLH inflammatory (OHI) index: OHI index has been reported to be more sensitive and specific than H score in patients with HLH in the setting of hematological malignancies. Zoref-Lorenz et al. have suggested that the utilization of the OHI index, sCD25 > 3,900 unit/μL, and ferritin > 1,000 ng/μL signifies the highest mortality and predicts hematologic malignancy-associated HLH with diagnostic prediction of 94% sensitivity and 72% specificity.

The *HiHASC 2023 consensus guideline* proposes a practical clinical tool for adult HLH: The *"three Fs"* mnemonic—*fever, falling blood counts,* and *raised ferritin*—as a prompt trigger for further investigation.

■ OTHER ORGAN SYSTEMS

Respiratory/renal/skin manifestations/coagulopathy/ophthalmological manifestations may be seen.

DIFFERENTIAL DIAGNOSIS

- MAS
- Sepsis
- Liver failure
- Multiple organ dysfunction syndrome
- Encephalitis
- Autoimmune lymphoproliferative syndrome (ALPS)
- Drug reaction with eosinophilia and systemic symptoms (DRESS)
- Kawasaki disease
- Cytophagic histiocytic panniculitis
- Thrombotic thrombocytopenic purpura (TTP)/hemolytic uremic syndrome (HUS)
- Drug-induced thrombotic microangiopathy/DITMA
- Transfusion-associated graft versus host disease

TREATMENT

Established Regimens

The *HLH94 protocol*, centered on immunochemotherapy with etoposide and dexamethasone, remains foundational for acute management.

The original HLH-94 protocol for HLH treatment includes an initial 8-week course of etoposide (150 mg/m^2 for adults, and 5 mg/kg for children <10 kg, twice weekly for the first 2 weeks, then weekly until week 8, with dose adjustments for liver or renal dysfunction), dexamethasone (starting at 10 mg/m^2/day for 2 weeks, then tapered), intrathecal methotrexate in cases of CNS involvement, and cyclosporine (dose-adjusted to reach therapeutic levels). Some advocate for the use of tacrolimus instead of cyclosporine due to lower nephrotoxicity **(Flowchart 1)**.

Emerging and Targeted Therapies

- *Emapalumab,* an anti-IFN-γ monoclonal antibody, is approved for refractory or relapsed primary HLH and, as of *June 2025,* also for MAS in Still's disease.
- Retrospective US data show emapalumab being used in rheumatologic-associated HLH cases, suggesting growing clinical utility beyond genetic HLH.
- *Other novel agents include*:
  - *Anakinra* (IL-1 receptor antagonist)
  - *Ruxolitinib* [Janus kinase (JAK) inhibitor]
  - *Alemtuzumab/Tocilizumab* (IL-6 receptor antagonist)

SPECIALIZED SETTINGS AND TRIGGERS

- A 2025 review discusses *CAR T-cell therapy-associated HLH* and compares its pathogenesis, clinical presentation, and management to cytokine release syndrome, underscoring the need for differential strategies.
- Similarly, flare-ups due to *immune checkpoint inhibitor therapy* have been reported, with some cases resolving successfully with corticosteroids.

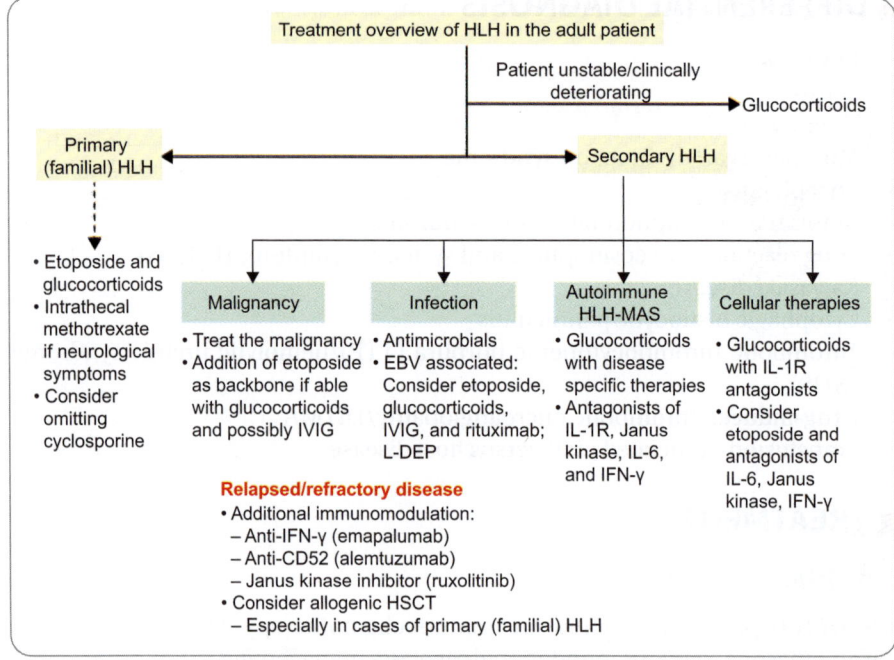

FLOWCHART 1: Overview of treatment considerations for hemophagocytic lymphohistiocytosis.
(EBV: Epstein–Barr virus; HLH: hemophagocytic lymphohistiocytosis; HSCT: hematopoietic stem cell transplant; IFN-γ: interferon gamma; IL-6: interleukin-6; IL-1R: interleukin-1 receptor; IVIG: intravenous immunoglobulin; L-DEP: PEG-asparaginase, liposomal doxorubicin, etoposide, and high-dose methylprednisolone; MAS: macrophage activating syndrome)

Courtesy: Created with Biorender.com

- In tuberculosis (TB)-associated HLH contexts, combination immunosuppression [steroids, intravenous immunoglobulin (IVIG), etoposide, and cyclosporine A] is integrated with anti-TB therapy, though data remain limited.

DIFFERENTIAL DIAGNOSIS

Prognosis and Outcomes

- *1-year survival* varies by setting: approximately 56% overall; better in rheumatologic-associated HLH (~74%) but poorer in malignancy-driven cases (~21%).
- A recent study cites 1-month mortality of 27.7% and *1-year survival around 50%*, reinforcing the high stakes and need for timely treatment.
- Delayed recognition remains a key barrier to improving outcomes.

Pediatric Perspective

- Children frequently present with infection-induced HLH.
- Relatively high recovery rates are seen with steroids and supportive care, but primary HLH without transplantation carries high mortality.

CONCLUSION

An entity of elevated, dysregulated inflammation, HLH can be conceptually divided into primary (or familial) and secondary HLH. Secondary HLH is commonly triggered by infections, malignancy, and rheumatologic conditions. It is a diagnostically challenging disease, with cytokine evaluation, pathogenic mutation testing, and inflammatory markers playing a role in supporting the diagnostic workup. The treatment largely depends on the underlying cause. The high mortality rate of the disease requires early and prompt recognition of clinical manifestations and appropriate workup, with early and adequate treatment.

FURTHER READINGS

1. Wu Y, Sun X, Kang K, Yang Y, Li H, Zhao A, et al. Hemophagocytic lymphohistiocytosis: current treatment advances, emerging targeted therapy and underlying mechanisms. J Hematol Oncol. 2024;17(1):106.
2. Konkol S, Killeen RB, Rai M. Hemophagocytic LymphohistiocytosisTreasure Island (FL): StatPearls Publishing; 2025.
3. Wikipdeia. Hemophagocytic lymphohistiocytosis. [online] Available from https://en.wikipedia.org/wiki/Hemophagocytic_lymphohistiocytosis [Last accessed November, 2025].
4. Cox MF, Mackenzie S, Low R, Brown M, Sanchez E, Carr A. Diagnosis and investigation of suspected haemophagocytic lymphohistiocytosis in adults: 2023 Hyperinflammation and HLH Across Speciality Collaboration (HiHASC) consensus guideline. Lancet Rheumatol. 2024;6(1):e51-e62.
5. Hines MR, von Bahr Greenwood T, Beutel G, Hays JA, Horne AC, Janka G, et al. Consensusbased guidelines for HLH in critically ill children and adults. Consensus-Based Guidelines for the Recognition, Diagnosis, and Management of Hemophagocytic Lymphohistiocytosis in Critically Ill Children and Adults. Crit Care Med. 2022;50(5):860-72.

CHAPTER 23

Approach to the Patient with Thrombocytopenia

Lovleen Bhatia, Vikas Sharma, Jhanvi Pawar

INTRODUCTION

It is defined as a platelet count less than normal range, typically <1,50,000/μL.

Mild: 100–150 × 10⁹/L, *Moderate*: 50–100 × 10⁹/L, *Severe*: <50,000/mm³

Patients with platelet counts of <5,000/μL–10,000/μL are at high risk for spontaneous, life-threatening hemorrhage. However, there is no absolute threshold for spontaneous bleeding due to thrombocytopenia **(Flowchart 1)**.

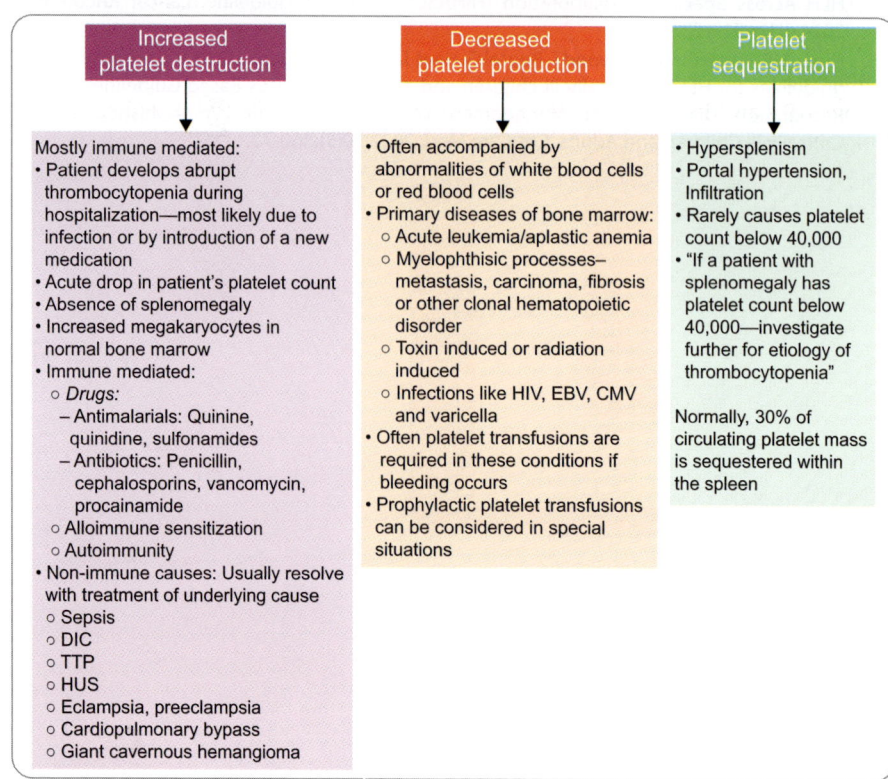

FLOWCHART 1: The causes of thrombocytopenia can be divided into three major groups.

In clinical settings always rule out two important causes first:
- *Pseudo-thrombocytopenia*:
  - *Platelet clumping*: In vitro platelet agglutination via antibodies (IgG >IgM and IgA), in the presence of hypocalcemia induced by blood collection in EDTA or when the blood sample is allowed to cool to room temperature.
  - *Platelet satellitism*: In vitro phenomenon in which platelets cling to white cells, particularly neutrophils in blood sample collected in EDTA vials.
  - Rather use blue top tube (sodium citrate) or green top (heparin) or prepare a smear from fresh blood by finger prick.
- *Infections*: HIV/Hepatitis C/Sepsis/EBV/CMV/Parvovirus 19

  Platelet histogram: It gives the platelet distribution curves
  Platelet size [in femtoliter (fL)] along x-axis
  Cell count: y-axis
  Normal, left skewed
  If cell size increases: Sharp rise and slow taper
  Sloping upward, with right skewing: Clumping, giant platelets **(Fig. 1)**
- *Mean platelet volume (MPV)*: It tells about average platelet size.
  Normal: 7.6–9.3 fL, *>12 fL*: Giant platelets
  Increased MPV: New platelets, immune thrombocytopenic purpura (ITP), hypersplenism
- *Platelet distribution width (PDW)*: It is the variation in platelet size.
  Normal: 9.4–16%, *increased PDW*: Activated platelets (generally giant platelets)
  Low MPV and PDW are suggestive of decreased bone marrow production.
- *Immature platelet fraction (IPF)*: Reticulated platelets, RNA staining, expressed as % of platelets
- *Platelet mass*: MPV × platelet count

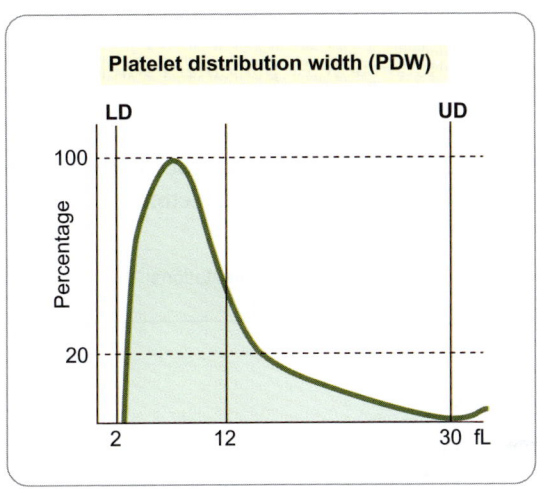

FIG. 1: Autoanalyzer reports.

ROLE OF PERIPHERAL BLOOD FILM

- *Normal peripheral blood film (PBF)*: ITP, HIT, drug-induced thrombocytopenia
- *Blasts/Hypogranular neutrophils*: MDS, AML
- *Schistocytes*: Thrombotic thrombocytopenic purpura (TTP), hemolytic uremic syndrome (HUS), disseminated intravascular coagulation (DIC), microangiopathic hemolytic anemia (MAHA)
- *Evan's syndrome*: Thrombocytopenia, micro-spherocytes, red cell agglutination
- *Increased neutrophils, toxic granules*: Sepsis, ITP, post-splenectomy
- *Lymphoid cells*: HIV, viral infections, lymphoproliferative disorders
- *Giant platelets + increased MPV*: Inherited macrothrombocytopenia, e.g., HARRIS syndrome
- *Plasmodium* species Plasmodium vivax (P. vivax), Plasmodium falciparum (P. falciparum)
- *Hypersegmented neutrophils + increased MPV*: B12 and folate deficiencies
- *Pelger Heut anomaly/Pseudo Pelger Heut*: Anomalies of white cell in MDS/B12 deficiency
- *ALD/cirrhosis*: Macrocytes, target cells, spur cells, and acanthocytes

PATHOBIOLOGY

Spontaneous hemorrhage does not occur unless counts are below 30,000/µL, increased chances in case of high-grade fever, sepsis, severe anemia.

Prophylactic Platelet Transfusions

- Patients with therapy-induced hypo-proliferative thrombocytopenia. PLADO trial demonstrates that low doses of platelets (110 billion/m² of body surface area) are safer and efficacious than larger doses
- In patients undergoing treatment for acute leukemia, recent clinical trials have supported prophylactic platelet transfusions when counts are below 5,000/µL or 10,000/µL **(Flowchart 2)**.
- Platelet count <10,000/µL
- In elective central venous catheter placement when counts are <20,000/µL elective diagnostic lumbar puncture counts <50,000/µL
- Prophylactic transfusion may be required for 7–10 days to maintain platelet count of 75,000–1 lakh in very high-risk procedures such as neurosurgery, ocular surgery, thyroid surgery, and prostatectomy

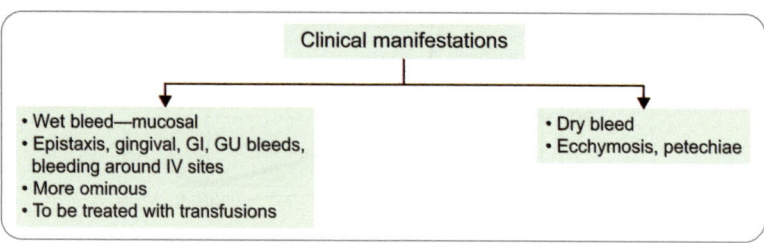

FLOWCHART 2: Clinical manifestation types.

- Platelets derived from single donor preferred over RDPs as they minimize the risk of alloimmunization preferred.
- *Contraindications:* Thrombocytopenia caused by TTP, HUS—as thrombosis occurs more frequently in these patients.

The Transfusion Refractory Patient

Patients who do not have predicted rise in their platelet count between 10,000/µL–12,000/µL for every unit of RDP. Analyze their count before next transfusion, 1 hour after that and 24 hours thereafter,
- If the counts rise after 1 hour and fall 24 hours later patient may have ongoing platelet consumption–severe sepsis, DIC, severe active hemorrhage or drug-mediated immune destruction.
- If significant rise not seen within 1 hour it suggests hypersplenism, presence of autoantibodies—ITP, alloantibodies or drug mediated immune destruction.

THROMBOCYTOPENIA IN SPECIFIC CONDITIONS

Thrombocytopenia in Sepsis

One of the most common causes of acute thrombocytopenia in hospitalized patients. It is due to the deposition of antigen-antibody complexes on platelet surface, which are then cleared from circulation when recognized by the Fc receptor of macrophages in spleen. It can also be due to DIC. Treatment is treating the underlying cause.

Drug-induced Thrombocytopenia

It can be immune mediated, the drug may be deposited on the platelet surface and antidrug antibodies lead to platelet clearance primarily in the spleen or the drug may bind to a protein on platelet surface and induce a neoantigen that is ultimately recognized by the immune system. Chemotherapy can also induce bone marrow suppression. In acute or subacute settings, it may be difficult to distinguish between drug induced thrombocytopenia and thrombocytopenia of infection (viral or bacterial). In critically ill patients both possibilities should be considered in the treatment plan.

Treatment: Best method is to stop all suspected offending drugs. Thrombocytopenia typically begins to resolve within days to a week of stopping the drug. In patients with profound thrombocytopenia (<10,000–15,000/µL) or at a high risk for bleeding, platelet transfusions are indicated. If ITP cannot be confidently excluded, and thrombocytopenia is life-threatening specific treatment for ITP may be initiated.

Heparin-induced Thrombocytopenia

Heparin-induced thrombocytopenia (HIT) should be suspected in any patient who develops thrombocytopenia while on heparin. A >50% decrease in platelet counts (even if in normal), especially on day 5 should raise the suspicion. It is limb and organ threatening thrombotic disease, with venous thrombosis more common than arterial thrombosis (in a 2:1).

Positive test for anti-heparin PF4 antibody by ELISA, confirmed by serotonin release assay.

UFH (2–5% patients) >> LMWH (0.7 % patients) >> Fondaparinux

Pathophysiology: P4 is released by platelets when activated. In some patients antibody mediated immune response occurs to PF 4 bound to heparin. They form complexes of Ig, heparin and PF4 which can accumulate on platelet surface and can activate platelets. Once activated platelets contribute to thrombosis. The activated platelet secretes more PF4 and the cycle continues **(Fig. 2)**.

- *Type 1 HIT*: No antibodies, resolves within 2 days. Platelet counts rarely fall below 100,000/μL
- *Type 2 HIT*: Anti-PF 4–heparin complex formation. Rapid and delayed onset occurs <5 days and >5 days after heparin.
- *Autoimmune HIT*: A severe subtype, where antibodies activate platelets even without heparin.
- *Refractory HIT*: It persists even weeks after heparin has been stopped **(Table 1)**.

No action if score <3. Otherwise, stop all heparin. Start new anti-coagulant. Send PF 4 antibodies assay.

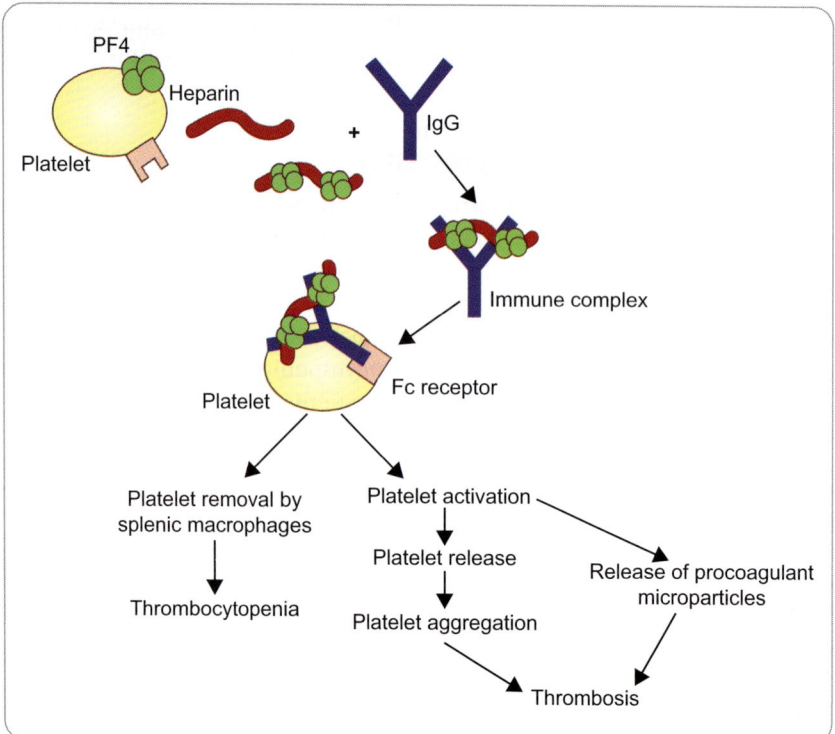

FIG. 2: Mechanism of heparin-induced thrombocytopenia (HIT), showing the formation of the heparin PF4-IgG immune complex and its consequences—platelet activation, aggregation, and thrombosis.
Source: Greinacher A. Clinical practice. Heparin-induced thrombocytopenia. N Engl J Med. 2015;373:252-61.

CHAPTER 23: Approach to the Patient with Thrombocytopenia

TABLE 1: 4Ts score—differentiates patients with heparin-induced thrombocytopenia (HIT) from those with other causes of thrombocytopenia.

50% fall in platelets	+2
5–10 days	+2
>10 days or <1 day	1
New thrombosis or DVT	+2
No other cause of thrombocytopenia	+2

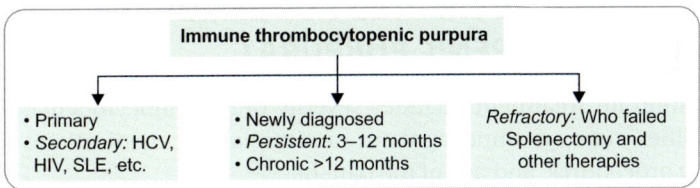

FLOWCHART 3: Immune thrombocytopenic purpura differentia classifications.

Score 0–3: Low probability; *Score 4-5*: Intermediate probability; *Score 6-8*: High probability

Treatment: Stop all heparin immediately, look for "Hidden heparin"—heparin flushes, heparin coated catheters, prothrombin complex concentrate, TPN products. Alternative anticoagulants—patients with HIT without thrombosis have 30% chance of developing a thrombus in the next 1 month. DOACs—with higher doses initially, direct thrombin inhibitor—argatroban, until the platelet counts normalize, bivalirudin, and fondaparinux.

Warfarin not recommended in acute HIT, when platelet counts return to normal, it should be slowly introduced and gradually increased to achieve an INR of 2–3 for 4-6 weeks duration. If patient had acute thrombosis attributable to HIT—minimum 3 months anticoagulation recommended.

IMMUNE THROMBOCYTOPENIC PURPURA

Definition

- Autoimmune destruction of platelets and impaired production, caused by circulating antiplatelet autoantibodies.
- Similar picture can also be seen in patients with AI diseases such as SLE, low-grade lymphoproliferative disorders, such as CLL and HIV infection **(Flowchart 3)**.

Clinical manifestations: Females > males, but can be seen in either sex and at any age. A chronic, recurring course is seen in adults, in contrast to pediatric patients who present with acute ITP. It can present with severe asymptomatic thrombocytopenia, excess mucocutaneous bleeding or life-threatening intracranial bleed **(Flowchart 2)**.

Diagnosis: It is a diagnosis of exclusion.

Thrombocytopenia (threshold of 1,00,000/μL), increased MPV, megakaryocytes on peripheral smear. Splenomegaly absent, unless ITP is due to an underlying disorder such as lymphoma. Bone marrow examination is usually not necessary in absence of abnormalities other than thrombocytopenia. If performed it shows normal or increased number of megakaryocytes.

Indications of bone marrow examination: Patients not responding to corticosteroids, relapsed cases, age >60 years.

WHO SHOULD BE TREATED FOR IMMUNE THROMBOCYTOPENIC PURPURA?

Consideration for treatment includes severity of thrombocytopenia, additional comorbidities, use of anticoagulant or antiplatelet medications, need for upcoming procedures, and age of the patient
- Asymptomatic patients with counts >30,000 μL can be followed without treatment.
- If platelet counts are <30,000/μL and asymptomatic or minor mucocutaneous bleeding.
- For patients with a platelet count at the lower end of this threshold, for those with additional comorbidities, on anticoagulant or antiplatelet medications, or upcoming procedures, and for elderly patients (>60 years old), treatment with corticosteroids may be appropriate.

First-line Treatment is a Course of Corticosteroids

In adults with newly diagnosed ITP, the ASH guideline panel recommends against a prolonged course (>6 weeks) of prednisone and in favor of a short course (≤6 weeks) and suggests prednisone (0.5–2.0 mg/kg/day). The ASH guideline panel suggests corticosteroids alone rather than rituximab and corticosteroids for initial therapy. Relapse is typical once therapy is tapered. *Mycophenolate mofetil* is also an emerging first-line treatment option.

IVIG: With corticosteroids should be used when a more rapid increase is required. Dose—1 g/kg/day for two consecutive days or 0.4 g/kg/day for five consecutive days, effects typically last for 2–4 weeks.

Second Line of Treatment

In adults with ITP lasting ≥3 months who are corticosteroid-dependent or have no response to corticosteroids, the ASH guideline panel suggests the following as potential second-line therapies:
- *Thrombopoietin receptor agonist:* They mimic the action of thrombopoietin to increase platelet production by binding to TPO receptor on megakaryocytes and hematopoietic stem cells. *Eltrombopag*—50 mg *per os* (po) daily, 25 mg in liver dysfunction, *avatrombopag*—20 mg po daily. They bind to the transmembrane domain of the EPO receptor. *Romiplostim*—2-3 μg/kg subcutaneously weekly then slowly escalated to 10 μg/kg/week. Competitively

binds to the receptor's extracellular domain. Effects appear by 2–3 weeks and disappears shortly after drug discontinuation.
- *Rituximab:* Anti-CD 20 antibody in a dose of 375 mg/m^2 IV weekly for 4 weeks
- *Splenectomy:* Durable (often lifelong) considered in refractory patients or those who want to avoid long term medication.
- *Fostamatinib:* A prodrug that converts to active form (R406), an oral inhibitor of spleen tyrosine kinase. Prevents the destruction of antibody coated platelets. Dosed at 100 mg bd, increase to 150 mg bd if platelet count remains <50,000/μL.
- *Anti-D immunoglobulin*: In patients who are unresponsive to or relapse after initial course of corticosteroids and therapy for refractory ITP, along with low-maintenance dose prednisone.

THROMBOTIC THROMBOCYTOPENIC PURPURA

Consumptive thrombocytopenia along with microangiopathic hemolytic anemia that is not associated with acute renal failure at presentation, DIC, or any other apparent cause. Classic pentad—thrombocytopenia, anemia, fever, neurologic symptoms, renal involvement—seen in <10%. Many patients have hemolytic anemia and thrombocytopenia **(Flowchart 4 and Fig. 3)**.

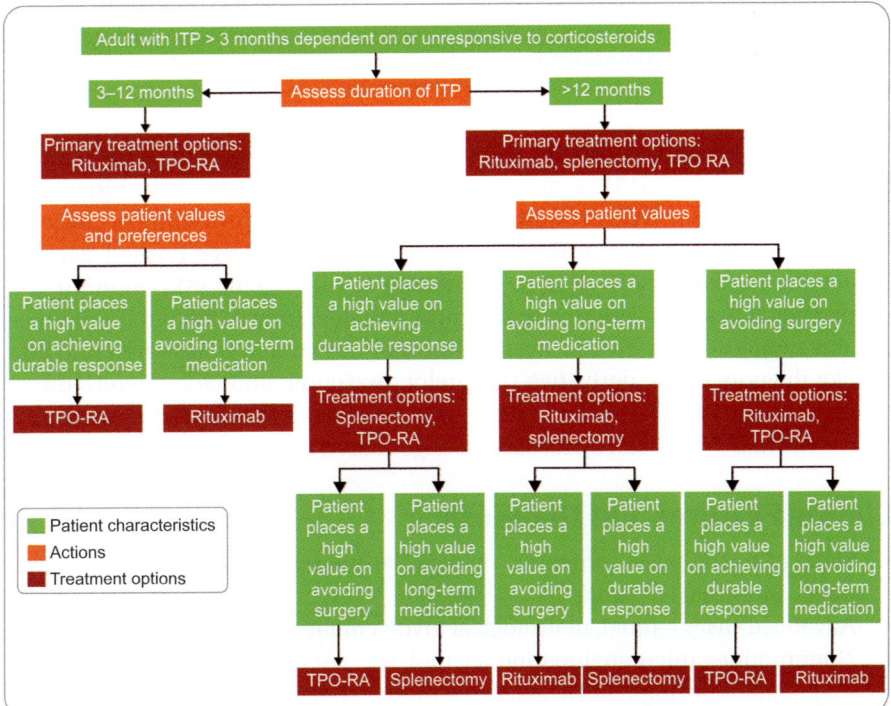

FLOWCHART 4: Conditional recommendation by American Society of Hematology 2019 guideline for immune thrombocytopenia.

Note: Selection of second-line therapy in adults with ITP should be individualized based on duration of disease and patient values and preferences. Other factors that may influence treatment decisions include frequency of bleeding sufficient to require hospitalization or rescue medication, comorbidities, compliance, medical and social support networks, cost, and availability of treatments. Patient education and shared decision-making is encouraged.

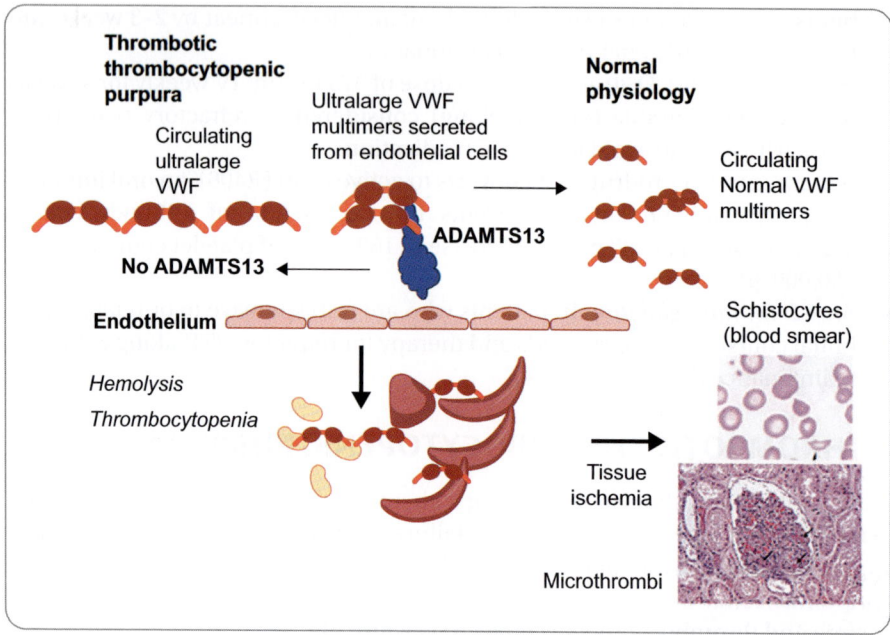

FIG. 3: Pathophysiology of thrombotic thrombocytopenic purpura (TTP)—deficiency of ADAMTS13 leads to accumulation of ultralarge von Willebrand factor multimers, causing platelet aggregation, microthrombi formation, hemolysis with schistocytes, thrombocytopenia, and tissue ischemia.

A disintegrin and metalloproteinase with a thrombospondin type 1 motif, member 13 (ADAMTS13), a metalloprotease, normally present in blood and cleaves multimers of vWF, preventing the formation of microvascular occlusions.
- *Adult onset TTP*: Autoantibodies against ADAMTS13 are formed causing acquired deficiency leading to circulating thrombogenic vWF multimers—platelet activation—microvascular thrombosis–mainly in terminal arterioles and capillaries—known as hyaline thrombi due to less fibrin content. Drug like thienopyridine derivative (ticagrelor, prasugrel, and clopidogrel), direct injury to the vascular endothelium—cyclosporin or tacrolimus can cause TTP.
  ○ Upshaw-Schulman syndrome—congenital ADAMTS13 deficiency

Clinical Features and Diagnosis
- Signs of thrombosis—phlebitis, myocardial infarction or stroke, abdominal pain – intestinal ischemia
- Advanced cases—renal, neurological involvement—somnolence, even coma.
- Nonimmune microangiopathic hemolytic anemia caused by red cell fragmentation—high S.LDH, elevated indirect bilirubin, low haptoglobin and increased reticulocyte count, PBF-fragmented RBCs (schistocytes >10% of RBCs), nucleated RBCs (precursors)
- Normal aPTT, PTI, TT, D-dimer
- ADAMTS13 assay—not recommended out of research settings. Levels below 10% highly suggestive, more than 30% against diagnosis **(Table 2)**.

TABLE 2: PLASMIC SCORE—tells about likelihood of severe ADAMTS13 deficiency.	
Parameter	Points
Platelet count <30 × 10⁹/L	1
Hemolysis (reticulocyte count >2.5%, haptoglobin undetectable, or indirect bilirubin > 2.0 mg/dL)	1
No active cancer	1
No history of solid-organ or stem-cell transplant	1
MCV <90 fL	1
INR <1.5	1
Creatinine <2.0 mg/dL	1

Score 0–4: Low risk for severe ADAMTS13 deficiency

Score 5: Intermediate risk for severe ADAMTS13 deficiency

Score 6–7: High risk for severe ADAMTS13 deficiency

Management: Plasmapheresis with plasma exchange for 1–2 weeks. It removes the pathogenic antibody from plasma and the normal plasma infused repletes the deficient ADAMTS13. Should be initiated as soon as possible, due to the risk of thrombotic complications. Patients respond within 3–5 days.

A glucocorticoid is initiated at the start to decrease antibody production. 1 mg/kg prednisone daily or methylprednisolone 1,000 mg daily for 3 days prior to starting prednisone

Caplacizumab: Anti von-Willibrand factor single variable domain immunoglobulin—inhibits interaction between ultra large vWF multimers and platelets. 10 mg subcutaneously daily during plasma exchange and 30 days afterward hastened resolution of acute TTP episode and reduced composite endpoint of TTP related death, recurrent TTP or a thromboembolic event. Best considered in patients who have neurologic or cardiac symptoms and in whom a very rapid response is needed to prevent impending catastrophic damage to vital organs.

HEMOLYTIC UREMIC SYNDROME

- *Definition:* Microangiopathic hemolytic anemia, caused by damage to endothelial cells leading to thrombosis in small blood vessels and fragmentation of red blood cells.
  - *Typical HUS*: Most common cause—Shiga toxin producing *Escherichia coli* (*E. coli*) infection; occurs few days after bloody diarrhea—toxigenic *E. coli* serotypes 157:H7 or O104:H4; Shiga toxin binds to and damages glomerular endothelium, localized thrombus formation, shearing of RBCs, renal failure
  - *Complement mediated HUS*: Inherited dysregulation of alternative complement cascade-deficiency of factor H, mutations in C3, factor B, CD46, and factor I preceded by URTI

- *Secondary HUS*: Caused by drugs or conditions that promote endothelial cell damage. E.g., calcineurin inhibitors (cyclosporin and tacrolimus), mitomycin C, cisplatin, bleomycin, autoimmune diseases, pregnancy, and cancers.
- *Management*: Aggressive antibiotic therapy for reducing spread of Shiga toxin. Neither plasmapheresis nor glucocorticoids seem to be helpful. Eculizumab, ravulizumab—inhibit the terminal steps of complement cascade. May be beneficial.

DISSEMINATED INTRAVASCULAR COAGULATION

- *Definition*: Acquired thrombohemorrhagic syndrome characterized by formation of diffuse micro—and macrovascular thrombi as a result of widespread uncontrolled activation of coagulation and progressive consumption of hemostatic factors such as platelets and clotting proteins with resultant risk of life-threatening hemorrhage and thrombosis.

  Urgent diagnosis and aggressive management of coagulopathy and underlying trigger of DIC is required as it is associated with mortality as high as 20–50%. Since no gold standard diagnostic test is available, keen attention on chemical status and lab abnormalities is required.

  Incidence is 1% of all hospital admissions of which 20% are in ICU.
- *Precipitating factors*:
  - Sepsis (gram negative sepsis, malaria, rickettsiae, and viruses)
  - Obstetrical calamities—preeclampsia, abruptio placenta, placenta previa, dead fetus, amniotic fluid embolism, and septic abortion
  - *Tissue damage*: Trauma, fat embolism, rhabdomyolysis, and acute pancreatitis
    AML M3
  - Mucin secreting adenocarcinoma
  - Snake bite
  - Large aneurysm, giant hemangioma intravascular hemolysis
- *Clinical features*: Uncontrolled bleeding in majority (64%). Skin, lungs, kidney, CNS. Purpura, ecchymosis, bleeding from venipuncture. Hemoptysis, hematuria, occult intra-abdominal bleed. Abdominal distress + signs of shock.
  - *Consumption tests*: Decreased platelets, increased PT and aPTT, decreased fibrinogen, increased FDP. All these tests may be normal in early phase.
  - Based on these there is a scoring system for DIC score **(Table 3)**
  - PT and aPTT can be normal in early phases (and in chronic DIC). So repeated values are more helpful.
  - Factor VIII and vWF are substantially increased, being acute phase reactants.
  - Fibrinogen is also an acute phase reactant. Therefore may not fall in severe cases. It is normal in 50% patients.
  - Schistocytes are seen in DIC, TTP, HUS, they must be interpreted in light of dynamic increase in PT/aPTT and fibrinogen and decreased platelets.
  - *Thromboelastography*: More useful in guiding therapy. On a TEG graph, maximum amplitude is most helpful. Value >60 indicates DIC.

TABLE 3: Disseminated intravascular coagulation (DIC) diagnostic scorecard and interpretation based on four laboratory parameters—platelet count, D-dimer/FDP, PT, and fibrinogen.

Platelet count	>100 = 0
	50–100 = 1
	<50 = 0
D-Dimer, FDP	Normal = 0
	Moderately increased = 2
	Severely increased = 3
Increased PT	<3 = 0
	3–6 = 1
	>6 = 2
Fibrinogen (g/L)	>1 = 0
	<1 = 1

Notes:
- Total score >5 = DIC
- <5 = repeat after 24 hours

Note: Continuous drop of platelets (even if >50,000) is more sensitive of DIC. D-Dimer is NOT sensitive or specific but when combined with FALLING platelets and other clotting factors it is more helpful and helps to differentiate from cirrhosis—

- *Differential diagnosis*: HIT, HELLP syndrome, rebalance hemostasis in cirrhosis, TTP/HUS.
- *Management*: Due to dynamic nature of the disease and combination of bleeds and thrombosis, patient's treatment may need tailoring as per need. Mostly we need to manage bleeding.
    - Treat the cause, e.g., sepsis with antibiotics.
    - Platelet infusion—to keep the platelet count >30,000/mm^3, definitely >50,000 to 1 lakh if surgical intervention needed.
    - FFP, cryoprecipitate, PCC for coagulation and other factors and rFVII as last resort may be used.
    - PRBC (to keep Hb >7 g/dL)
    - Anti-fibrinolytics rarely only in severe, refractory bleeding after other measures are exhausted.
    - Thrombotic patient (especially in chronic DIC)—use of heparin, antithrombin, APC, rhTM, TFPI is debatable. Heparin preferably LMWH may be used where thrombosis predominates.

THROMBOCYTOPENIA IN PREGNANCY

It occurs in 7–10 % of pregnancies.

Gestational thrombocytopenia (incidental thrombocytopenia of pregnancy): 75% cases. Mild, asymptomatic thrombocytopenia in late pregnancy, counts usually do not fall below 75,000/μL. Resolves spontaneously post delivery.

Preeclampsia: 15–20 % cases thrombocytopenia as part of HELLP syndrome (thrombocytopenia, microangiopathic hemolytic anemia and markedly-elevated liver function tests). If these syndromes do not resolve within 3 days post-delivery, alternative diagnosis ITP and TTP should be considered.

Preeclampsia versus TTP: The diagnosis of TTP can be difficult to make because many symptoms are identical to those of preeclampsia. The diagnosis of TTP is more certain if thrombocytopenia develops early during pregnancy (<20 weeks). If no improvement is seen by the third postpartum day, standard treatment for TTP including plasma exchange are recommended.

Immune thrombocytopenic purpura: Found in 3–4 % of normal pregnancies. Antiplatelet IgG antibodies can cross placenta and lead to thrombocytopenia in fetus. Counts >30,000/μL are considered safe in early stages of pregnancy and for vaginal delivery, >80,000/μL acceptable for caesarean section.

Management: Glucocorticoids, IVIG, and rituximab.

VASCULITIS-ASSOCIATED THROMBOCYTOPENIA

- Autoimmune diseases such as SLE, RA, and others can cause thrombocytopenia.
- Immune thrombocytopenic purpura like process that occurs in patients with a propensity for development of autoantibodies
- Some patients with active vasculitis and inflammation consume circulating platelets by promoting their adherence to damaged vessel wall
- *Treatment*: immunosuppression

Dilutional Thrombocytopenia

It occurs very rarely in massive transfusions.

Post-transfusion Purpura

- Due to sensitization to platelet alloantigen—HPA1A
- Week after transfusion
- Treatment IVIG or plasma exchange

Congenital Thrombocytopenia

- Autosomal dominant—May-Heggllin anomaly; Sebastian syndrome
- Autosomal recessive—Bernard-Soulier disease; Fanconi anemia, gray platelet syndrome, thrombocytopenia with absent radius
- X-linked Wiskott-Aldrich syndrome, *GATA 1* gene related, and FLNA related

CONCLUSION

Thrombocytopenia, defined as a platelet count less than the normal range, is categorized into three major causes: increased platelet destruction, decreased platelet production, and platelet sequestration. The clinical approach requires first ruling out pseudothrombocytopenia, an in vitro phenomenon like platelet clumping. The peripheral blood film provides essential clues; for instance, schistocytes suggest conditions like TTP, HUS, or DIC. Key specific conditions include ITP, an autoimmune condition often treated with corticosteroids; HIT, a prothrombotic condition requiring immediate cessation of heparin; and TTP, a life-threatening microangiopathy that needs urgent plasma exchange. DIC, a thrombohemorrhagic syndrome, is managed by treating the underlying cause, such as sepsis. In all cases, management aims to prevent spontaneous, life-threatening hemorrhage, which is a high risk at very low platelet counts.

FURTHER READINGS

1. Larry JJ, Fauci Anthony S, Kasper Dennis L, Hauser Stephen L, Longo Dan L, Joseph L, et al. Harrison's Manual of Medicine. 20th edition. New York: McGraw-Hill Education; 2020.
2. Goldman L, Schafer AI. Goldman-Cecil Medicine. 26th edition. Philadelphia: Elsevier. 2020.
3. Krishnan K, Dala Bl, Dasgupta A, Malhotra P, Varma N. PGI Textbook of Laboratory and Clinical Hematology. 1st edition. Mumbai: Bhalani Publishing House; 2024.

SECTION 9

Hepatology

CHAPTER 24

Acute-on-Chronic Liver Failure

Ashish Bhagat

INTRODUCTION

Acute-on-chronic liver failure (ACLF) is a clinical syndrome that has gained significant attention in hepatology over the last two decades. It is characterized by the acute deterioration of pre-existing chronic liver disease, usually cirrhosis, and is associated with organ failure and high short-term mortality. While there is unanimity in the recognition of clinical entities of acute liver failure (ALF) and decompensated cirrhosis, there is heterogeneity in the concept of ACLF. Nevertheless, all authorities recognize ACLF as a distinct clinical syndrome with an ominous clinical course and prognosis. Because of its rapid progression and high fatality, ACLF is considered a medical emergency. ACLF is a severe form of acutely decompensated cirrhosis, associated with a 28-day mortality rate of 20% or more (vs. 5% or less among patients with acutely decompensated cirrhosis without ACLF). Therefore, it is important for the physicians to identify the patients of chronic liver disease presenting with ACLF to prognosticate and triage them for intensive care and liver transplantation and predict futility of care.

DEFINITION

Different international liver societies have provided definitions of ACLF, reflecting regional variations in the causes of chronic liver disease. Alcoholic cirrhosis constitutes 50–70% of all the underlying liver diseases of ACLF in the Western countries, whereas hepatitis-related cirrhosis constitutes about 10–15% of all cases.

Asian Pacific Association for the Study of the Liver

Acute-on-chronic liver failure is defined as an acute hepatic insult manifesting as jaundice and coagulopathy, complicated within 4 weeks by ascites and/or encephalopathy in a patient with previously diagnosed or undiagnosed chronic liver disease. The primary precipitating event, the acute hepatic insult, should be hepatic in origin.

Acute event in ACLF could be hepatotropic and nonhepatotropic viruses, reactivation of hepatitis B (overt or occult) or hepatitis C other infectious agents afflicting the liver. Noninfectious events could be alcohol, hepatotoxic drugs/herbs, flare of autoimmune hepatitis or Wilson's disease, and surgical intervention for variceal bleed. The AARC [Asian Pacific Association for the Study of the Liver (APASL) ACLF Research Consortium] score is applied to patients diagnosed as having ACLF using the APASL criteria to determine short-term mortality.

European Association for the Study of the Liver–Chronic Liver Failure Consortium

Acute-on-chronic liver failure is described as acute decompensation of cirrhosis associated with organ failure and high short-term mortality. Both patients with prior decompensation and those without are included in the definition of ACLF. Severe organ failure as per the European Association for the Study of the Liver–Chronic Liver Failure Consortium (EASL-CLIF-C) criteria is essential to define ACLF. The number of organ failures according to the CLIF-C organ failure score that are simultaneously present is associated with an increasing case fatality rate at 28 days. The CLIF-C ACLF score and ACLF grade are used to predict mortality. It emphasizes identifying the most common precipitants, which include proven bacterial infection, alcohol-related hepatitis, gastrointestinal hemorrhage with hemodynamic instability, flare of hepatitis B virus (HBV) infection, hepatitis E virus infection, and recent use of drugs known to cause cerebral failure and kidney failure.

American Association for the Study of Liver Diseases

The American Association for the Study of Liver Diseases (AASLD) considers the dysfunction of four organ systems (brain, kidneys, heart, and lungs). Curiously, liver and coagulation are not considered, and kidney, circulatory, and respiratory failures are defined by the physician's response to the problem, namely the need for renal replacement therapy, inotropes, or mechanical ventilation, respectively. The NACSELD (North American Consortium for the Study of End-Stage Liver Disease) score is determined by the number of organ system failures (and therefore ranges from 1 to 4); ACLF is defined by a NACSELD score of 2 or more, with a maximum of 4.

Despite these variations in definitions of ACLF, it is generally accepted that there is acute worsening of the liver status from the baseline with systemic inflammation, organ failure, and high mortality.

■ ETIOLOGY

Acute-on-chronic liver failure develops when an acute precipitating factor impacts a patient with chronic liver disease. Common triggers include the following:
- *Infections*: Spontaneous bacterial peritonitis, pneumonia, urinary tract infections, and sepsis are the most frequent precipitants.
- *Alcoholic hepatitis*: Excessive and prolonged alcohol consumption can cause severe liver inflammation on the background of cirrhosis.

- *Viral hepatitis reactivation*: Reactivation of hepatitis B or superimposed hepatitis A/E infection or nonhepatotropic viruses may trigger ACLF.
- *Drug-induced liver injury (DILI)*: Hepatotoxic drugs [antituberculosis drugs, antiepileptics, nonsteroidal anti-inflammatory drugs (NSAIDs)], herbs, or complementary and alternative medicines (CAMs) may cause acute hepatic insult.
- *Gastrointestinal bleeding*: Massive variceal or nonvariceal bleeding contributes to circulatory dysfunction and precipitates ACLF.
- *Ischemic hepatitis or toxins*: Reduced liver perfusion due to shock or toxic exposure may trigger acute injury.

In some patients, no clear precipitant is found, indicating underlying immune or metabolic disturbances.

PATHOPHYSIOLOGY

The pathogenesis of ACLF involves complex interactions between liver injury, systemic inflammation, and multiorgan dysfunction.

Systemic inflammation: Systemic inflammatory response, characterized by a predominantly proinflammatory cytokine profile, causes the transition from stable cirrhosis to ACLF. Acute insult activates the immune system, leading to excessive release of proinflammatory cytokines and chemokines, leading to "cytokine storm" and widespread tissue injury. Proinflammatory cytokines are believed to mediate hepatic inflammation, apoptosis, and necrosis of liver cells; cholestasis; and fibrosis. The clinical picture of both ACLF and septic shock is strikingly similar, characterized by progressive vasodilatory shock and multiple organ failure.

Immune paralysis: After initial hyperinflammation, immune dysfunction occurs, predisposing patients to infections. ACLF is a state of severe functional failure of neutrophils in a proportion of patients with cirrhosis and alcoholic hepatitis, and these defects are associated with an increased risk of infection, organ failure, and mortality.

Circulatory changes: Increased nitric oxide (NO) and vasodilation cause systemic hypotension, while renal vasoconstriction precipitates hepatorenal syndrome. Inflammation and oxidative stress also induce the production of NO, which appears to cause the circulatory and renal disturbances of liver failure. There is evidence that the mediators of inflammation (e.g., proinflammatory cytokines, NO, and oxidative stress) could modulate the effect of hyperammonemia in precipitating encephalopathy. The liver plays a prominent role in the metabolism of asymmetric dimethyl-L-arginine (ADMA), an endogenous inhibitor of NO synthase. Hepatocellular damage is a main determinant of elevated ADMA concentration in advanced alcoholic cirrhosis. By inhibiting NO release from vascular endothelium, ADMA might oppose the peripheral vasodilation caused by excessive NO production in severe cirrhosis. Plasma ADMA and stereoisomer symmetric dimethylarginine (SDMA) are significantly high in patients with alcoholic hepatitis and nonsurvivors.

ORGAN FAILURES

Organ failure is the defining criterion of the EASL definition and the most important determinant of clinical course in ACLF. With the increasing number of failing organs, mortality rises exponentially.

Liver: Severe jaundice and coagulopathy

Kidney: Acute kidney injury or hepatorenal syndrome

Brain: Hepatic encephalopathy

Lungs: Acute respiratory distress syndrome

Circulatory system: Shock and cardiac dysfunction

It is important to understand that ACLF is not limited to liver failure alone but represents a multisystem disorder.

CLINICAL FEATURES

Patients with ACLF often present with:
- *Jaundice*: Rapid increase in serum bilirubin levels
- *Ascites and edema*: Worsening portal hypertension and fluid retention
- *Hepatic encephalopathy*: Confusion, altered behavior, drowsiness, or coma
- *Coagulopathy*: Easy bruising, bleeding from gums, or gastrointestinal bleeding
- Signs of infection or sepsis
- *Renal impairment*: Oliguria, elevated creatinine
- *Respiratory distress*: Hypoxemia or pneumonia
- *Hemodynamic instability*: Hypotension and tachycardia
- The syndrome progresses quickly, and without intervention, mortality rises steeply within 28 days.

DIAGNOSIS

Diagnosis is based on clinical presentation, laboratory investigations, and severity scoring systems.

Investigations

- *Liver function tests*: Marked elevation of bilirubin, deranged international normalized ratio (INR), and elevated liver enzymes
- *Renal profile*: Serum creatinine and urea levels to detect kidney injury
- *Complete blood count*: Leukocytosis, anemia, and thrombocytopenia
- *Cultures*: Blood, urine, and ascitic fluid to detect infections
- *Imaging*: Ultrasound or computed tomography (CT) scan to assess cirrhosis, ascites, and portal hypertension
- *Other markers*: Inflammatory cytokines (experimental) and arterial ammonia levels

Diagnostic Criteria

In a patient of chronic liver disease, organ failures as included in the EASL-CLIF-C criteria should be used for the diagnosis of ACLF. The failure of one or more of the six major organ systems according to the EASL-CLIF-C criteria should be used to define the severity of ACLF and the risk of 28-day mortality.

Model for End-Stage Liver Disease (MELD) score: Used to predict prognosis and transplant prioritization

MANAGEMENT

The management of ACLF is challenging and requires a multifaceted approach.
- *General supportive care*:
  - Admission to an intensive care unit
  - Oxygen therapy or ventilatory support
  - Fluid and electrolyte balance
  - Nutritional support (high-protein diet unless encephalopathy is severe)
- *Treatment of precipitating factors*:
  - *Infections*: Broad-spectrum antibiotics, followed by targeted therapy
  - *Alcoholic hepatitis*: Corticosteroids in selected cases
  - *Viral reactivation*: Nucleos(t)ide analogs for HBV reactivation
  - *Drug-induced injury*: Withdrawal of offending drug, use of antidotes if available
  - *Variceal bleeding*: Endoscopic band ligation, vasoactive drugs, and blood transfusions
- *Organ support*:
  - *Renal replacement therapy*: Dialysis for kidney failure
  - *Vasopressors*: For circulatory collapse
  - *Mechanical ventilation*: For respiratory failure
- *Specific liver support*: Artificial liver support systems [e.g., MARS (molecular adsorbent recirculating system)] may provide temporary stabilization, though survival benefits are limited.
- *Liver transplantation*:
  The definitive treatment for ACLF with poor prognosis.
  Early referral and evaluation are critical, as short-term mortality without transplantation is extremely high.

PROGNOSIS

Acute-on-chronic liver failure has a very poor natural course. Mortality ranges between 30 and 70% within 28 days, depending on the number of organ failures. Prognosis is worse in patients with:
- Higher bilirubin and INR
- Multiple organ failure
- Uncontrolled infections
- Delay in initiating treatment
  Early recognition and transplantation significantly improve survival.

PREVENTION

Since ACLF often results from preventable triggers, several strategies are crucial:
- Vaccination against hepatitis viruses
- Strict control of alcohol use
- Avoidance of hepatotoxic drugs
- Early treatment of infections
- Routine monitoring in patients with cirrhosis

CONCLUSION

Acute-on-chronic liver failure is a distinct and severe clinical syndrome with high morbidity and mortality. It occurs when an acute hepatic insult precipitates rapid deterioration in patients with chronic liver disease, leading to systemic inflammation, multiorgan failure, and a poor prognosis. Management requires early recognition, aggressive supportive therapy, treatment of precipitating factors, and timely referral for liver transplantation. As the global burden of liver disease rises, understanding ACLF and improving therapeutic strategies are essential to reduce mortality and improve the quality of life in affected patients.

SUGGESTED READINGS

1. Moreau R, Jalan R, Gines P, et al. Acute-on-chronic liver failure is a distinct syndrome that develops in patients with acute decompensation of cirrhosis. Gastroenterology. 2013;144(7):1426-37, 1437.e1-9.
2. Sarin SK, Kedarisetty CK, Abbas Z., et al. Acute-on-chronic liver failure: consensus recommendations of the Asian Pacific Association for the Study of the Liver (APASL) 2014. Hepatol Int. 2014;8(4):453-71.
3. Arroyo V, Moreau R, Kamath PS, et al. Acute-on-chronic liver failure in cirrhosis. Nat Rev Dis Primers. 2016:2:16041.
4. Hernaez R, Kramer JR. Acute-on-Chronic Liver Failure. Clinical Liver Disease. 2020;24(2): 241-61.
5. Gustot T, Fernandez J, Garcia E, et al. (2015). Clinical Course of acute-on-chronic liver failure syndrome and effects on prognosis. Hepatology. 2015l;62(1):243-52.
6. Piano S, Angeli P. Pathophysiology and Management of ACLF: The Role of Inflammation and Organ Failure. Journal of Hepatology. 2021;75(4):989-1004.
7. Northup PG, Garcia-Tsao G, Intagliata NM, et al. AASLD Guidance on acute-on-Chronic Liver Failure: Diagnostic and Management Strategies. Hepatology. 2021;74(3):1611-44.

SECTION 10

Infectious Disease

CHAPTER 25

Long COVID

Pradeep Agarwal, Ramesh Kumar, Yashraj Saini

INTRODUCTION

The coronavirus disease 2019 (COVID-19) pandemic has resulted in an increasing population who have recovered from severe acute respiratory syndrome coronavirus 2 (SARS-CoV-2) infection. A significant number of them continue to experience a broad spectrum of symptoms beyond the acute phase of illness described in literature using terms such as "PASC (postacute sequelae of COVID-19)" and "chronic COVID." Even years after infection, some patients continue to experience symptoms and reduction in quality of life, asserting that this postillness condition remains a significant public health challenge.

"Long COVID is defined as new, persistent, or relapsing symptoms—or symptom clusters of COVID-19, varying in severity, duration, and across systems—at least 12 weeks after the initial COVID-19 infection."

Various definitions have been proposed, but there is a consistent recognition across these frameworks affirming the existence and clinical significance of the condition. The SARS-CoV-2 continues to circulate widely, and long COVID remains a significant and ongoing challenge to global public health **(Table 1)**.

TABLE 1: Definitions of long COVID by major health authorities.		
Name	**Definition**	**Attribution**
Long COVID	Signs, symptoms, and conditions that continue or develop after initial SARS-CoV-2 infection and last >4 weeks	US Centers for Disease Control and Prevention (CDC)
Postacute sequelae of COVID-19 (PASC)	Ongoing, relapsing, or new symptoms or clinical conditions present at 30 or more days after SARS-CoV-2 infection	National Institutes of Health (NIH)
Post-COVID-19 condition	Symptoms presenting 3 months from the onset of COVID-19 that last for at least 2 months and cannot be explained by other diagnoses	World Health Organization (WHO)
Post-COVID syndrome	Symptoms that are unexplained by an alternative diagnosis and persist for >12 weeks after acute COVID-19	UK National Institute for Health and Care Excellence (NICE)

EPIDEMIOLOGY AND RISK FACTOR

True prevalence of long COVID is hard to define due to varying definitions, clinical criteria, and analysis methods, but globally, pooled prevalence is estimated at 21% and in India, estimated at 27.2%.

Risk Factors
- Age 18–79 years
- Female population
- Individuals with higher body mass index
- Smokers at higher risk
- Higher prevalence in individuals with acute COVID illness requiring hospitalization, intensive care unit (ICU) care, and severe acute COVID infection
- Pre-existing conditions—diabetes mellitus, depression
- Inadequate recovery or rest after COVID-19
- Unvaccinated

PATHOPHYSIOLOGY

The pathogenesis of long COVID remains poorly understood, with no single, clearly outlined etiology. However, accumulating evidence suggests that multiple overlapping mechanisms contribute to clinical features seen in affected individuals **(Fig. 1)**.

Probable mechanisms include persistent viral reserves in tissues triggering immune activation, autoimmune-like response leading to chronic inflammation, circulating microclots impairing oxygen delivery to tissues, immune dysregulation, with or without reactivation of latent viruses [i.e., Epstein–Barr virus and human herpesvirus 6 (HHV-6)], and dysfunctional neurological signaling. Emerging research suggests that additional factors, such as endothelial dysfunction, virus-mediated cellular injury, microbiota dysbiosis, reduced peripheral serotonin levels, complement dysregulation, and genetic link (involving the *FOXP4* gene), remain under investigation and research.

Similarities between long COVID and other postviral chronic illnesses suggest a potentially common underlying mechanism triggered by various infectious conditions **(Tables 2 and 3)**.

Approaches to Systematizing Symptom Patterns in Long COVID

Due to the heterogeneity of symptoms and distribution, a structured symptom categorization is needed to identify, detect cases early and risk stratification, and address functional, diagnostic, and pathophysiological needs.
- *Organ system-based classification:* Grouping symptoms by organ system enhances clinical clarity. General symptoms include fatigue, postexertional malaise (PEM), and appetite or weight changes. Cardiopulmonary symptoms such as dyspnea, palpitations, and orthopnea are common. Neurological

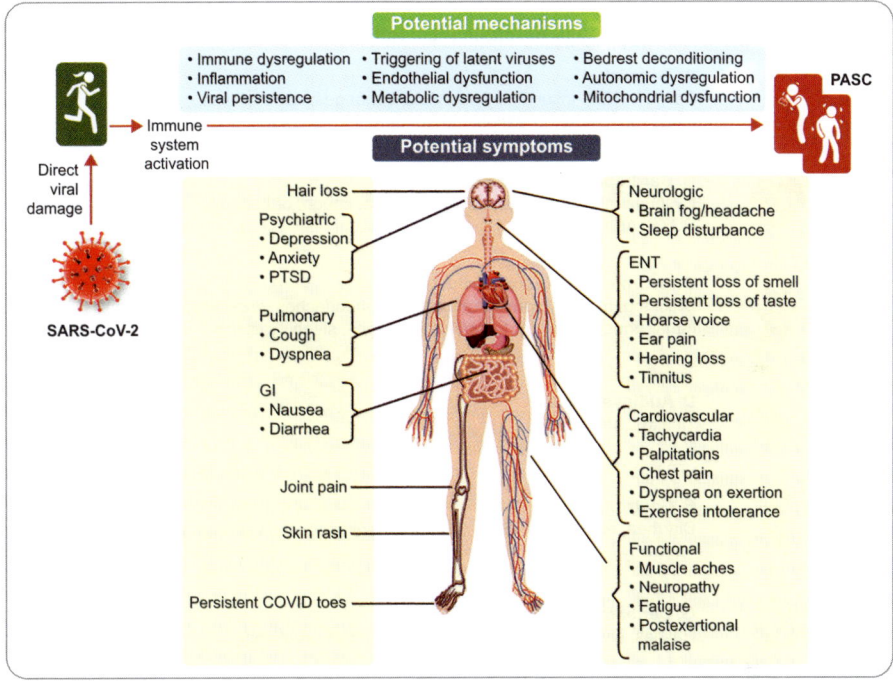

FIG. 1: COVID mechanisms and symptoms.
(COVID: coronavirus disease; ENT: ear, nose, and throat; GI: gastrointestinal; PASC: postacute sequelae of COVID-19; PTSD: post-traumatic stress disorder; SARS-COV-2: severe acute respiratory syndrome coronavirus 2)

TABLE 2: Impact level and symptoms.

Impact level	Symptoms
High impact	Fatigue/PEM, cognitive issues, dyspnea
Moderate impact	Myalgia, chest pain, tinnitus, insomnia
Low impact	Mild rashes, mild GI discomfort

(GI: gastrointestinal; PEM: postexertional malaise)

TABLE 3: Frequency and symptoms.

Frequency	Symptom
Common (>20%)	Fatigue, PEM, dyspnea, myalgia, brain fog, anosmia
Moderate (5–20%)	Headache, palpitations, insomnia, tinnitus, GI symptoms
Rare (<5%)	Autoimmune sequelae, peripheral edema, vision changes

(GI: gastrointestinal; PEM: postexertional malaise)

and neuropsychiatric features include cognitive dysfunction, neuropathy, dysautonomia, and sleep disturbances. Other frequently affected systems include the audiovestibular, gastrointestinal, musculoskeletal, dermatologic, and immune/inflammatory systems **(Fig. 2)**.

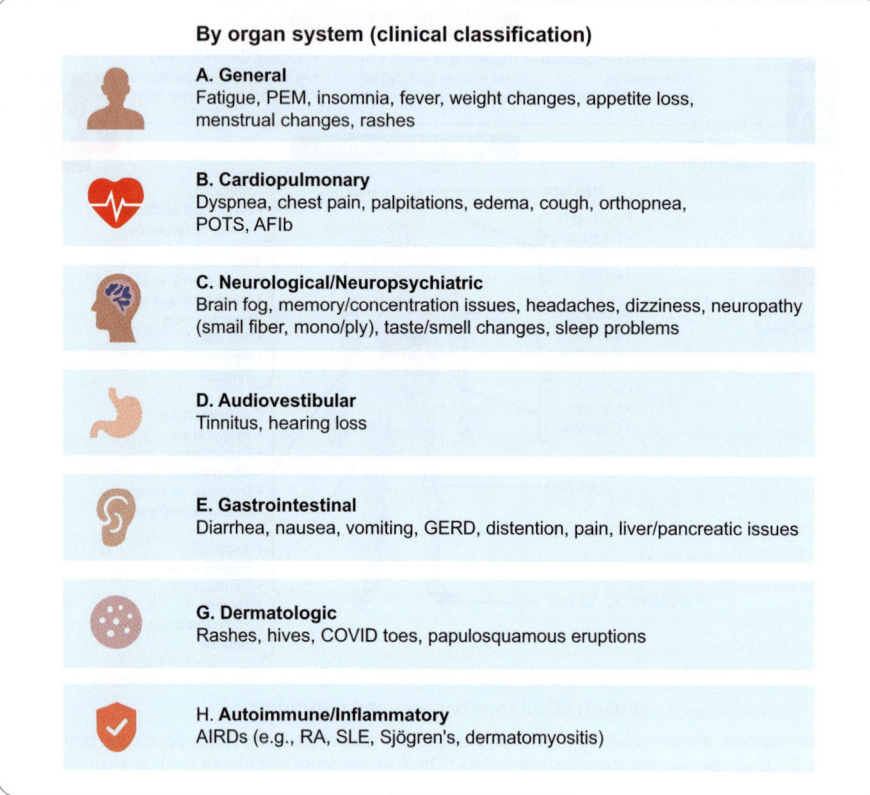

FIG. 2: Organ system-based classification.
(AFib: atrial fibrillation; GERD: gastroesophageal reflux disease; PEM: postexertional malaise; POTS: postural orthostatic tachycardia syndrome; RA: rheumatoid arthritis; SLE: systemic lupus erythematosus)

- *Functional impact approach:* This patient-centered model assesses how symptoms disrupt daily life. High-impact symptoms like cognitive dysfunction or breathlessness cause significant impairment, while moderate-impact symptoms affect quality of life without full disability. This approach aids in prioritizing care.
- *Diagnostic and clinical priority framework:* Symptom triage based on urgency is key. Acute signs such as chest pain or unexplained dyspnea require immediate evaluation to rule out serious conditions like pulmonary embolism or myocarditis. Less urgent symptoms (e.g., fatigue, insomnia) may be managed conservatively.
- *Phenotypic subtypes of PASC:* Clustering analyses have identified reproducible PASC phenotypes, including cardiorenal, respiratory–sleep–anxiety, musculoskeletal–neurologic, and digestive–respiratory subtypes. These patterns may reflect distinct pathophysiologic end types, guiding future personalized treatment **(Box 1)**.

CHAPTER 25: Long COVID

> **BOX 1: Phenotypic subtypes of PASC.**
> - *Subphenotype 1*: Cardiorenal classified as primarily having cardiac and pulmonary symptomatology, acute renal failure, anemia, and fluid/electrolyte disturbances
> - *Subphenotype 2*: Respiratory, sleep, and anxiety classified as primarily having respiratory symptoms, sleep disorders, anxiety issues, headaches, and chest pain
> - *Subphenotype 3*: Musculoskeletal and nervous. Classified as primarily having musculoskeletal pain, headaches, and sleep disorders
> - *Subphenotype 4*: Digestive and respiratory. Primarily digestive and respiratory conditions
>
> (PASC: postacute sequelae of COVID-19)

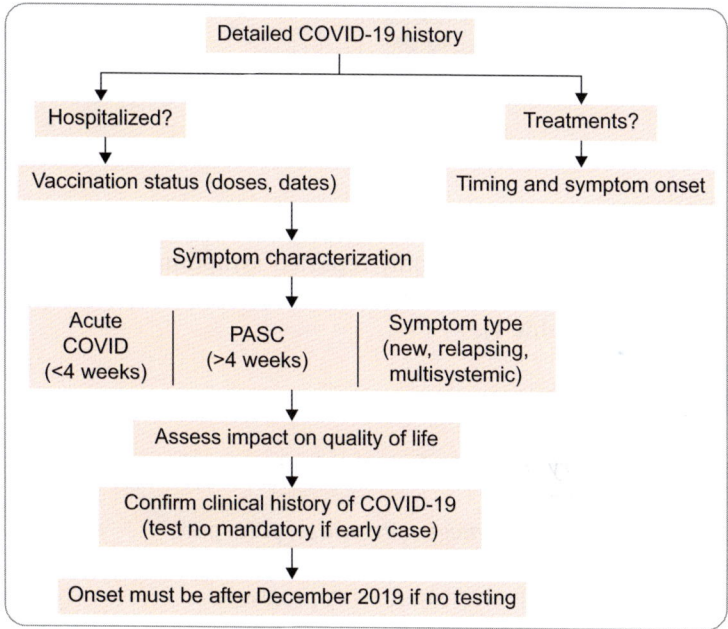

FLOWCHART 1: COVID-19 history.
(COVID-19: coronavirus disease 2019; PASC: postacute sequelae of COVID-19)

Clinical Assessment for Long COVID

In a patient with suspected long COVID, a detailed history of COVID-19 infection is essential. History should include whether the patient was hospitalized, what treatment was administered, ICU requirement, and vaccination status. Long COVID symptoms can be distinguished from those of acute COVID-19 by their persistence or new onset beyond the initial 4-week period of infection, often presenting with fluctuating, multisystem involvement that cannot be explained by an alternative diagnosis.

COVID-19 illness by assessing the timing, duration, and nature of symptoms; whether symptoms are new, relapsing, or persistent; whether multiple organ systems are affected; and impairment on quality of life. A positive test of COVID-19 is not mandatory, but onset must be after December 2019 **(Flowchart 1 and Fig. 3)**.

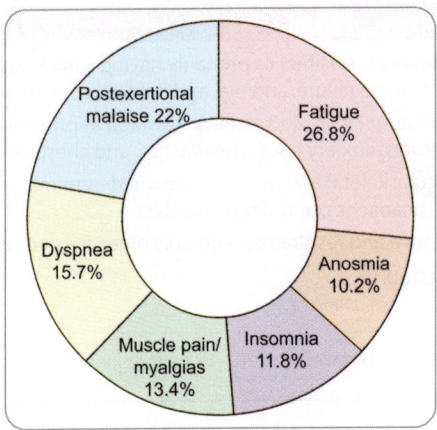

FIG. 3: Symptom distribution.

Fatigue

Fatigue is one of the most commonly reported symptoms, affecting 26.3% of patients. It is often persistent, severe, not alleviated by rest, exertion sensitive, and functionally limiting **(Table 4)**.

Management

- *General principles*:
  - *Multidisciplinary care,* including physicians, therapists, and mental health professionals
  - *Energy conservation strategies:* Prioritize, plan, pace
  - *Avoid high-intensity exercise,* which may worsen PEM
- *Rehabilitation*: Titrated return-to-activity programs
- *Supportive measures*:
  - Treat comorbidities (e.g., insomnia, depression, nutritional deficiencies)
  - No pharmacologic therapy is currently approved specifically for PASC-related fatigue. Management remains individualized and supportive.

Pulmonary Sequelae of Long COVID

Dyspnea (Shortness of Breath)

Long COVID can present as exertional breathlessness, orthopnea, or, at times, at rest. It can also be associated with chest discomfort, chest tightness, wheezing, or cough. Symptoms may persist beyond the acute infection and significantly impair daily function and quality of life.

It is described as sensations of air hunger, chest tightness, or needing to "consciously breathe" or "work harder" to breathe—often in the absence of any other objective findings. In certain cases, this can be altered breathing patterns or dysfunctional breathing.

TABLE 4: Clinical features, evaluation, and management.

Clinical characteristic	Clinical assessment		
Often described as "flat battery" sensation, reduced functional capacity, and symptom exacerbation after exertion. It commonly exists with exertional dyspnea, orthostatic intolerance, and neurocognitive dysfunction *Diagnostic criteria (adapted from ME/CFS)* Consider a long COVID-related fatigue syndrome if the following are present: • Persistent fatigue impairing function for ≥6 months • PEM (described as crashing) • Nonrestorative sleep *Plus at least one of*: • Cognitive impairment • Orthostatic intolerance *Functional assessment*: • Fatigue assessment scale (measures fatigue severity) • WHO disability assessment schedule (assess impact on daily function)	• Detailed history including symptom onset, pattern, and PEM • Physical examination to identify contributory conditions • Use of symptom diaries and validated scales		
	Test	**Purpose**	**Potential Alternative Diagnoses**
	CBC	Anemia or infection	Iron-deficiency anemia, leukocytosis
	TSH	Thyroid function	Hypo-/hyperthyroidism
	Vitamin B12	Nutritional deficiency	B12 deficiency anemia, neuropathy
	Vitamin D	Nutritional deficiency	Vitamin D deficiency
	CMP	Electrolytes, renal/hepatic status	Kidney/Liver disease
	HbA1c	Glucose control	Diabetes
	HIV, RPR, hepatitis C	Chronic infection	HIV, syphilis, hepatitis C
	Laboratory tests: Additional tests for persistent fever (blood cultures, urine analysis, and stool studies) *Differential diagnosis*: Anemia, thyroid dysfunction, sleep disorders (e.g., insomnia, apnea), mood disorders, chronic infections, diabetes or metabolic syndrome, autonomic dysfunction (e.g., POTS), cardiopulmonary disease, and ME/CFS		

(CBC: complete blood count; ME/CFS: myalgic encephalomyelitis/chronic fatigue syndrome; PEM: postexertional malaise; POTS: postural orthostatic tachycardia syndrome; RPR: rapid plasma regain; TSH: thyroid-stimulating hormone; WHO: World Health Organization)

Possible etiologies:
- *Pulmonary sequelae:* Persistent inflammation, fibrosis, and small airway disease
- *Cardiovascular involvement:* Reduced cardiopulmonary reserve, myocarditis, myocardial injury, and microvascular dysfunction
- *Autonomic dysfunction:* Postural orthostatic tachycardia syndrome (POTS)
- *Thromboembolic disease:* Pulmonary embolism (reported with elevated incidence for up to 110 days post-COVID-19, particularly in patients with severe illness or comorbidities)

Clinical evaluation
- Vital signs, including orthostatic vitals
- Pulse oximetry at rest and during exertion
- Cardiac auscultation and examination of the lower extremities for edema
- Pulmonary auscultation to assess for crackles, wheezing, or signs of consolidation **(Table 5)**
  - *Altered breathing pattern/dysfunctional breathing:* In the absence of significant pulmonary pathology—
    - Chest tightness ("COVID squeeze")
    - Shallow, inefficient breathing
    - A sensation of needing to consciously initiate each breath

Management

Strategies are guided by the etiology, emphasis on symptomatic relief, rehabilitation, improving quality of life, and exclusion of life-threatening pathology.
- *Pulmonary etiologies:*
  - Treat underlying asthma or COPD (e.g., bronchodilators and inhaled corticosteroids)
  - In patients with suspected interstitial lung disease or pulmonary fibrosis, consider antifibrotic therapy or pulmonary rehabilitation.
- *Thromboembolic disease*: Anticoagulation per standard venous thromboembolism (VTE) guidelines (extended-duration anticoagulation in select post-COVID populations, particularly with persistent risk factors)
- *Dysfunctional breathing*:
  - *Breathing retraining*: Techniques such as diaphragmatic breathing, paced respiration, and nasal breathing patterns
  - *Respiratory physiotherapy*: Targeted interventions to normalize breathing patterns and improve endurance
  - *Digital support*: Guided breathing and rehabilitation platforms
  - *Psychological support*: Cognitive behavioral therapy (CBT) or integrative therapy if anxiety contributes to breathing symptoms **(Table 6)**.

TABLE 5: Investigations.	
Test/Tool	**Purpose**
Sit-to-stand test	Detect oxygen desaturation or orthostatic intolerance
6-minute walk test	Evaluate exertional hypoxia or tachycardia
In-clinic spirometry	Support diagnosis of obstructive lung disease
Chest X-ray	Rule out persistent parenchymal disease or pneumonia
PFT	Rule out asthma, COPD, or restrictive patterns
High-resolution CT chest	In posthospitalized patients or those with persistent symptoms
CT pulmonary angiogram	Evaluate for pulmonary embolism (in high risk)
Transthoracic echocardiogram	To rule out cardiac etiology
(COPD: chronic obstructive pulmonary disease; PFT: pulmonary function testing)	

TABLE 6: Differential diagnosis, evaluation, and management of COVID-19.

Differential diagnosis	Evaluation	Management

Conditions to rule out include:
• COVID reinfection or relapse
• Pneumonia
• Obstructive or restrictive lung parenchymal disease
• GERD-related cough
• Cardiac causes (i.e., heart failure)
	• *History*: Character and duration of cough, associated symptoms
	• *Physical examination*: Respiratory and cardiovascular systems
	• *Investigations*:
	  ○ Chest X-ray or CT
	  ○ Spirometry with bronchodilator testing
	  ○ Inflammatory markers
		• Antitussives
		• Inhaled corticosteroids ± bronchodilators
		• *GERD therapy*: PPI, lifestyle modification

(GERD: gastroesophageal reflux disease; PPI: proton pump inhibitor)

Cough

In long COVID, cough is defined as a persistent or new-onset cough lasting ≥4 weeks after initial COVID-19 infection, without active infection or another identifiable etiology.

Cough in long COVID may be due to residual airway inflammation, hyperresponsiveness, gastroesophageal reflux, or pulmonary fibrosis.

Cough may present as:
- Dry cough (most common)
- Productive cough
- Postviral hypersensitivity cough

Cardiovascular Sequelae of Long COVID

The American College of Cardiology (ACC) and Journal of the American College of Cardiology (JACC) Expert Consensus proposed a structured approach for management of cardiovascular manifestations of PASC, including classification: PASC-cardiovascular disease (PASC-CVD) (with objective CVD) and PASC-cardiovascular syndrome (PASC-CVS) (with cardiovascular symptoms but no identifiable disease).

Cardiovascular symptoms such as chest pain, exertional dyspnea, palpitations, tachycardia, and exercise intolerance/fatigue are frequently reported in individuals with long COVID. These symptoms may reflect cardiovascular pathologies such as myocardial injury, myocarditis, and pericardial involvement or can occur in the absence of objective findings, suggesting autonomic dysfunction or cardiopulmonary deconditioning.

Cardiopulmonary deconditioning: Following acute COVID-19 infection, especially in patients with prolonged bed rest, illness, or inactivity, there is reduced cardiac preload, leading to decreased stroke volume and compensatory increase in heart rate even during mild exertion in the absence of any identifiable structural

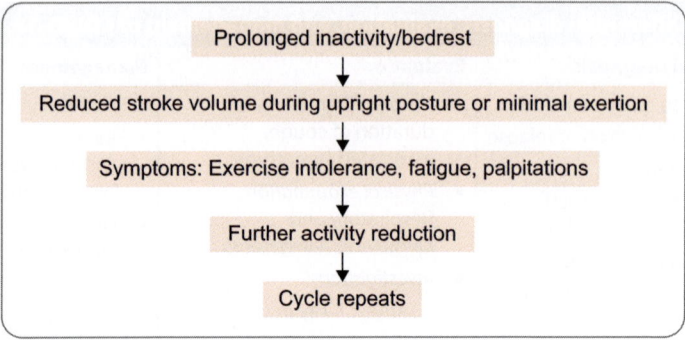

FLOWCHART 2: Downward spiral of deconditioning: A potential mechanism of exercise intolerance and excessive tachycardia in COVID-19.

pathology. Symptoms include exercise intolerance, fatigue, tachycardia out of proportion to exertion, and even orthostatic symptoms **(Flowchart 2)**.

Classification of Cardiovascular Sequelae

PASC-CVD: Symptoms (e.g., chest pain, dyspnea, and palpitations) attributable to identifiable cardiovascular pathology such as myocarditis, myocardial injury, pericarditis, heart failure, or thromboembolic disease.

PASC-CVS: Cardiovascular symptoms persist despite normal diagnostic testing. These may reflect autonomic dysregulation, microvascular dysfunction, or deconditioning.

Evaluation:
- For all symptomatic patients, "Triad Testing":
    - 12-lead electrocardiogram (ECG)
    - High-sensitivity cardiac troponin
    - Transthoracic echocardiogram

If any of these tests are abnormal or clinical suspicion is high (e.g., exertional symptoms, syncope, and abnormal vital signs), advanced imaging and further cardiopulmonary evaluation are required.
- *Advanced investigations:* Refer to **Table 7**

TABLE 7: Advanced investigations of COVID-19.	
Cardiopulmonary exercise testing (CPET)	Identify exertional limitations due to cardiovascular, pulmonary, or deconditioning pathology
Ambulatory ECG monitoring	Assess for arrhythmias
Cardiac MRI	Gold standard for evaluating myocarditis and myocardial inflammation
CT pulmonary angiogram	Evaluate for pulmonary embolism (if high suspicion/raised markers)

Management:
- *Myocarditis and myocardial injury*: Diagnosis is based on symptoms (e.g., chest pain, fatigue, and palpitations), elevated troponin, and imaging (e.g., cardiac MRI demonstrating late gadolinium enhancement)
  - Physical activity restriction for ≥3-6 months
  - Initiate standard guideline-directed medical therapy for left ventricular dysfunction
  - Avoid immunosuppression unless biopsy-proven myocarditis with active inflammation
- *Pericarditis*: Present as pleuritic chest pain, pericardial rub, or effusion on imaging
  Treatment:
  - Nonsteroidal anti-inflammatory drugs (NSAIDs) and colchicine
  - Corticosteroids in refractory or recurrent cases
  - Monitor for signs of tamponade if effusion is present.
- *Microvascular and endothelial dysfunction*: If angina-like chest pain occurs but normal epicardial coronary arteries are present, microvascular ischemia may be suspected.

Approach: Empirical antianginal therapy
- *Return-to-activity protocol*: According to the Journal of the American College of Cardiology (JACC) guidelines, a graded return-to-activity program is suggested for patients with exertional symptoms, deconditioning.
- Begin with recumbent/semirecumbent exercise (rowing, swimming, and recumbent cycling), 5-10 min/day.
- Increase duration by 1-2 min/week, maintaining the ability to speak in full sentences during activity.
- Monitor for postexertional symptom exacerbation (PESE); avoid rapid escalation of intensity.
- For orthostatic intolerance, maintain exercises that avoid upright posture until tolerance improves.

Neurological Sequelae of Long COVID

Brain Fog

Brain fog is characterized by deficits in attention, memory, executive functioning, and mental clarity. It is among the most common reported neurological symptoms, described as cognitive slowing, difficulty concentrating/focusing, or a feeling of mentally "clouded" and mental fatigue. These symptoms can be persistent and cause significant impairment, in work and daily activities, and worsen by physical exertion or multitasking.

Diagnostic evaluation: To differentiate postviral neurocognitive sequelae from neurodegenerative or psychiatric disorders

Bedside cognitive screening:
- *Mini–mental state examination (MMSE)*: Screens for global cognitive function and dementia.

- *Montreal cognitive assessment (MoCA)*: Detects mild cognitive impairment and frontal lobe dysfunction.
- *Hopkins verbal learning test (HVLT)*: Assesses short-term memory loss and recall performance.

Laboratory evaluation:
- Rule out anemia, hypothyroidism, and electrolyte imbalances.
- *Rule out alternate infectious etiologies*: Infectious screen [human immunodeficiency virus (HIV), rapid plasma reagin (RPR), and hepatitis C]
- Vitamin levels (D, B1, B6, and B12)—detect vitamin deficiencies

Imaging and neurophysiology:
- Brain MRI (with and without contrast)—recommended in patients with red flags or worsening symptoms
- Electroencephalogram (EEG)—in cases where encephalopathy or seizures are suspected
- Expanded neuropsychological testing—for persistent or occupationally limiting symptoms

Management strategies are supportive and focus on symptom improvement, functional recovery, and occupational symptoms recovery.

Nonpharmacologic approaches:
- Energy conservation and pacing techniques
- Cognitive aids
- Avoidance of multitasking
- Formal neuropsychological referral in patients unable to resume prior occupational or cognitive roles

Pharmacologic considerations (investigational treatments but limited evidence)
- *Guanfacine*: 1 mg PO at bedtime, titrated to 2 mg after 1 month
- *N-acetylcysteine (NAC)*: 600 mg daily **(Table 8)**

Psychiatric and Sleep Sequelae of Long COVID

- Psychiatric and sleep disturbances, manifesting as mood disorders, anxiety, post-traumatic stress disorder (PTSD), insomnia, and poor sleep quality, are prevalent with a significant impact on quality of life.
- Patients usually present with anhedonia, low motivation, fatigue, restlessness, concentration difficulties, irritability, guilt, sleep disturbances, being easily startled with or without somatic symptoms, i.e., body aches.
- Patients with sleep dysfunctions usually present as unrefreshing sleep, vivid dreams or nightmares, fatigue, daytime dysfunction or sleepiness, and brain fog.
- Possible mechanisms for the above include genetic vulnerability, hormonal imbalance, social and environmental stressors, and immune-mediated dysregulation post COVID-19 **(Tables 9A and B)**.

TABLE 8: Various symptoms and their management.

Symptom	Clinical description	Evaluation	Management
Headache	New onset or exacerbation of pre-existing migraine or tension-type headaches (due to neuroinflammation or trigeminovascular system activation)	• History (timing, triggers, and patterns) • Neurologic examination, including cranial nerves • If red flags are present. Rule out secondary causes (e.g., stroke, intra-cranial mass) via MRI	• Migraine prophylaxis • Conventional analgesics and abortive agents (avoid overuse of medications to prevent rebound headache)
Dizziness and vertigo	• Episodic dizziness, lightheadedness, vertigo (spinning sensation), and imbalance • May be due to central (neurological), peripheral (vestibular), or cardiovascular (autonomic) causes	• History and examination (e.g., nystagmus, postural BP, neurologic signs) • Orthostatic vitals (to assess for POTS or orthostatic hypotension) • Dix–Hallpike maneuver (to assess for BPPV) • Cardiac evaluation if arrhythmias are suspected	• Audiology referral for vestibular deficits and vestibular rehabilitation • Hydration and salt intake if orthostatic intolerance • Avoid fall risks
Peripheral neuropathy and small fiber neuropathy	• Paresthesia (burning, tingling, pins and needles) • Hyperalgesia • Allodynia • Dysautonomia (palpitations, dry eyes/mouth, and sweating abnormalities)	• *Neurologic examination*: Deep tendon reflexes, Phalen test, Tinel signs • EMG, NCV • *Labs*: CBC, TSH, ANA, HbA1c, HIV, EBV, hepatitis C, Lyme serologies, vitamins B12/D	• *First-line*: Gabapentin (300–1,200 mg TID), pregabalin (25–75 mg daily), duloxetine, venlafaxine • *Adjunctive*: α-Lipoic acid (≥300 mg), acetyl-l-carnitine (500–1,000 mg TID); vitamin repletion
Tinnitus and hearing loss	New onset or worsening of pre-existing/persistent tinnitus or sensorineural hearing loss (SNHL)	• Audiology testing • Consider MRI of the internal auditory canals for persistent unilateral symptoms	• Tinnitus retraining therapy • Corticosteroid therapy (SNHL)
Loss of taste and smell	• Reported in ~5% of patients, post infection • Females and those with severe symptoms or nasal congestion recover more slowly	• Rule out chronic sinusitis, allergic rhinitis • Cranial nerve examination and MRI if focal neurological signs/deficits	• Olfactory retraining • Intranasal corticosteroid spray/drops/rinses (select cases)

(ANA: antinuclear antibody; BP: blood pressure; BPPV: benign paroxysmal positional vertigo; CBC: complete blood count; EBV: Epstein–Barr virus; EMG: electromyography; HIV: human immunodeficiency virus; MRI: magnetic resonance imaging; NCV: nerve conduction velocity; POTS: postural orthostatic tachycardia syndrome; TSH: thyroid-stimulating hormone)

TABLES 9A AND B: Evaluation and management.

9A. Diagnostic evaluation

Mental health screening tools	Sleep assessment
• *PHQ-9*: Depression assessment • *GAD-7*: Anxiety screening • *PTSD checklist for DSM-5*: PTSD symptom evaluation	• *Epworth sleepiness scale*: Evaluate daytime somnolence • *STOP-bang questionnaire*: screen for obstructive sleep apnea • *Polysomnography*: For diagnostic clarification • Assess for underlying psychological factors, including coexisting depression or PTSD

9B. Management

Mental health disorder	Insomnia and sleep dysfunction
Whole-person, multidisciplinary care is recommended: • *Nonpharmacologic intervention*: Cognitive behavioral therapy (CBT) as a first line for depression, anxiety, and PTSD • *Pharmacologic management*: Antidepressants tailored to psychiatric diagnosis (e.g., SSRIs for major depressive disorder) or • Referral to mental health professionals • Assess for suicidality or risk to others	*Nonpharmacologic*: • Sleep hygiene (structured routines established, reduce caffeine and stimulant intake) • Short naps as needed • Melatonin may help in selected patients (rule out other causes before initiating) • *Pharmacologic options (use shortest effective duration—preferably <4 weeks)*: Such as benzodiazepines, benzodiazepine receptor agonists, etc. • Treat comorbid conditions (i.e., obstructive sleep apnea) with positive airway pressure therapy

[DSM-5: Diagnostic and Statistical Manual of Mental Disorders, Fifth Edition; GAD-7: Generalized Anxiety Disorder-7; PHQ-9: Patient Health Questionnaire-9; PTSD: post-traumatic stress disorder; SSRIs: selective serotonin reuptake inhibitors; STOP: snoring, tiredness, observed apnea, pressure (high blood pressure) questionnaire]

Postural Orthostatic Tachycardia Syndrome in Long COVID

Postural orthostatic tachycardia syndrome is characterized as an exaggerated heart rate response to standing, typically defined as a rise of ≥30 beats/min (or ≥120 bpm) within 10 minutes of standing, without orthostatic hypotension. Probable etiologies are sympathetic overactivation, baroreflex impairment, and abnormal autonomic response **(Table 10)**.

Persistent or recurrent disease: Symptoms of PASC can persist for weeks to years and can be episodic. They may resolve temporarily and recur, especially in response to physiological or psychological stressors, reinfection, or subsequent illness.

Admission criteria: Hospitalization is warranted when there is:
- Worsening hypoxia
- New thromboembolic complications (e.g., PE)
- Acute cerebrovascular events
- Myocardial infarction

TABLE 10: Approach and therapy.

Diagnostic approach	Nonpharmacological interventions	Pharmacological therapy
• *Vital signs*: Orthostatic measurements to detect variation in heart rate and hypotension • *NASA 10-minute lean test*: To evaluate for POT physiology • *Autonomic reflex testing*: For suspected generalized dysautonomia • *COMPASS-31*: To assess autonomic symptom burden and need for further testing • *Exclude mimics*: Differential diagnoses such as vasovagal syncope, adrenal insufficiency, and structural cardiovascular disease	• *Graded exercise therapy*: Begin with recumbent exercises (e.g., rowing and recumbent cycling) • Follow a POTS-specific program such as the Levine Protocol, emphasizing slow incline progression and aerobic reconditioning • *Hydration and salt loading*: Liberal oral fluid intake • Increased sodium intake under guidance • *Compression garments*: Waist-high stockings or abdominal binders to reduce venous pooling • *Physical counterpressure maneuvers*: Leg crossing, squatting, and isometric contraction during symptomatic episodes • *Lifestyle measures*: Avoidance of prolonged standing, hot environments	• Used when nonpharmacological measures are insufficient or the symptom burden is high *Drugs such as*: • Midodrine • Propranolol • Fludrocortisone • Ivabradine • IV saline (in acute condition)

(NASA: National Aeronautics and Space Administration; POTS: postural orthostatic tachycardia syndrome; IV: intravenous; COMPASS: composite autonomic symptom score)

Postvaccination symptomatology: A detailed clinical history should differentiate symptoms attributable to COVID-19 vaccination versus prior infection. Current literature is inconclusive regarding whether postvaccine syndromes share pathophysiology with long COVID.

Recurrent COVID infections: Data from a large cohort study demonstrated that patients with multiple SARS-CoV-2 infections have higher all-cause mortality and an increased likelihood of persistent symptoms at 6 months compared to those without prior infections.

Monitoring: Regular follow-up (e.g., every 4–6 weeks) to ensure adequate symptom control, supportive care, and timely referral as needed.

Complications: Long COVID can result in significant functional, physical, psychological, cognitive, and psychosocial disability.

Prognosis: A nonrepresentative longitudinal cohort study revealed that a majority of patients still report at least one long COVID symptom 2 years after acute infection. Fatigue, pain, and memory impairment were the most prevalent long-term complaints.

Prevention:
- *Nirmatrelvir-ritonavir (paxlovid)*: Data from a US Veterans Affairs cohort showed that this antiviral reduces the risk of developing long COVID. One study reported a relative risk of 0.74 with an absolute risk reduction of 4.51% in patients treated during the acute phase.
- *Vaccination*: A meta-analysis of 11 studies concluded that COVID-19 vaccination was associated with reduced risk of developing PASC in over half of the studies, supporting its role as a preventive measure.

FURTHER READINGS

1. Centers for Disease Control and Prevention. (2023). Post-COVID conditions. [online]. Available from https://www.cdc.gov/coronavirus/2019-ncov/long-term-effects/ [Last accessed October, 2025].
2. National Institutes of Health (NIH). RECOVER initiative—Researching covid to enhance recovery. [online]. Available from: https://recoverCOVID.org/ [Last accessed October, 2025].
3. World Health Organization. A clinical case definition of post-COVID-19 condition by a Delphi consensus. Geneva: World Health Organization; 2021.
4. National Institute for Health and Care Excellence (NICE). COVID-19 rapid guideline: managing the long-term effects of COVID-19. NICE Guideline [NG188]; 2022.
5. Lopez-Leon S, Wegman-Ostrosky T, Perelman C, Sepulveda R, Rebolledo PA, Cuapio A, et al. More than 50 long-term effects of COVID-19: a systematic review and meta-analysis. Sci Rep. 2021;11(1):16144.

CHAPTER 26: Tuberculosis and Other Infections in Uncontrolled Diabetes Mellitus

BL Bhardwaj, Rajbir Singh, Prabhpreet Kaur, Kanchan Bhardwaj, RS Bhatia

■ INTRODUCTION

Persistent hyperglycemia is a risk factor for precipitation as well as activation of infection, including tuberculosis (TB), especially in the elderly/malnourished/immunosuppressed persons, mostly inflicting eyes, skin, buccal cavity, chest, genitourinary system, gastrointestinal system, etc. Hyperglycemia or uncontrolled diabetes mellitus also predisposes to TB and is also considered a risk factor for its activation. The centuries-old association has seen diabetes mellitus in <10% of cases of TB hospital admissions, which has increased to 10% in TB patients over the age of 40 years who have diabetes mellitus at present in India.

Radiological diagnosis of TB among diabetic patients in Korea varied from 9.6 to 12.8%, whereas the 2002 Imphal study revealed the prevalence of pulmonary TB in 100 diabetic patients as 27% radiologic diagnosis and 60% sputum positivity. The risk of TB in diabetes mellitus increases 3.4 times, directly related to uncontrolled hyperglycemia of a longer duration. Relative risk is higher among younger age groups, i.e., 9.88% (30–39 years), 4.72% (40–49 years), and 1.76–2.3% (above 49 years). TB among male diabetics is 2.2 times more than female diabetics. Both bronchial and pleuropulmonary involvements are known to occur. Multiple lobe involvement can occur; lower lung fields are commonly affected in diabetes mellitus. The duration of diabetes mellitus has no correlation with the occurrence of TB, but the risk of developing multidrug-resistant (MDR)-TB is higher; various types of lesions of TB in diabetes mellitus are listed in **Table 1**.

TABLE 1: Tubercular diseases and a variety of tubercular lesions in diabetes mellitus.	
Tuberculosis	• Minimal • Moderate • Advanced
Tuberculosis lesions	• Cavitary • Homogenous opacities • Heterogeneous opacities • Pleural effusion • Consolidation • Fibrosis

PATHOGENESIS

Tuberculosis is mainly transmitted via droplet nuclei. A higher prevalence of pulmonary TB in diabetes mellitus is attributed to an existing inadequate substrate for immunity formation due to disturbed protein metabolism. At the same time, higher chances of infection are due to low opsonic index, reduced antibacterial activity, poor tissue resistance, reduced collagen synthesis, impaired defensive function of reticulo-endothelial (RE) cells, and increased availability of tissue glycerol as a substrate that enhances the growth of TB bacilli. Prognosis is not favorable, and doctors must be vigilant to suspect infection in cases with uncontrolled hyperglycemia. Keeping the fasting blood sugar level at 100 mg/dL is the prudent target. Diagnosis and management with anti-TB drugs for an appropriate duration with maintenance of glucose status are rewarding and are not dependent on the type of hypoglycemic therapy [insulin or oral hypoglycemic agents (OHAs)] used.

EFFECT OF UNCONTROLLED PERSISTENT DIABETES MELLITUS

Bacterial chest infections are increased in the presence of hyperglycemia, and this is attributed to reduced availability of NADPH, producing decreased production of superoxide anion along with depressed respiratory burst, which would contribute to impaired chemotaxis, phagocytosis, and intracellular killing of microorganisms by granulocytes and mononuclear cells in diabetes mellitus. Similarly, impaired ability of alveolar macrophages in inhibiting fungal spore germination would enhance azygomytosis.

Comorbidities and altered pulmonary functions in two-third cases of diabetes mellitus, influence of obesity, muscle weakness, and congestive heart failure add to the agony. Reduced lung columns (in insulin-dependent diabetes mellitus), pulmonary elastic recoil, impaired pulmonary diffusion, and pulmonary epithelial permeability along with abnormal ventilatory response to hypoxia can cause unexpected cardiorespiratory arrest in diabetic patients, possibly due to increased sleep-related breathing disorder produced as a result of autonomic neuropathy. Diabetic patients (1) have reduced diffusion capacity for carbon monoxide, (2) have increased vascular injury (pulmonary microangiopathy), and (3) also contribute independently to airflow obstructive disease (due to systemic inflammation and endothelial dysfunction). Further, it is worsened by smoking, poor glycemic control, and other cardiopulmonary comorbidities.

Reduced gradient between pulmonary wedge pressure and serum colloid oncotic pressure may produce cerebral edema, which may cause neurogenic pulmonary edema due to increased permeability during acidosis. Acute respiratory distress syndrome (ARDS) can also occur because of cardiogenic pulmonary edema while treating diabetic ketoacidosis, which may produce alveolar hypoventilation due to hypokalemia and hypophosphatemia because of severe muscular weakness.

Bronchial asthma may rarely coexist with diabetes mellitus. Nevertheless, exacerbation of bronchospasm may occur in bronchial asthma during hypoglycemia. Diabetic autonomic neuropathy, on the other hand, reduces bronchial hyperreactivity possibly because of depressed cholinergic bronchomotor tone. Diabetic neuropathy hand persistent transudative pleural effusion due to left ventricular dysfunction may produce transient vocal cord paralysis. Pulmonary thromboembolism may get precipitated due to dehydration in a case of diabetic ketoacidosis. Tuberculosis can involve the tongue, palate, and draining lymph nodes. These lesions are painful, and histopathology reveals nonspecific inflammation with necrosis. Caseation is seen in deeper parts of the lesion where *Mycobacterium tuberculosis* may be demonstrable. Hyperglycemia enhances infection and inflammation by impairing chemotaxis, phagocytosis, and intracellular killing of microorganisms by granulocytes and mononuclear cells. In the oral cavity, it alters secretions in gingiva and salivary glands, which decreases pH, and along with microvascular damage, causes host tissue damage. Therefore, dental plaque, candidal infections, halitosis, periodontal infections, and tooth abscesses enhance the risk of caries and severely affect the gingival health. This further increases the risk of systemic diseases. Therefore, care of oral/periodontal hygiene is of utmost importance.

Metabolic disorders and lung involvement require elaborated diagnostic procedures to establish the diagnosis. At the same time, these facilities may not be available at all centers or may not be affordable for all patients. Hence, the clinical acumen used is rewarding. Achieving and maintaining 100 mg/dL levels of glucose in the blood wisely stand for a fruitful outcome.

CONCLUSION

Diabetes mellitus and chest infections including TB are directly related in case of uncontrolled hyperglycemia due to higher susceptibility, sustenance, and reduced bactericidal activity and tissue resistance because of the inability of granulocytes, mononuclear cells, and even alveolar macrophages to contain infection. The sibling risk factor of hyperglycemia, further influenced by obesity, smoking, alcohol intake, and lack of exercise, adds to cardiopulmonary dysfunctions. Comorbidities and diabetic ketoacidosis would add agony to the existing problem. Maintenance of fasting blood glucose as/around 100 mg/dL would prevent as well as help in the early recovery of accompanying chest disorders in diabetes mellitus. Uncontrolled diabetes mellitus precipitates comorbidities, especially in the form of infections. It also delays the diagnosis of TB. Misuse of corticosteroids in diabetic patients during COVID-19 has yielded a number of systemic infections, including TB and malignant disorders, due to suppression of immunity. Further treatment outcome in TB is also affected by uncontrolled sugar levels in diabetes mellitus. Metformin has shown a potential prophylactic value.

FURTHER READINGS

1. Bhatia RS, Singh H. Cardiopulmonary complications in diabetes; Pee Pee Publ. Cardiopulmonary Topic. 2008;15:123-9.
2. Sarkar M, Sarkar J. Transmission of Mycobacterium tuberculosis. JAPI. 2025;73:91-6.
3. Bhatia RS. Metabolic disorders and lungs. In: BB Thakur. (Ed); PG Med API; 2002;16:125-29.
4. Shingo T, Nishmora F. Diabetes mellitus and periodontitis. Japan Dental Sci Rev. 2024;60:15-21.
5. PA Mahesh, et al. Respiratory Medicine. Word Scientific Singapore. 2024.

CHAPTER 27

Decoding the Mystery Fever: A Practical Guide to Pyrexia of Unknown Origin: A Simple Approach to Acute Febrile Illness

K Vengadakrishnan

■ INTRODUCTION

Fever is a challenge for any physician. Short-duration fever needs early decision, precise laboratory investigations, and prompt treatment. Untreated and missed diagnosis leads to complications, morbidity, and mortality. Clinical experience plays a major role in the current scenario of atypical presentation.

■ PRESENT SCENARIO

A variety of infections can lead to fever and viral (flu virus, dengue), bacterial [respiratory infections, urinary tract infection (UTI), leptospirosis, and enteric fever], and other infections (malaria and rickettsial infections).

■ GENERAL APPROACH

A thorough history and clinical examination along with routine laboratories, specific laboratories as appropriate, and empirical treatment with the best possible initial antimicrobial therapy is the best guide to management. We have discussed three case scenarios for a better understanding of difficulties in managing acute febrile illness.

■ CLINICAL SCENARIO 1

A 35-year-old female housewife presents with an intermittent, high-grade fever for 5 days and a dry cough for 3 days. She reports no other systemic complaints, and her past medical history is insignificant. Two days ago, her family physician prescribed azithromycin 500 mg and paracetamol, but the fever has persisted. On examination, she is conscious and oriented, with a normal pharynx and no skin rash or icterus. Her vital signs are pulse rate (PR) 76 beats/min, blood pressure (BP) 100/70 mm Hg, temperature (temp) 102°F, and respiratory rate (RR) 18 breaths/min. Her systemic examination is normal. As per the scenario, the provisional diagnosis could be malaria, enteric fever, dengue fever, or pneumonia. Investigations revealed hemoglobin—9.8 g%, total count (TC)—4,700 (P 50, L 42, E1), platelets —120,000, blood urea nitrogen (BUN)—14 mg%, creatinine—0.9 mg%, QBC MP (quantitative buffy coat for malarial parasite)—negative, serum glutamic-oxaloacetic transaminase (SGOT)—72, serum glutamic-pyruvic transaminase (SGPT)—94, alkaline phosphatase (ALP)—140, total bilirubin—1.8 mg%, direct bilirubin—0.8 mg%, total protein—8.2 mg%, serum albumin—4.6 mg%, and international normalized ratio (INR)—1.1. Chest X-ray (CXR) is normal, ultrasound of abdomen shows mild hepatomegaly, and cultures are awaited. The final diagnosis is narrowed down to enteric fever. The patient was treated with Ceftriaxone and her condition improved.

Clinical Pearls in Acute Fever and Cough
- Not all coughs are primary respiratory.
- Have clues to viral or bacterial.
- Look for warning symptoms or signs.
- Judicious antibiotic use

CLINICAL SCENARIO 2

A 46-year-old female housewife presents with a 4-day history of fever, pain in the right hypochondrium, and vomiting. Associated symptoms include headache, body pain, and decreased appetite. She reports no history of dysuria, cough, or rigors and has no significant past medical illnesses. On clinical examination, her eyes are congested, and her temperature is only 100°F. She exhibits no neck stiffness and has a dry tongue. Her vital signs are PR 110 beats/min (tachycardic), RR 18 breaths/min, and BP 114/80 mm Hg. The cardiovascular system (CVS) and respiratory system (RS) examinations are normal, and the only abdominal finding is nonspecific epigastric tenderness. As per the scenario, the provisional diagnosis could be malaria, leptospirosis, or viral hepatitis. Investigations revealed hemoglobin—12.2 g%, TC—13,460 (P 82, L 14, E4), platelets— 64,000, BUN—42 mg%, creatinine—2.2 mg%, QBC MP—negative, SGOT—120, SGPT—148, ALP—480, total bilirubin—4.8 mg%, direct bilirubin—3.2 mg%, total protein—7.2 mg%, serum albumin—3.8 mg%, and INR—2.3. CXR is normal, ultrasound of abdomen shows moderate hepatomegaly and minimal ascites, and cultures are awaited. The final diagnosis was narrowed down to leptospirosis. She was treated with doxycycline and her condition improved.

Learning Points
- Fever with gastrointestinal (GI) symptoms
- Clinical clues to localization
- Identify early warning signs
- Ideal empirical antibiotic therapy

CLINICAL SCENARIO 3

A 54-year-old male, a known diabetic for 8 years with a recent HbA1c 8.1 and hypertensive for 5 years, presents with a 5-day history of high-grade fever. He also reports concurrent dysuria and increased urinary frequency. For the past 2 days, he has developed a productive cough with greenish sputum, denying hemoptysis or dyspnea. He has no past history of hospitalization. 2 days prior, his family physician started him on Levofloxacin 500 mg daily along with paracetamol and expectorants, but the high-grade fever spikes persisted, leading to his hospitalization. On examination, he is conscious, oriented, well hydrated, and without skin rash or icterus. Vital signs are concerning: PR 110 beats/min, BP 110/74 mm Hg, temp 102°F, and RR 24 breaths/min. Physical examination reveals fine crackles over the left infrascapular area and mild tenderness over the left hypochondrium. As per the scenario, the provisional diagnosis could be UTI or pneumonia. Investigations revealed hemoglobin—11.4 g%, TC—18,200 (P 88, L 8, E4), platelets—170,000, BUN—32 mg%, creatinine—1.3 mg%, QBC MP—negative, urinalysis—plenty of pus cells, no casts or RBCs, SGOT—184, SGPT—124, ALP—132, totalbilirubin—0.8 mg%, direct bilirubin—0.6 mg%, totalprotein—7.8 mg%, serum albumin—4.8 mg%, and INR—1.0. CXR is normal, ultrasound of abdomen shows mild hepatomegaly and mild increase in renal cortical echoes, and cultures are awaited.

The patient was initially started on ceftriaxone, levofloxacin, intravenous (IV) fluids, and supportive treatment. Despite this regimen, the patient continued to have high-grade fever spikes. On the following day, his condition deteriorated. He became dyspneic (RR 36) and was hypotensive with a BP of 94/60 mm Hg. RS examination revealed bilateral crackles. The arterial blood gas (ABG) analysis showed significant hypoxemia (PO_2 54.1), and a CXR showed perihilar shadows. The patient was subsequently diagnosed with sepsis and acute respiratory distress syndrome (ARDS) and was shifted to the intensive care unit (ICU). Blood and urine cultures confirmed the etiology, growing *E. coli* [extended-spectrum beta-lactamase (ESBL)] with a colony count of more than 100,000. The patient eventually responded to Imipenem therapy.

PITFALLS IN INITIAL MANAGEMENT

In the initial management of a patient, certain pitfalls could have been avoided. In a diabetic patient presenting with a UTI and lung signs, sepsis should be immediately considered. Even if laboratory results show high counts and pyuria with only a high-normal creatinine and increased BUN, the clinical picture is paramount. A key mistake is the choice of an antibiotic. If sepsis is suspected, one must think of virulent organisms and choose broad-spectrum coverage initially, with a plan to de-escalate if required after culture results. Also, a normal CXR does not mean everything is fine or rule out severe systemic infection, as sepsis can progress rapidly.

CONCLUSION

Managing a patient with an acute febrile illness effectively relies fundamentally on a proper history and clinical signs, which should always guide the treatment plan. It is imperative not to treat based solely on laboratory results because of the potential for false positives. Similarly, in the case of false-negative reports, we must always judge the situation by the patient's clinical signs and response to treatment. Consequently, a revision of the treatment plan is mandatory, and we must be prepared to escalate or de-escalate care as the clinical picture demands.

FURTHER READINGS

1. Salvi S, Apte K, Madas S, Barne M, Chhowala S, Sethi T, et al. Symptoms and medical conditions in 204 912 patients visiting primary health-care practitioners in India: a 1-day point prevalence study (the POSEIDON study). Lancet Glob Health. 2015;3(12):e776-84.
2. Aggarwal S, Walia K. Treatment guidelines for antimicrobial use in common syndromes 2019, 2nd edition. [online] Available from https://www.icmr.gov.in/icmrobject/custom_data/pdf/resource-guidelines/Treatment_Guidelines_2019_Final.pdf [Last accessed October, 2025].
3. Bhargava A, Ralph R, Chatterjee B, Bottieau E. Assessment and initial management of acute undifferentiated fever in tropical and subtropical regions. BMJ. 2018;363:k4766.
4. Mørch K, Manoharan A, Chandy S, Chacko N, Alvarez-Uria G, Patil S, et al. Acute undifferentiated fever in India: a multicentre study of aetiology and diagnostic accuracy. BMC Infect Dis. 2017;17(1):665.
5. Chrispal A, Boorugu H, Gopinath KG, Chandy S, Prakash JAJ, Thomas EM, et al. Acute undifferentiated febrile illness in adult hospitalized patients: the disease spectrum and diagnostic predictors - an experience from a tertiary care hospital in South India. Trop Doct. 2010;40(4):230-4.

Postexposure Prophylaxis for HIV, Hepatitis B, and Hepatitis C

Raminderpal Singh Sibia

INTRODUCTION

- *Risk in healthcare and beyond*: Despite adherence to standard precautions, healthcare personnel and the general population remain at the risk of exposure to bloodborne pathogens—HIV, hepatitis B, and hepatitis C—through needlestick injuries, contact with contaminated body fluids, mucocutaneous exposure, and sexual contact.
- *Urgency of postexposure prophylaxis (PEP)*: Exposure to these viruses constitutes a *medical emergency*. Timely initiation of *PEP—ideally within 1–2 hours—*is critical, as efficacy declines rapidly with delay.
- *Safety net*: Structured *postexposure management protocols* are vital for occupational and nonoccupational exposures alike, reinforcing workplace safety, infection control, and public health preparedness.

HIGHLIGHTING THE NEED

Needlestick injuries remain a major concern, accounting for an estimated *37.6% of occupationally acquired hepatitis B, 39% of hepatitis C,* and *4.4% of HIV* infections among healthcare workers.

Who is at Risk?

Professions with a high risk of exposure include nursing staff, emergency care providers, doctors, medical students, and laboratory technicians. Health facility cleaning staff, mortuary staff, and clinical waste handlers are also at an increased risk **(Tables 1 and 2)**.

Average Risk after Exposure

The average risk of acquiring HIV infection following different types of occupational exposure is low compared to HBV or HCV **(Table 2)**.

Despite adequate precautions, exposure may occur that places the healthcare personnel at risk of acquiring bloodborne infection. Nonoccupational exposure, like unprotected sex or sexual assault, may also occur.

CHAPTER 28: Postexposure Prophylaxis for HIV, Hepatitis B, and Hepatitis C

TABLE 1: Body fluid differences.

Body fluids considered "at risk"	Body fluids considered "not at risk"
Blood	Tears
Semen	Sweat
Vaginal secretions	Urine and feces
Synovial, pleural, pericardial, peritoneal, and amniotic fluids	Saliva
Other fluids contaminated with blood	Sputum
	Vomitus

TABLE 2: Average risk of acquiring HIV infection following different types of occupational exposure.

Exposure route	HIV transmission rate
Blood transfusion	>98%
Perinatal	20–40%
Sexual intercourse	0.1–10%
Oral	0.01%
Needlestick injury	0.3%
Mucous membrane splash	0.09%

(HBV: hepatitis B virus; HCV: hepatitis C virus; HIV: human immunodeficiency virus)

TABLE 3: Baseline laboratory investigations.

Timing	In person taking PEP (standard regimen)	In persons not taking PEP
Baseline	HIV, HCV, anti-HBsAg*, complete blood count, and serum transaminases	HIV, HCV, and anti-HBsAg*

*HIV, HBV, and HCV testing of exposed staff within 6 days of an accidental exposure to blood (AEB) is recommended (baseline sero status).
Offer an HIV test in case of an AEB, as a positive HIV status may indicate the need to discontinue PEP.
The decision to test for HIV or not should be based on the informed consent of the exposed person.
Exposed persons not taking PEP need to be counseled for repeat testing of HIV, HCV, and anti-HBsAg at 6, 12, and 24 weeks from the date of exposure.
(anti-HBsAg: hepatitis B surface antibody; HBV: hepatitis B virus; HCV: hepatitis C virus; HIV: human immunodeficiency virus; PEP: postexposure prophylaxis)

REPORTING

All sharps injuries and mucosal exposures must be reported to the immediate supervisor and to the Casualty Medical Officer to evaluate the injury **(Table 3)**.

MANAGEMENT OF VIRUS-SPECIFIC EXPOSURE

Exposure to HIV-infected Source

Management of Exposure Site (First Aid)
Immediately wash the exposed area with water and soap and rinse. In mucous splash, irrigate the exposed eye and rinse the mouth thoroughly using water or saline several times. Do not use antiseptics, scrubs, or disinfectants.

Establish Eligibility for Postexposure Prophylaxis
Exposed personnel must be assessed for the severity of exposure and risk of transmission following an AEB.
- *Categories of exposures*: Categories of exposure are given in **Table 4**.
- *Assessing the HIV status of the source of exposure*: A baseline rapid HIV test should be done before starting PEP. However, PEP, where indicated, should be initiated within 72 hours of exposure and should not be delayed waiting for the results of HIV testing. A positive HIV test result helps in the decision to start PEP, but a negative result does not exclude HIV infection (too low antibody titers to detect in the window period from 21 to 28 days).
- *Assessment of the exposed individual*: The exposed individuals should be screened for pre-existing HIV infection. HIV-positive patients should not receive PEP.

Counseling for Postexposure Prophylaxis
Psychological support as well as appropriate information about the risks and benefits of PEP should be explained, as PEP is not mandatory. He/she should be counseled on safe sexual practices till both the baseline and 3-month HIV tests are negative.

Assessing Need for Postexposure Prophylaxis
It is decided based on exposure code and source code **(Table 5)**.

TABLE 4: Categories of exposure (or classification of exposure severity).	
Category	
Mild	• Exposure to mucous membrane/nonintact skin with small volumes (EC1) • Subcutaneous injection with a small-bore needle
Moderate	• Exposure to mucous membrane with large volumes (EC2) • Percutaneous exposure with a solid needle (EC2)
Severe	• Percutaneous exposure with large volumes (EC3) • For example, high-caliber needle, deep wound, and material previously used intravenously/arterially

TABLE 5: Postexposure prophylaxis (PEP) recommendations based on exposure code and source code.

Exposure code	Source code	PEP recommendation
EC1	SC 1	Not warranted
EC1	SC 2	Yes
EC2	SC 1	Yes
EC2	SC 2	Yes
EC3	SC 1/2	Yes

Notes: HIV-positive sources—
- *SC1*: Low titer exposure with high CD4 count, usually >350 cells/mm^3 (asymptomatic).
- *SC2*: High titer exposure with low CD4 count, usually <200 cells/mm^3 (advanced disease).

As PEP has its greatest effect if begun within 2 hours of exposure, it should be started as soon as possible, preferably within 72 hours in healthcare workers. It is given for a period of 28 days. In cases of sexual assault, PEP should be given to the exposed person as a part of the overall package of postsexual assault care.

The preferred PEP regimen in adults is a fixed-dose combination (FDC) of tenofovir (300 mg), lamivudine (300 mg), and dolutegravir (50 mg), one tablet per day. Alternative regimens include tenofovir, lamivudine, lopinavir/ritonavir or tenofovir, lamivudine, efavirenz.

The compliance rate for the Tenofovir, Lamivudine, and Dolutegravir (TLD) regimen is very high, as it causes minor side effects like nausea, diarrhea, headache, and fatigue. Stop drugs if the patient develops jaundice, a generalized rash, or severe depression/psychosis/suicidal tendencies, especially with efavirenz.

Follow-up

Both clinical and laboratory monitoring must be done in PEP. An exposed person should be monitored for signs of HIV seroconversion, like nonspecific flu-like symptoms, generalized lymphadenopathy, and mucocutaneous eruptions/ulcers. It occurs in 50–70% of acute HIV patients, almost always between 3 and 6 weeks of exposure. Avoid blood donation, pregnancy, and breastfeeding.

Baseline HIV, HBsAg, anti-HCV, complete blood count (CBC), and liver function test (LFT) are done within 6 days of AEB. Follow-up laboratory monitoring in the form of HIV, HBsAg, and anti-HCV is done at 6, 12, and 24 weeks. If the HIV test is negative at 6 months, no further testing is recommended.

Additionally, CBC (for patients on zidovudine), fasting blood sugar/random blood sugar (FBS/RBS) (for patients on dolutegravir), and serum creatinine may be done at 2–4 weeks.

Exposure to a Hepatitis B-infected Source

- Treatment after exposure varies based on the vaccination status of the exposed individual and the HBV status of the patient.

TABLE 6: Postexposure management of healthcare personnel (HCP) after occupational exposure.

HCP status	Postexposure testing		Postexposure prophylaxis		Postvaccination serologic testing
	Source patient (HBsAg)	HCP testing (anti-HBs)	HBIG	Vaccination	
Documented responder after complete series	No action needed				
Documented nonresponder after two complete series	Positive/ Unknown	–	HBIG × 2 separated by 1 month	–	N/A
	Negative	No action needed			
Response unknown after complete series	Positive/ Unknown	<10 mIU/ mL	HBIG × 1	Initiate revaccination	Yes
	Negative	<10 mIU/ mL	–	Initiate revaccination	Yes
	Any result	≥10 mIU/ mL	–	–	–
Unvaccinated/ Incompletely vaccinated or vaccine refusers	Positive/ Unknown	–	HBIG × 1	Complete vaccination	Yes
	Negative	–	None	Complete vaccination	Yes

(anti-HBs: hepatitis B surface antibody; HBIG: hepatitis B immune globulin; HBsAg: hepatitis B surface antigen)

- If an individual suffers a needle stick and is unvaccinated, a vaccination series should be initiated along with hepatitis B immunoglobulins (dose = 0.06 mL/kg).
- If an individual has been vaccinated and has a documented response (anti-HBs ≥ 10 mIU/mL) to the vaccine, then no treatment is required after exposure **(Table 6; Flowchart 1)**.

Exposure to a Hepatitis C-infected Source

- *Hepatitis C virus*: No treatment has been shown to prevent infection for workers exposed to HCV.
- Recommendations center on following workers after the injury and monitoring of HCV ribonucleic acid (RNA) in the serum.
- *Recommendations include*: Begin testing for HCV antibodies and alanine aminotransferase (ALT) levels immediately after the event.
- Repeat testing at 6 weeks, 3 months, and 6 months.

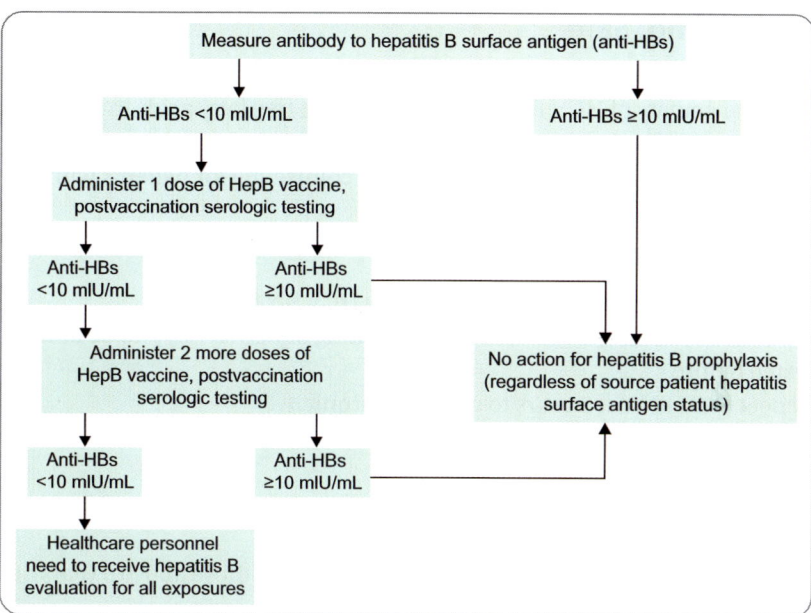

FLOWCHART 1: Pre-exposure evaluation for healthcare personnel previously vaccinated with complete HepB vaccine series.

Management of Hepatitis B and Hepatitis C in Pregnant Women and Infants Born to Them

Pregnancy with hepatitis C:
- A 7.2% risk of perinatal transmission
- Risk increases to 12.1% in pregnant people with HIV

Pregnancy with anti-HCV +ve: Document HCV viremia

Evaluate for the presence of cirrhosis:
- *Ultrasound sonography (USG) abdomen*
- *Aspartate aminotransferase to platelet ratio index (APRI) and fibrosis-4 (FIB-4) are helpful to rule out cirrhosis, but may be falsely elevated [minor elevations in AST (aspartate aminotransferase) and ALT, dilutional thrombocytopenia]*

FibroScan contraindicated:
- Defer treatment till completion of breastfeeding
- Counseling the patient is of vital importance.
- No DAA is approved by the Food and Drug Administration (FDA) for use in pregnancy
  Trials underway
  The HIP-2 study is investigating the safety and efficacy of sofosbuvir-velpatasvir (SOF/VEL)
- A prospective observational study in India that provided LDV/SOF treatment after the first trimester to pregnant patients with chronic hepatitis C saw a 100% cure rate at 12 weeks post-treatment and no congenital abnormalities.

Breastfeeding: Safe
- Breast milk contains much lower levels of HCV RNA than blood.
- The viral activity of HCV RNA is reduced by the free fatty acids in breast milk.
- It is thought to be inactivated in the infant's digestive tract.
- Guidelines advise standard breastfeeding counseling for patients with HCV.

Exposed Infant
- Test exposed infants at 2–6 months using HCV RNA NAT.
- No antibody testing till 18 months (circulating maternal Ab)—to be done if not tested before
- Repeat HCV RNA at 3 years to confirm chronicity.
- Treat children >3 years with DAAs; no cure for <3 years
- Pediatric patients
- Sofosbuvir/ledipasvir and sofosbuvir plus ribavirin are approved for children as young as 3 years of age.
- Sofosbuvir + Velpatasvir is approved by the FDA for those above 6 years of age.
- Full dose if body weight > 30 kg
- Half dose if body weight < 30 kg

Pregnancy with hepatitis B:
- Hepatitis B virus DNA to be quantified in the third trimester (24–28 weeks)
- The World Health Organization (WHO) recommends that pregnant women testing positive for HBV infection (HBsAg positive) with an HBV DNA ≥ 5.3 $\log_{10}$ copies/mL (≥200,000 IU/mL) to receive tenofovir prophylaxis from the 28th week of pregnancy until at least birth to prevent mother-to-child transmission of HBV **(Flowchart 2)**.
- Treat if meeting criteria

Rationale for TDF use:
- Substantial protective effect of using antiviral prophylaxis in preventing mother-to-child transmission in infants born to HBV-infected women
- Tenofovir disoproxil fumarate (TDF) has a high genetic barrier to resistance.
- There was a low risk of maternal HBV flare after TDF discontinuation.
- Entecavir is NOT recommended in pregnancy.
- Tenofovir to be used in pregnancy and preferred in women of child-bearing age
- TDF dose—300 mg OD

Approach: To Treat or Not Based on Noninvasive Assessment
- *Cirrhosis*: Treat irrespective of ALT or HBV DNA levels—concomitant management of complications of cirrhosis.
- *Significant fibrosis*: Treat if HBV DNA > 2,000, irrespective of ALT levels. Monitor if HBV DNA **(Flowchart 3)**.

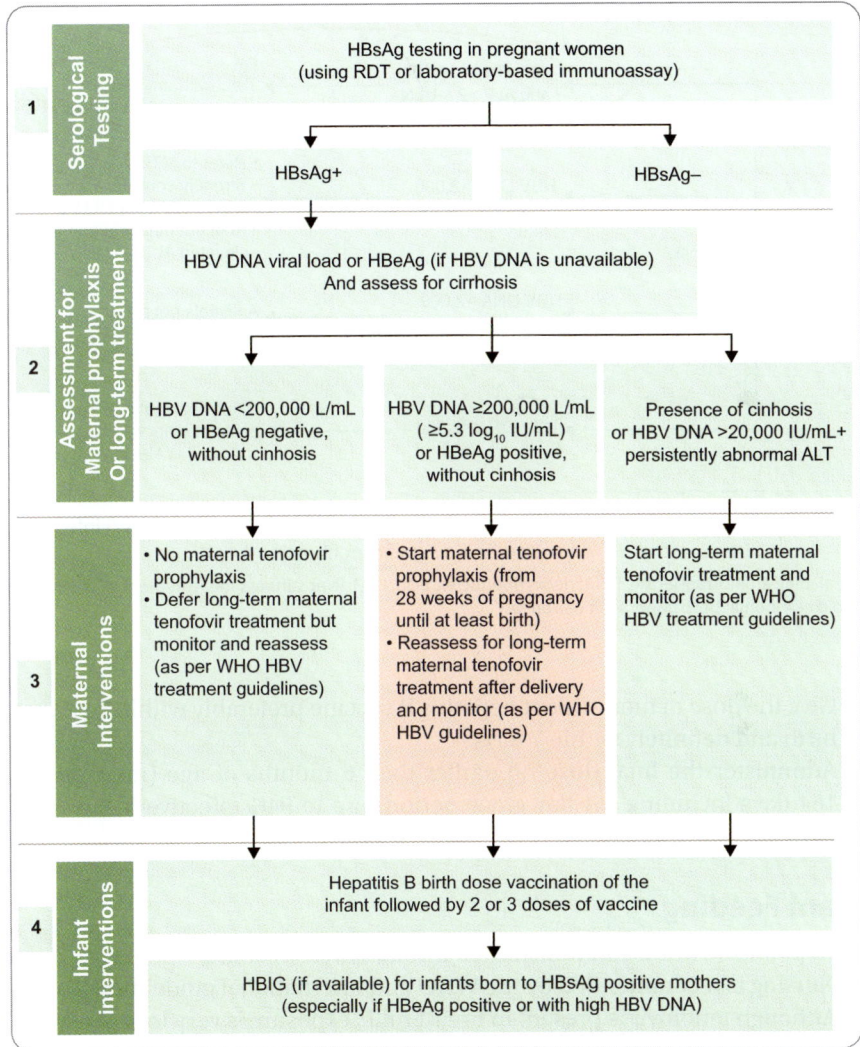

FLOWCHART 2: Summary algorithm on HBV testing of pregnant women to prevent mother-to-child transmission of HBV.

(HBsAg: hepatitis B surface antigen; HBV: hepatitis B virus)

Management of Infants Born to Women With Hepatitis B Virus Infection

- Administer HBIG (100 IU I/M) and single-antigen vaccine in separate limbs at birth.
- Preferably within 12 hours of birth and certainly within 48 hours. (Efficacy decreases markedly if given more than 48 hours after birth.)
- *Complete vaccine series with four total doses*: 0, 2, 4, and 6 months

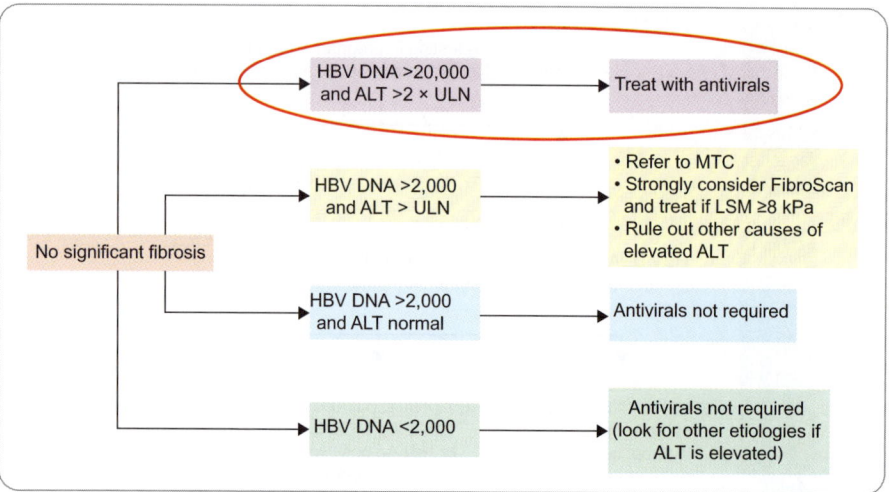

FLOWCHART 3: Algorithm for antiviral treatment of chronic hepatitis B virus (HBV) infection in patients with no significant fibrosis.

(ALT: alanine aminotransferase; DNA: deoxyribonucleic acid; LSM: liver stiffness measurement; MTC: medullary thyroid carcinoma; ULN: upper limit of normal)

- Give the dose of monovalent hepatitis B vaccine preferably within 24 hours of birth and definitely within 7 days.
- Administer the final dose no earlier than 6 months of age (minimum age 164 days including a 4-day grace period), up to 94% effective in preventing perinatal transmission.

Infant Feeding
- Hepatitis B virus is not transmitted through breastfeeding.
- Nursing is recommended by the WHO and international guidelines.
- Although tenofovir is present in breast milk, exposure is very low.

Postvaccination Serologic Testing
- Recommended for infants and children born to women with hepatitis B infection.
- Confirms whether the child has developed immunity or has been infected with HBV.
- Postvaccination serologic testing (PVST) should include HBsAg and anti-HBs only.
- PVST should occur between 9 and 12 months of age or 1–2 months after vaccine series completion, if the series is delayed.
- Tests for antibodies to hepatitis B core antigen (anti-HBc) should not be ordered (passively acquired maternal antibodies that are detectable in HBV-exposed infants up to 24 months of age)

FURTHER READINGS

1. Park K. Park's Textbook of Preventive and Social Medicine, 25th edition. Bhopal: Banarsidas Bhanot; 2018.
2. Gladwin M, Trattler W. Clinical Microbiology Made Ridiculously Simple, 6th edition. MedMaster.
3. Jameson JL, Fauci AS, Kasper DL, Hauser SL, Longo DL, Loscalzo J. Harrison's Principles of Internal Medicine, 20th edition. New York: McGraw-Hill Education; 2020.
4. Török E, Cooke F, Moran E. Oxford Handbook of Infectious Diseases and Microbiology, 2nd edition. Oxford: Oxford University Press; 2016.

CHAPTER 29

Complicated Vivax Malaria

Kripa Anna, Vikas Loomba

INTRODUCTION

Malaria remains a global health challenge, with an estimated 263 million cases and 597,000 deaths in 2023. Most deaths (96%) occur in Africa due to *Plasmodium falciparum*, the species traditionally regarded as the most lethal. India contributes ~3% of the global malaria burden but carries a disproportionate share of *Plasmodium vivax*, accounting for nearly half of urban malaria cases.

Once considered the agent of "benign tertian malaria," *P. vivax* is increasingly recognized as a cause of severe disease. Large prospective studies indicate 3–23% of vivax cases present with severe malaria, with case fatality rates of 0.8–1.6%.

In a study conducted in our institution over a period of 1 year, 283 patients of acute febrile illness were enrolled. Out of the 283 patients, 20 were diagnosed with malaria (17 were *P. vivax* and three were *P. falciparum*). Of the cases of vivax malaria, 11 (65%) were complicated, underscoring *P. vivax* as a significant cause of severe malaria.

PATHOPHYSIOLOGY OF COMPLICATED MALARIA

The pathogenesis of severe malaria involves parasite biology, host immunity, and inflammatory responses. Traditionally, *P. falciparum* has been the prototype for severe disease. Its hallmark is sequestration of infected erythrocytes in microvasculature, mediated by parasite surface proteins binding to endothelial receptors such as *endothelial protein C receptor (EPCR)* and *intercellular adhesion molecule 1 (ICAM-1)*. This causes microvascular obstruction, endothelial dysfunction, coagulation abnormalities, and local tissue hypoxia. In cerebral malaria, blood–brain barrier disruption is well documented.

In contrast, *P. vivax* has long been considered "benign" due to its restriction to reticulocytes. However, growing evidence now highlights multiple mechanisms contributing to severe *vivax* malaria. These include exaggerated host immune responses with higher cytokine levels [*tumor necrosis factor-α (TNF-α) and interferon-γ (IFN-γ)*] relative to parasite density, leading to endothelial injury and complications such as acute respiratory distress syndrome (ARDS). Severe anemia arises from destruction of both infected and uninfected erythrocytes, dyserythropoiesis, and splenic clearance. Thrombocytopenia is frequent, mediated by immune destruction and platelet consumption. Splenic pathology is prominent, with congestion and increased clearance of reticulocytes.

Unique to *vivax* malaria are hypnozoites in the liver, which trigger relapses, causing recurrent systemic inflammation and cumulative morbidity. Thus, while *falciparum* severity is driven by sequestration and microvascular pathology, *vivax* severity stems from immune-mediated injury, hematological dysfunction, and relapse-driven cumulative burden.

CLINICAL SPECTRUM OF COMPLICATED MALARIA

The clinical spectrum of severe *P. vivax* malaria largely overlaps with that of *P. falciparum*, as defined by WHO severity criteria.

A key distinction lies in the *parasite index*. WHO thresholds for hyperparasitemia (>200,000/µL for *P. falciparum*) are not appropriate for *P. vivax*, which preferentially invades reticulocytes—a small subset of circulating red cells. Hence, even in severe illness, peripheral parasitemia is typically low (<2%), and cases requiring intensive care unit (ICU) admission have been documented with parasite counts as low as 500/µL **(Table 1)**.

TABLE 1: World Health Organization (WHO) criteria for severe Plasmodium vivax malaria.

Criterion	Definition
Impaired consciousness	Glasgow Coma score < 11/15
Prostration	Generalized weakness such that person is unable to sit, stand or walk without assistance
Multiple convulsions	More than two episodes within 24 hours
Acidosis	A base deficit of >8 mEq/L or plasma bicarbonate < 15 mmol/L or venous plasma lactate ≥ 5 mmol/L. Manifests clinically as respiratory distress (rapid, deep, and labored breathing)
Hypoglycemia	Blood glucose < 40 mg/dL
Severe malarial anemia	Hemoglobin < 7 g/dL and hematocrit < 20%
Renal impairment	Plasma or serum creatinine > 3 mg/dL or blood urea > 20 mmol/L
Jaundice	Serum bilirubin > 3 mg/dL
Pulmonary edema	Radiologically confirmed or O_2 saturation < 92% on room air, respiratory rate (RR) > 30 breaths/min, with chest indrawing and crepitations
Significant bleeding	Recurrent or prolonged bleeding from nose, gums, venepuncture sites, hematemesis, or melena
Shock	*Compensated*: Capillary refill ≥ 3 s or temperature gradient on leg, no hypotension. Decompensated: systolic blood pressure (SBP) < 80 mm Hg

DIAGNOSIS OF MALARIA

Malaria diagnosis relies on microscopy, rapid diagnostic tests (RDTs), and polymerase chain reaction (PCR), each with distinct advantages and limitations.

Microscopy of Giemsa-stained smears remains the *WHO gold standard*. It enables species identification, parasite staging, and parasite density estimation, essential for assessing severity (>5% RBCs infected). *Specificity is high (97–100%)*, but *sensitivity is moderate (~72–93%)*, particularly at low parasitemia, mixed infections, or early ring stages, and results depend on operator expertise. If initial smears are negative, repeat testing is recommended at each febrile episode every 12–24 hours for three sets before excluding malaria.

Rapid diagnostic tests are rapid and practical for point-of-care use, with *sensitivity 79–99%* and *specificity 88–96%*. They provide quick results but cannot quantify parasitemia or stage parasites. *False positives may result from persistent antigenemia, while pfhrp2/3 (plasmodium falciparum histidine rich protein 2/3) deletions can cause false negatives.*

Polymerase chain reaction offers the highest *sensitivity (>95–99%)*. It detects low-density or mixed infections, confirming species with high accuracy. However, it is resource-intensive and largely restricted to research and epidemiological settings.

In our institutional study of 20 malaria patients, 14 were RDT-positive and 13 smear-positive, with seven overlapping. This shows that while smear remains the gold standard, RDTs and PCR can enhance detection, particularly in low-parasitemia cases.

TREATMENT

Severe malaria is life-threatening, with untreated *mortality approaching 100%*. Prompt parenteral therapy and supportive care reduce mortality to 10–20%. Risk factors include:
- Organ dysfunction
- High parasitemia
- Multiple organ involvement
- Age extremes
- Comorbidities
- Delayed care

Parenteral therapy: All severe malaria cases, regardless of species, should receive *intravenous artesunate* (2.4 mg/kg at admission, at 12 hours, 24 hours, and then once a day). Treatment should continue for at least 24 hours or until the patient can tolerate oral therapy. Artesunate is preferred over quinine due to lower mortality and simpler administration.

Follow-on oral therapy: Once clinically improved and able to take oral drugs, patients should complete a full course of ACT (artesunate + amodiaquine, artemether + lumefantrine, or dihydroartemisinin + piperaquine). Avoid mefloquine-containing ACTs in patients with prior impaired consciousness. Alternatives include artesunate + clindamycin/doxycycline or quinine + clindamycin/doxycycline. Doxycycline is avoided in children <8 years and pregnancy.

Manifestation	Management
Coma (cerebral malaria)	Maintain airway, place patient on side, exclude other causes (e.g., hypoglycemia and meningitis); intubate if necessary
Hyperpyrexia	Administer tepid sponging, fanning, cooling blanket, and paracetamol
Convulsions	Maintain airways; treat with IV/rectal diazepam, lorazepam, midazolam, or IM paraldehyde. Check blood glucose
Hypoglycemia	Check blood glucose, correct and maintain with glucose infusion. Intervene if BS < 40 mg/dL
Severe anemia	Transfuse with screened fresh whole blood
Acute pulmonary edema	Prop up at 45°, oxygen and diuretic, stop IV fluids, intubate if needed
Acute kidney injury	Exclude prerenal causes, check fluid balance/urinary sodium; if renal failure, use hemofiltration/hemodialysis
Spontaneous bleeding and coagulopathy	Transfuse fresh whole blood (or cryoprecipitate, FFP, platelets); give vitamin K injection
Metabolic acidosis	Exclude/treat hypoglycemia, hypovolemia, and septicemia. If severe, add hemofiltration/hemodialysis
Shock	Suspect septicemia, send cultures; give parenteral broad-spectrum antimicrobials, correct hemodynamics

(BS: blood sugar; FFP: fresh frozen plasma; IM: intramuscular; IV: intravenous)

Plasmodium vivax/Plasmodium ovale anti-relapse therapy: Primaquine should be administered in a total dose of 7 mg/kg, either as 0.5 mg/kg daily for 14 days or 1 mg/kg daily for 7 days, to prevent relapses (by eliminating liver hypnozoites). Alternatively, tafenoquine [if glucose-6-phosphate dehydrogenase (G6PD)-normal] can be used. Avoid antirelapse therapy in pregnancy and G6PD deficiency **(Table 2)**.

OUTCOME

Mortality from *P. vivax* is generally low. Meta-analyses estimate overall mortality at *0.01% (0–0.07%)* in all cases and up to 0.56% (0.35–0.92%) among hospitalized patients, with another review reporting a case-fatality rate of 0.3%. In our institutional study, no deaths were documented; all 20 patients were discharged.

CONCLUSION

The traditional view of *P. falciparum* as the sole cause of severe malaria and *P. vivax* as "benign" is outdated. *P. vivax* is now recognized to cause life-threatening complications, and clinical management must be guided by severity rather than species. Any patient fulfilling WHO criteria for severe malaria requires urgent parenteral artesunate, irrespective of species, followed by completion with oral ACTs. Radical cure with primaquine or tafenoquine is essential to prevent relapse. Rapid recognition and treatment of severity, not species, determines patient outcomes.

FURTHER READINGS

1. Badiane A, Thwing J, Williamson J, Rogier E, Diallo MA, Ndiaye D. Sensitivity and specificity for malaria classification of febrile persons by rapid diagnostic test, microscopy, parasite DNA, histidine-rich protein 2, and IgG: Dakar, Senegal 2015. Int J Infect Dis. 2022:1;121:92-7.
2. Singhasenee P, Tangpukdee N, Krudsood S, Niyom SL, Chancharoenthana W, Matsee W, et al. Factors associated with severe plasmodium vivax malaria: a 15-year retrospective study. Southeast Asian J Trop Med Public Health. 2024:9;55(3).
3. WHO. (2025). WHO guidelines for malaria. [online] Available from https://www.who.int/publications/i/item/guidelines-for-malaria [Last accessed October, 2025].
4. Mehkri MI, Arahalli A. Severe Malaria Due to Vivax: The Underestimated Culprit. Indian J Pharm Pract. 2025;18(1):122-4.
5. Kojom Foko LP, Arya A, Sharma A, Singh V. Epidemiology and clinical outcomes of severe Plasmodium vivax malaria in India. J Infect. 2021;82(6):231-46.

CHAPTER 30

Controversial Updates in Community-acquired Pneumonia

Ben Cherian Mathew, Vikas Loomba

INTRODUCTION

Community-acquired pneumonia (CAP) is an acute infection of the lung parenchyma occurring outside of healthcare settings without recent exposure. It remains one of the leading causes of morbidity and mortality worldwide. Globally, lower respiratory tract infections, including CAP, are the most frequent infectious cause of death, with an estimated over 3 million deaths reported in 2019, accounting for significant hospital admissions and healthcare costs. India is responsible for 23% of the global burden of CAP and 36% of the regional burden, as per the World Health Organization. It is estimated that approximately 4 million CAP cases occur annually in India, with 20% requiring hospitalization. The annual incidence rate of CAP in India is between 5 and 11 per 1,000 people. The mortality rate for CAP is under 5% among outpatients, about 10% for hospitalized patients, and can surpass 30% for those in intensive care units.

DEFINITION

Community-acquired pneumonia is defined as an acute lung infection involving the alveoli that occurs in a patient without recent healthcare exposure. Pneumonia developed in a nursing home facility also is considered in CAP. It consists of clinical spectrum from pneumonia in a healthy patient to necrotizing or multilobar disease with septic shock.

According to guidelines of British Thoracic Society, CAP is defined as:
- Symptoms and signs of an acute lower respiratory tract illness (cough and at least one of the other lower respiratory tract symptom)
- New focal chest signs on examination
- New radiographic shadowing for which no other explanation
- At least one systemic feature (either a symptom complex of sweating, fevers, shivers, aches, and pains and/or temperature of 38°C or more).
- The illness is the primary reason for hospital admission.
- No other explanation for the illness, which is treated as CAP with antibiotics.

ETIOLOGY

Many pathogens cause CAP, including bacteria, viruses, and fungi **(Table 1)**.

DIAGNOSTIC TESTING FOR COMMUNITY-ACQUIRED PNEUMONIA

Sputum Gram Stain and Culture for Diagnosis of Community-acquired Pneumonia

Obtaining sputum gram stain and culture routinely in CAP patients on outpatient department (OPD) basis is not always recommended. However, if the patient is admitted who is categorized as severe CAP, intubated or previously infected, or empirically treated for methicillin-resistant *Staphylococcus aureus* (MRSA) or *Pseudomonas aeruginosa* or prior hospitalization and received parenteral antibiotics within the last 90 days, sputum culture is indicated. Obtaining a valid sputum specimen remains a challenging effort and often yields poor results.

- Should blood culture be done in all CAP patients?
  Blood cultures are not usually taken in CAP unless patient is admitted with severe CAP or:
  - Empirically treated for MRSA or *P. aeruginosa,* or
  - Prior hospitalization within the last 90 days and received parenteral antibiotics
- *Relevance and frequency of doing chest X-rays (CXRs) in patients with CAP*:
  Chest X-rays are required during admission to confirm the diagnosis, assess the extension, and rule out other causes such as pleural effusion, pulmonary edema, and heart failure. Repeat CXR is not recommended once diagnosis of CAP is confirmed.
  - *Repeat CXRs only indicated if*:
    - Clinical deterioration of patient—new onset of fever, hypoxia, and hemodynamic instability.

TABLE 1: Classification of common pathogens.	
Gram-positive agents	*Streptococcus pneumoniae, Staphylococcus aureus,* Group A streptococci, and other streptococci
Gram-negative agents	*Haemophilus influenzae, Moraxella catarrhalis,* and *Enterobacteriaceae*
Atypical agents	*Legionella, Mycoplasma, Chlamydia pneumoniae,* and *Chlamydia psittaci*
Viruses	Rhinovirus, influenza, severe acute respiratory syndrome coronavirus 2 (SARS-CoV-2), and other respiratory viruses such as parainfluenza, respiratory syncytial virus, and human metapneumovirus

Note: Worldwide, *Streptococcus pneumoniae,* and *Haemophilus influenzae* are still the leading causes of acute bacterial pneumonia.

- No improvement in clinical condition of patient after 48–72 hours of treatment.
- Evaluation of complications such as pleural effusion, empyema, lung abscess, and pneumothorax.
- Follow-up CXRs after 6–8 weeks of discharge in high-risk patients like above 50 years of age, smokers, and those who are at risk of lung malignancy or chronic lung disease.

- *C-reactive protein (CRP) and procalcitonin (PCT) in CAP*:
  - Both CRP and PCT will be elevated in bacterial CAP while CRP will be elevated in all kinds of CAP.
  - CRP will be useful for monitoring severity and response to treatment.
  - Baseline CRP is done at the time of admission and is repeated typically after 3 or 4 days of starting the treatment.
  - If patient is clinically improving, no further CRP monitoring is needed.
  - PCT will be useful for distinguishing between bacterial versus viral though not confirmatory and guiding antibiotic therapy and can be repeated after 48 hours to monitor the efficacy of the treatment.
  - A fall in PCT > 80% from its peak or < 0.25 ng/mL can be considered for limiting antibiotics.
  - However, PCT is not a diagnostic tool marker, sensitivity of PCT to detect bacterial infection ranges from 38 to 91%, indicating that PCT alone cannot be justified to decide on antibiotics treatment.
- *Newer modalities in diagnosis of CAP*: Newer modalities include methods such as multiplex PCR testing, ultrasonography of lungs.
  - With multiplex PCR testing, it is possible to adjust antibiotics rapidly for unsuspected antibiotic-resistant pathogens. This helps in reducing adverse outcomes in CAP which usually happens due to 48–72 hours of waiting for culture reports and treating with inappropriate antibiotic therapy. PCR testing for viral etiology [e.g., influenza, severe acute respiratory syndrome coronavirus 2 (SARS-CoV2)] should be performed based on seasonality and local guidelines. However, the cost of PCR testing and availability are the limiting factors of tests.
  - Ultrasonography of lung has shown to be a good diagnostic tool with high accuracy to rule in or out CAP. USG also helps to avoid radiation exposure by CXR. Addition of lung ultrasound aids in improving confidence in diagnosis of CAP and leads to significant treatment modification and portability of USG makes it more favorable diagnostic tool. However, USG can take more time to perform and is difficult to visualize the entire lungs unlike CXR. CXR can also detect tumors or mediastinal abnormalities. Hence, USG can be used as a diagnostic tool but should not replace CXR to confirm the diagnosis
  - CT chest helps in early diagnosis of CAP and to rule out other causes such as heart failure, pulmonary embolism, and to visualize site of bronchoscopy or image guided sampling.

SEVERITY ASSESSMENT OF COMMUNITY-ACQUIRED PNEUMONIA PATIENTS

Assessment of severity of CAP patients is done using either by CURB65 scoring or Pneumonia Severity Index (PSI). They help to categorize patients into low, intermediate, or high risk of death **(Table 2)**.

CURB65 Score for Mortality Risk Assessment in Hospital

CURB65 score is calculated by giving 1 point for each of the following prognostic features:
- Confusion (abbreviated Mental Test score 8 or less, or new disorientation in person, place, or time)
- Blood urea nitrogen > 20 mg/dL
- Raised respiratory rate ≥ 30 breaths/min
- Low blood pressure (systolic 90 mm Hg or less or diastolic 60 mm Hg or less)
- Age 65 years or more.

Pneumonia Severity Index

The PSI scoring system is more efficient in grading severity among pneumonia patients than CURB65 scoring. PSI scoring includes 20 variables consisting of age, coexisting illness, abnormal physical, and laboratory findings. Based on score patients are classified into 1 of the 5 different classes with **(Table 3)** following mortality rates.

PATIENTS ADMITTED WITH SEVERE COMMUNITY-ACQUIRED PNEUMONIA HAVE A SEPARATE CRITERIA

At least one major or at least three minor criteria to categorize as severe CAP **(Box 1)**.
- When to start antibiotics in CAP?
    - Rule of thumb is "Do not delay antibiotics" while waiting for imaging and investigation reports if clinical suspicion is high of pneumonia **(Tables 4 and 5)**.
- *Corticosteroids in severe CAP:*
    - There was evidence of use of corticosteroids with antibiotics compared to antibiotics alone treating in severe CAP of CURB65 score of 3–5, showed reduced mortality rates and hospitalization time **(Table 6)**.

TABLE 2: Admission of patients with community-acquired pneumonia.			
Score	Severity	Mortality risk	Recommendations
0–1	Mild	< 3%	Outpatient treatment
2	Moderate	3%–15%	Hospital admission to ward
3–5	Severe	> 15%	Admission to intensive care unit

TABLE 3: Pneumonia severity index (PSI) classes, scores, and associated mortality rates.

Class	Score	Mortality rates
2	≤ 70	0.6%
3	71–90	2.8%
4	91–130	8.2%
5	> 130	29.2%

Note: PSI scoring rate also helps in lowering the admission rates for 2 and treated on OPD basis. Class 3 above are ideally admitted and evaluated.

BOX 1: Criteria for severe community-acquired pneumonia (ATS/IDSA).

Major criteria:
- Respiratory failure requiring intubation and mechanical ventilation
- Septic shock requiring vasopressors

Minor criteria:
- Respiratory rate ≥ 30 breaths/min
- PaO_2/FiO_2 ratio ≤ 250
- Multilobar infiltrates
- Confusion/Disorientation
- Uremia (BUN ≥ 20 mg/dL)
- Leukopenia (WBC < 4,000 cells/uL)
- Thrombocytopenia (< 1 lakh cells/uL)
- Hypothermia (< 36°C)
- Hypotension requiring aggressive fluid resuscitation

(ATS: American Thoracic Society; BUN: blood urea nitrogen; IDSA: Infectious Disease Society of America; PaO_2/FiO_2: Arterial oxygen pressure/fraction of inspired oxygen; WBC: white blood cell)

TABLE 4: Treatment of community-acquired pneumonia (CAP).

Clinical scenario	When to start antibiotics?
Severe CAP/Sepsis/ICU	Immediately within 1 hour
Hospitalized stable CAP	At least within 4 hours of arrival
Outpatient CAP	At the time of diagnosis
Suspected viral	Can withhold review with biomarkers

- However, they are also reasonable for increased chances of hyperglycemia and increased risk of secondary infections in less severe pneumonia. Corticosteroids may not be beneficial in viral pneumonia.
- Currently IV hydrocortisone is considered for severe CAP due to potential mortality benefits but further studies are needed to determine specific dosing and types of corticosteroids for different groups of patient.

TABLE 5: Antibiotic stewardship.		
Clinical scenario	Choice of antibiotics	Alternatives
OPD CAP	Amoxicillin 500 mg thrice daily	Macrolide-azithromycin, clarithromycin or Tetracyclines-doxycycline
Hospital admitted CAP	Amoxicillin + Macrolide	
Severe CAP	IV β-lactamase like amoxicillin-clavulanate + macrolide (azithromycin)	2nd or 3rd generation cephalosporin + macrolide or Injection piperacillin-tazobactum, ceftazidime + Avibactam, carbapenems like meropenem and Vancomycin/Teicoplanin/Linezolid in case of MRSA

(CAP: community-acquired pneumonia; MRSA: methicillin-resistant *Staphylococcus aureus*)

TABLE 6: How long antibiotics should be given?	
Type	Duration
Low or moderate severity CAP	5–7 days
High Severity CAP needing ICU	7–10 days
Pseudomonas or aspiration pneumonia	14 days
Necrotizing pneumonia due to MRSA or Gram-negative enteric bacilli pneumonia CAP	14–21 days

(CAP: community-acquired pneumonia; MRSA: methicillin-resistant *Staphylococcus aureus*)

Alternative like dexamethasone is preferred if hydrocortisone is not suitable **(Table 7)**.

FOLLOW-UP OF COMMUNITY-ACQUIRED PNEUMONIA CASES AFTER DISCHARGE

Refer to **Table 7**.

PREVENTION IS BETTER THAN CURE! (TABLE 8)

Smoking cessation: Smoking cessation advice should be offered to all patients with CAP who are current smokers to improve quality of life and reduce morbidities.

CHAPTER 30: Controversial Updates in Community-acquired Pneumonia

TABLE 7: Follow-up is obligatory to monitor further condition of CAP patients.

Type of review	Duration after discharge	Scenarios	Intervention
Early	48–72 hours	To check resolution of symptoms (fever, cough), oxygen requirement, adherence to antibiotics	Readmit and re-evaluate if worsening
After completion of antibiotics	• 5–7 days in mild-moderate CAP cases • Up to 10 days in severe CAP cases	Reassessment of clinical condition—fever, HR, BP, RR, O_2 saturation	If clinically stable no need to further evaluate
Intermediate	2–4 weeks	Meant for slow recovery, COPD, DM, CKD or other comorbidities	Evaluation of ongoing symptoms such as cough, hemoptysis, fatigue, chest pain
Radiological	6–8 weeks	In high-risk patients like age > 50 years, smokers, chronic lung disease like COPD, suspicion of malignancy or TB, unexplained weight loss, persisting or deteriorating condition	Confirm resolution and exclude underlying cancer or structural lung diseases
Delayed/ Extended	12–14 weeks	Mainly for elderly patients	Unresolving cases, bronchoscopy or/and HRCT chest done to rule out TB, chronic lung disease, malignancy, etc.

(BP: blood pressure; CAP: community-acquired pneumonia; CKD: chronic kidney disease; COPD: chronic obstructive pulmonary disease; DM: diabetes mellitus; HR: heart rate; O_2: Oxygen; RR: respiratory rate; TB: Tuberculosis)

TABLE 8: Vaccination is a key prevention in patients at risk of community-acquired pneumonia (CAP).

Group	Pneumococcal vaccine	Influenza vaccine	Other vaccines
• Healthy adults • Age 50 years or older	Not previously vaccinated—1 dose of either PCV15/ PCV20/ PCV21 followed by 1 dose of PPSV23 after 1 year	Annual flu shot	COVID-19, Tdap once in adulthood and then Td booster once in every 10 years
19–49 years with comorbidities	Not previously vaccinated—1 dose of either PCV15/PCV20/ PCV21 followed by 1 dose of PPSV23 after 1 year (8 weeks in immunocompromised adults)	Annual flu shot	COVID-19, Tdap

Continued

Continued

Group	Pneumococcal vaccine	Influenza vaccine	Other vaccines
Immunocompromised adults such as HIV, cancer, transplants, asplenia, long-term steroids	1 dose PCV13 followed by PPSV23 (after 8 weeks in immunocompromised). PCV 20 and PCV 21 which are US FDA approved instead of PCV13 will be available in India in future	Annual flu shot	COVID-19, Tdap, Hib in asplenia/transplant
> 65 years	1 dose PCV13 followed by PPSV23 (after 1 year). PCV 20 and PCV 21 which are US FDA approved instead of PCV13 will be available in India	Annual flu shot	COVID-19, Tdap

(PCV: pneumococcal conjugate vaccine; PPSV: pneumococcal polysaccharide vaccine; Tdap: tetanus, diphtheria, acellular pertussis; Td: tetanus, diphtheria)

CONCLUSION

Smoking cessation advice should be offered to all patients with CAP who are current smokers to improve quality of life and reduce morbidities.

FURTHER READINGS

1. Rider AC, Frazee BW. Community-acquired pneumonia. Emerg Med Clin North Am. 2018;36(4):665-83.
2. Ferreira-Coimbra J, Sarda C, Rello J. Burden of community-acquired pneumonia and unmet clinical needs. Adv Ther. 2020;37(4):1302-18.
3. Vikhe VB, Faruqi AA, Patil RS, Reddy A, Khandol D. A systematic review of community-acquired pneumonia in Indian adults. Cureus. 2024;16(7):e63976.
4. Lim WS, Baudouin SV, George RC, Hill AT, Jamieson C, Le Jeune I, et al. British Thoracic Society guidelines for the management of community acquired pneumonia in adults: Update 2009. Thorax. 2009;64:iii1-55.
5. Regunath H, Oba Y. Community-Acquired Pneumonia. StatPearls, Treasure Island (FL): StatPearls Publishing; 2025.

SECTION 11

Nephrology

CHAPTER 31

Clinician's Approach to Secondary Hypertension

RBS Manian

INTRODUCTION

Hypertension remains one of the most common and impactful cardiovascular risk factors worldwide, affecting hundreds of millions of adults and contributing to high rates of morbidity and mortality. Most patients are diagnosed with primary (essential) hypertension, a condition with multifactorial causes that develops gradually over time. However, in a smaller but clinically significant proportion of individuals, elevated blood pressure results from an identifiable, often correctable medical condition or medication effect. This form is known as secondary hypertension.

Secondary hypertension is not merely an academic distinction. Unlike primary hypertension, which requires long-term risk factor control and pharmacological therapy, secondary hypertension carries the potential for complete reversal if its root cause is detected and appropriately treated. Failing to recognize this form may expose patients to unnecessary polypharmacy, persistent uncontrolled blood pressure, and preventable cardiovascular complications.

This chapter critically examines the definition, epidemiology, pathophysiology, causes, clinical features, diagnostic strategies, treatment options, prognosis, preventive measures, and emerging research on secondary hypertension while highlighting the importance of timely identification and management.

DEFINITION AND OVERVIEW

Secondary hypertension is defined as persistently elevated blood pressure that arises as a direct consequence of an underlying medical condition or pharmacological agent, as opposed to primary hypertension, which has no single identifiable cause. Common culprits include renal disorders, endocrine abnormalities, vascular malformations, sleep-related breathing disorders, and drug-induced mechanisms.

The clinical relevance of this distinction lies in its curative potential. Whereas essential hypertension requires lifelong therapy to control blood pressure and reduce cardiovascular risk, secondary hypertension can often be controlled—or even resolved—by treating its source. For example, excising a hormone-secreting adrenal tumor or correcting renal artery stenosis (RAS) may restore blood pressure to normal without the need for long-term pharmacotherapy.

■ EPIDEMIOLOGY AND PREVALENCE

Secondary hypertension is less common than primary hypertension, yet its prevalence is not trivial. Epidemiological studies estimate that 2–10% of adult hypertensive patients have a secondary form. The proportion is significantly higher in certain subgroups, such as:
- *Resistant hypertension*: Patients whose blood pressure remains uncontrolled despite the use of three or more antihypertensive drugs, including a diuretic
- Young individuals (<30 years) presenting with severe hypertension without typical risk factors
- Older patients (>55 years) who develop sudden, new-onset hypertension

Among pediatric populations, secondary hypertension is the predominant form, often due to renal or congenital vascular anomalies.

Though the absolute percentage is modest compared to essential hypertension, the clinical importance of secondary forms cannot be overstated: Recognition prevents years of uncontrolled blood pressure, reduces cardiovascular risk, and allows targeted treatment.

■ PATHOPHYSIOLOGY

The mechanisms leading to secondary hypertension vary widely, depending on the underlying etiology. A few illustrative pathways include the following:
- *RAS*: Narrowing of one or both renal arteries reduces renal perfusion. The kidney interprets this as hypotension, activating the renin–angiotensin–aldosterone system (RAAS). This leads to sodium retention, vasoconstriction, and chronic hypertension.
- *Renal parenchymal disease*: Chronic kidney disease (CKD) impairs sodium excretion and disturbs intravascular volume regulation. This fluid overload, combined with increased sympathetic drive, elevates blood pressure.
- *Endocrine causes*:
  - *Primary hyperaldosteronism (Conn's syndrome)*: Excess aldosterone enhances sodium and water retention while causing potassium loss, resulting in volume expansion and hypertension.
  - *Cushing's syndrome*: High cortisol levels act on mineralocorticoid receptors, mimicking aldosterone's effects.
  - *Pheochromocytoma*: Catecholamine-secreting adrenal tumors lead to episodic surges of vasoconstriction, tachycardia, and severe hypertension.
  - *Thyroid and parathyroid disorders*: They alter vascular tone, cardiac output, and calcium homeostasis.
- *Medication-induced hypertension*: Drugs such as nonsteroidal anti-inflammatory drugs (NSAIDs), corticosteroids, oral contraceptives, antidepressants, and stimulants can elevate blood pressure via mechanisms like sodium retention, sympathetic activation, or increased systemic vascular resistance.

In essence, the pathophysiology is inseparable from the primary disease, underscoring the importance of tailored diagnostic evaluation.

CAUSES OF SECONDARY HYPERTENSION

- *Renal causes*:
  - *CKD*: It is the most frequent renal cause. CKD alters sodium balance and stimulates RAAS.
  - *RAS*: Either atherosclerotic (older adults) or fibromuscular dysplasia (younger women)
  - *Polycystic kidney disease*: Structural damage disrupts renal function, driving hypertension.
- *Endocrine causes*:
  - *Primary hyperaldosteronism*: Now recognized as a more common cause than previously thought, especially in resistant hypertension
  - *Cushing's syndrome*: Cortisol excess, often from adrenal adenomas or long-term steroid therapy
  - *Pheochromocytoma and paragangliomas*: Rare but dangerous, with hallmark episodic hypertension
  - *Thyroid dysfunction*: Both hyper- and hypothyroidism can elevate blood pressure through different mechanisms
  - *Hyperparathyroidism*: Excess parathyroid hormone alters calcium dynamics, affecting vascular smooth muscle
- *Other medical causes*:
  - *Coarctation of the aorta*: Congenital narrowing leads to upper-body hypertension.
  - *Obstructive sleep apnea (OSA)*: Nocturnal hypoxia heightens sympathetic tone and blood pressure.
- *Medication-related causes*:
  - Estrogen-containing contraceptives, particularly older high-dose formulations
  - NSAIDs, which impair renal sodium handling and vasodilatory prostaglandins
  - Glucocorticoids, decongestants, antidepressants, antipsychotics, and chemotherapy agents

CLINICAL PRESENTATION AND SYMPTOMS

Unlike primary hypertension, which typically develops insidiously, secondary hypertension may have a sudden onset and is often resistant to therapy. Key clinical clues include:
- Severe or abrupt rise in blood pressure, especially in young patients or those over 55 years with no prior history
- Resistance to three or more antihypertensive medications
- Hypokalemia (suggestive of hyperaldosteronism)
- No family history of hypertension

Symptoms may be general or disease-specific:
- Headaches, chest pain, confusion, or vision changes (due to hypertensive urgency or emergency)
- Palpitations, sweating, and episodic anxiety (pheochromocytoma)
- Muscle weakness or cramps (aldosterone excess)
- Polyuria and fatigue (renal disease)
- Snoring and daytime sleepiness (sleep apnea)

Recognizing these associations is crucial for early suspicion.

DIAGNOSTIC APPROACH

Clinical Suspicion
- Onset before the age of 30 years or after 55 years
- Resistant hypertension
- Electrolyte abnormalities, particularly hypokalemia
- Lack of traditional risk factors such as obesity or family history

Investigations
- *Laboratory studies*:
  - *Renal function*: Serum creatinine, glomerular filtration rate (GFR), and urinalysis
  - *Electrolytes*: Potassium and calcium
  - *Hormonal assays*: Plasma renin activity, aldosterone, cortisol, and thyroid function tests
- *Imaging*:
  - Renal ultrasound and Doppler
  - Computed tomography/magnetic resonance imaging (CT/MRI) of the adrenal glands
  - Echocardiography or CT angiography for coarctation
- *Specialized tests*:
  - Plasma or urinary metanephrines for pheochromocytoma
  - Polysomnography for sleep apnea
  - Adrenal venous sampling in suspected hyperaldosteronism

A stepwise, hypothesis-driven approach prevents unnecessary testing while ensuring that rare but treatable causes are not missed.

TREATMENT STRATEGIES

The cornerstone of therapy is addressing the underlying cause. Approaches include the following:
- *Renal causes*:
  - Angioplasty/stenting or surgical revascularization for RAS
  - Optimized CKD management with RAAS blockade and dialysis when necessary

- *Endocrine causes*:
  - Surgical removal of adrenal tumors
  - Mineralocorticoid receptor antagonists (spironolactone and eplerenone) for hyperaldosteronism
  - Medical or surgical therapy for Cushing's syndrome, thyroid disorders, or hyperparathyroidism
- *Sleep apnea*: Continuous positive airway pressure (CPAP) therapy plus weight management
- *Drug-induced hypertension*: Withdrawal or substitution of offending agents
- *Symptomatic control*: While definitive therapy is pursued, antihypertensive medications [angiotensin-converting enzyme (ACE) inhibitors, angiotensin II receptor blockers (ARBs), calcium channel blockers, diuretics, and beta-blockers] are used.

Lifestyle measures remain vital—dietary sodium restriction, weight reduction, regular exercise, smoking cessation, and moderation of alcohol amplify treatment success.

PROGNOSIS AND OUTCOMES

The prognosis of secondary hypertension depends heavily on timely recognition and treatment. Early intervention can lead to:
- Complete resolution of hypertension (e.g., curative surgery for adrenal tumors)
- Improved blood pressure control, even when not fully reversible
- Reduction in long-term risks of myocardial infarction, stroke, renal failure, and death

Delayed or missed diagnosis, however, may allow irreversible end-organ damage to develop, leaving patients with permanent hypertension and higher cardiovascular risk.

PREVENTION

While many causes cannot be entirely prevented, certain measures lower risk:
- Adopting healthy lifestyle practices (balanced diet, reduced sodium, physical activity, and tobacco and alcohol moderation)
- Managing chronic diseases such as diabetes, kidney disease, and sleep apnea
- Cautious use of medications known to elevate blood pressure, with regular monitoring

Prevention is thus closely tied to primary care vigilance and patient education.

CURRENT RESEARCH AND FUTURE DIRECTIONS

Secondary hypertension remains an evolving field. Recent advances include:
- Molecular diagnostics for detecting subtle genetic and hormonal abnormalities
- Improved imaging techniques for renal and adrenal pathology

- Personalized medicine, tailoring therapies to the individual's hormonal or genetic profile
- Interdisciplinary care models, integrating cardiology, nephrology, endocrinology, and surgery for resistant cases

Such innovations promise earlier detection, less invasive treatment, and better long-term outcomes.

CONCLUSION

Secondary hypertension, though less common than primary hypertension, represents a critical subset of hypertensive disease with unique clinical implications. Defined by its identifiable and often reversible causes, it differs fundamentally from essential hypertension in prognosis and management.

Early suspicion—guided by clinical red flags, targeted investigations, and interdisciplinary collaboration—can lead to curative treatments, prevent complications, and reduce the global burden of cardiovascular disease. For clinicians, the challenge lies not only in lowering numbers on a blood pressure chart but also in seeking and treating the hidden causes that, once addressed, can transform patient outcomes.

Secondary hypertension, in short, is a reminder that not all hypertension is created equal—and in medicine, looking deeper often saves lives.

FURTHER READINGS

1. Hegde S, Suresh MS, Kumar P. Secondary Hypertension. [Internet] Treasure Island (FL): StatPearls Publishing; 2023. Available from https://www.ncbi.nlm.nih.gov/books/NBK544305/ [Last accessed October, 2025].
2. Taler SJ. Secondary causes of hypertension. Prim Care. 2008;35(3):489-500.
3. Sarathy H, Anand S, Maddukuri P. Evaluation and management of secondary hypertension. Med Clin North Am. 2022;106(2):269-83.
4. Mayo Clinic. (2022). Secondary hypertension: symptoms and causes. [online] . Available from https://www.mayoclinic.org/diseases-conditions/secondary-hypertension/symptoms-causes/syc-20350679 [Last accessed October, 2025].
5. Cleveland Clinic. (2025). Secondary hypertension: causes and symptoms. [online] Available from https://my.clevelandclinic.org/health/diseases/21128-secondary-hypertension [Last accessed October, 2025].

CHAPTER 32

Hyponatremia and Hypernatremia: Emergency Management Updates

Kalyan Mitra

▮ INTRODUCTION AND EPIDEMIOLOGY

Hyponatremia and hypernatremia represent two of the most common electrolyte disorders observed in both hospital and community settings. Hyponatremia is defined as a serum sodium concentration < 135 mEq/L, while hypernatremia is defined as that > 145 mEq/L. Epidemiological studies reveal striking differences in prevalence across patient populations: Mild hyponatremia is found in 22% of geriatric ward patients, 6% of nongeriatric wards, and 17% of intensive care unit (ICU) admissions. Severe hyponatremia (sodium < 125 mEq/L) affects 4.5% of geriatric ward patients, 0.8% of nongeriatric inpatients, and >10% of ICU cases. In ambulatory populations, hyponatremia affects between 4 and 7%, with nursing home residents showing a prevalence of 18.8%. Both disorders are clinically important because they are linked to poor prognosis, increased morbidity, longer hospital stays, and higher mortality rates. For example, patients with preoperative hyponatremia undergoing cardiac surgery have higher complication rates and mortality, while even mild outpatient hyponatremia carries a nearly two-fold increase in mortality risk. Similarly, both community-acquired and hospital-acquired hyponatremia predict worse outcomes in patients. Hypernatremia, although less common, is equally serious: Its presence in surgical and critically ill patients correlates strongly with increased perioperative morbidity and mortality. The studies also emphasize that hyponatremia is not always just a marker of disease severity but may contribute causally to adverse outcomes. Similarly, hypernatremia often indicates severe illness or impaired access to water. Thus, sodium disorders serve as both biomarkers of disease and direct contributors to pathophysiological decline.

▮ ETIOLOGY AND PATHOPHYSIOLOGY

Sodium concentration in plasma is tightly regulated by osmolality, which reflects the total solute concentration of water. Effective osmolality is controlled through thirst and arginine vasopressin [antidiuretic hormone (ADH)]. When osmolality rises, ADH promotes water retention; when it falls, ADH secretion decreases, promoting water excretion. Disruption in this homeostasis underlies both hyponatremia and hypernatremia. Hyponatremia is classified based on volume status: Hypovolemic—decreased total body sodium with proportionally greater water loss. Causes include gastrointestinal loss, renal salt wasting, adrenal insufficiency, or diuretic use. Euvolemic—total body water is increased, but sodium content remains normal. It is most often due to syndrome of inappropriate antidiuretic hormone secretion (SIADH), but also seen in hypothyroidism and adrenal insufficiency. Hypervolemic—total body water increases more than sodium, often due to cirrhosis, heart failure, or renal disease. Hypernatremia usually reflects net water loss rather than sodium gain. Causes include gastrointestinal or renal fluid losses, restricted access to water, diabetes insipidus, or excessive sodium intake (iatrogenic). Risk groups include infants, elderly patients, and the critically ill. Pathophysiologically, hypernatremia causes cellular dehydration and brain shrinkage, which can lead to vascular rupture, intracranial bleeding, and severe neurological consequences **(Flowchart 1)**.

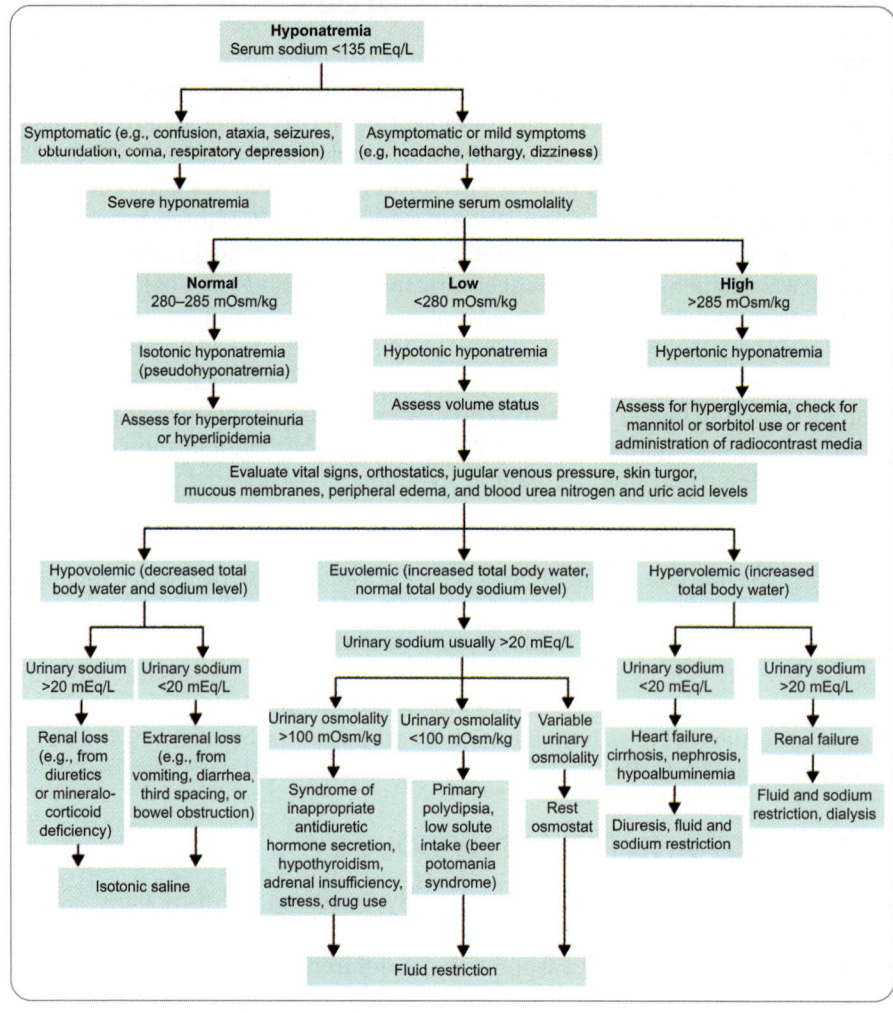

FLOWCHART 1: Algorithm for the evaluation of hyponatremia.

DIAGNOSTIC APPROACH TO HYPONATREMIA

The diagnostic process begins with assessing symptom severity and the rate of sodium decline. Rapid drops can produce seizures, coma, or status epilepticus, while gradual declines may be asymptomatic. Physicians must evaluate hydration and volume status using vital signs, jugular venous pressure, edema, and mucous membranes. A careful history is critical. Relevant details include comorbidities, recent surgery, medications [diuretics, selective serotonin reuptake inhibitors (SSRIs), and carbamazepine], alcohol or illicit drug use, and high-endurance athletic activity. Laboratory evaluation should include a metabolic panel, urine sodium and creatinine, serum osmolality, thyroid and adrenal function, and, in selected cases, brain natriuretic peptide or uric acid excretion. Pseudohyponatremia—due to hyperglycemia, hyperlipidemia, or laboratory artifact—should always be excluded. The workup differentiates hypovolemic, euvolemic, and hypervolemic hyponatremia **(Table 1)**.

TABLE 1: Differential diagnosis and treatment of hyponatremia.

Condition	Diagnosis	Treatment
Pseudohyponatremia—hyperglycemia (e.g., in diabetic ketoacidosis)	Elevated glucose levels [>400 mg/dL (22.2 mmol/L)], elevated anion gap	Insulin, intravenous fluids, isotonic saline
Pseudohyponatremia—hyperlipidemia	Elevated total and low-density lipoprotein cholesterol levels	Statin therapy
Pseudohyponatremia—hyperproteinemia (e.g., in multiple myeloma)	Serum and urinary monoclonal protein, bone marrow biopsy, and lytic bone lesions detected on radiography	Chemotherapy
Pseudohyponatremia—laboratory errors	Repeat sodium levels	–
Hypovolemic hyponatremia—cerebral salt wasting	Diagnosis of exclusion (e.g., head injuries, intracranial hemorrhage); urinary sodium >20 mEq/L	Isotonic or hypertonic saline
Hypovolemic hyponatremia—diuretic use	Clinical; urinary sodium >20 mEq/L	Stop diuretic therapy
Hypovolemic hyponatremia—gastrointestinal loss (e.g., diarrhea, vomiting)	Clinical; urinary sodium <20 mEq/L	Intravenous fluids
Hypovolemic hyponatremia—mineralocorticoid deficiency (e.g., Addison's disease)	Low aldosterone and morning cortisol levels, hyperkalemia, increased plasma renin level, low or increased adrenocorticotropic hormone level (cause-dependent), urinary sodium > 20 mEq/L, positive results on cosyntropin stimulation test, 21-hydroxylase autoantibodies (Addison's disease), computed tomography of adrenal glands to rule out infarction	Steroid replacement therapy

Continued

Continued

Condition	Diagnosis	Treatment
Hypovolemic hyponatremia—osmotic diuresis	Elevated glucose level, mannitol use	Correct glucose level, stop mannitol use
Hypovolemic hyponatremia—renal tubular acidosis	Urinary osmolar gap, increased urinary pH, urinary sodium > 25 mEq/L, fractional excretion of bicarbonate > 15–20%, hyperchloremic acidosis, decreased serum bicarbonate level, potassium abnormalities (type dependent)	Correct acidosis, sodium bicarbonate
Hypovolemic hyponatremia—salt-wasting nephropathies	Urinary sodium > 20 mEq/L	Correct the underlying cause
Hypovolemic hyponatremia—third spacing (e.g., bowel obstruction, burns)	Clinical; computed tomography	Intravenous fluids relieve obstruction
Euvolemic hyponatremia—3,4-methylenedioxymethamphetamine ("Ecstasy") use	Urine drug screen	—
Euvolemic hyponatremia—beer potomania syndrome	Excessive alcohol consumption, low serum osmolality	Therapy to decrease alcohol use and nutritional counseling to increase protein intake
Exercise-associated hyponatremia	Clinical	Isotonic or hypertonic saline, depending on symptoms
Glucocorticoid deficiency	Low aldosterone, morning cortisol, and ACTH; hyperkalemia, increased plasma renin	Steroid replacement therapy
Hypothyroidism	Elevated TSH, low free thyroxine	Thyroid replacement therapy
Low solute intake	Clinical	Increase sodium intake
Nephrogenic SIADH	Same as SIADH, with low vasopressin levels	Fluid restriction, loop diuretics
Psychogenic polydipsia	History of schizophrenia with excessive water intake	Psychiatric therapy
Reset osmostat	Free water challenge test, normal fractional excretion of uric acid	Treat the underlying disease
SIADH	Decreased osmolality, urinary osmolality > 100 mOsm/kg, euvolemia, urinary sodium > 20 mEq/L, absence of thyroid disorders or hypocortisolism, normal renal function, no diuretic use	Fluid restriction, consider vaptans

Continued

Continued

Condition	Diagnosis	Treatment
SIADH secondary to medication use	SIADH with the use of causative agent	Stop causative medication
Water intoxication	Clinical; excessive water intake	Diuresis
Heart failure	Clinical (e.g., jugular venous distention, edema), elevated BNP, echocardiography, urinary sodium < 20 mEq/L	Diuretics, ACE inhibitors, beta blockers
Hepatic failure/cirrhosis	Elevated liver function tests, ascites, elevated ammonia, biopsy, urinary sodium < 20 mEq/L	Furosemide (Lasix), spironolactone, transplant
Nephrotic syndrome	Urinary protein, urinary sodium < 20 mEq/L	Treat the underlying cause
Renal failure (acute or chronic)	Blood urea nitrogen-to-creatinine ratio, glomerular filtration rate, proteinuria, urinary sodium >20 mEq/L	Correct underlying disease with ACE inhibitors or angiotensin receptor blockers

(ACE: angiotensin-converting enzyme; ACTH: adrenocorticotropic hormone; BNP: brain natriuretic peptide; SIADH: syndrome of inappropriate antidiuretic hormone secretion; TSH: thyroid-stimulating hormone).

TYPES OF HYPONATREMIA AND TREATMENTS

- *Hypovolemic hyponatremia*: Often due to vomiting, diarrhea, renal salt-wasting, or adrenal insufficiency. Diagnostic markers include urine sodium < 20 mEq/L in extrarenal losses and >20 mEq/L in renal causes. Treatment involves isotonic saline repletion and addressing the underlying etiology. Salt tablets may be used in select cases.
- *Euvolemic hyponatremia*: It is commonly caused by SIADH, hypothyroidism, or glucocorticoid deficiency. Diagnosis is supported by low serum uric acid, normal blood urea nitrogen (BUN)-to-creatinine ratio, and urine sodium > 20 mEq/L. Management focuses on fluid restriction, maintaining adequate protein and salt intake, and treating the underlying condition. Failure of fluid restriction is predicted by urine osmolality > 500 mOsm/kg or urine output < 1.5 L/day.
- *Hypervolemic hyponatremia*: It is associated with cirrhosis, heart failure, or renal failure. Effective arterial blood volume is reduced, triggering excess ADH release and impaired water excretion. Treatment includes sodium and fluid restriction, diuretics, and disease-specific management **(Table 2)**.

SEVERE SYMPTOMATIC HYPONATREMIA

Severe symptomatic hyponatremia develops rapidly (within 24 hours) with sodium levels < 120 mEq/L and presents with coma, seizures, or respiratory failure. Immediate correction is critical to prevent cerebral edema and herniation. Recommended treatment includes hypertonic (3%) saline, delivered as either

SECTION 11: Nephrology

TABLE 2: SORT: Key recommendations for practice.			
Clinical recommendation	Evidence rating	References	Comments
In patients with severe symptomatic hyponatremia, the rate of sodium correction should be 6–12 mEq/L in the first 24 hours and 18 mEq/L or less in 48 hours	C	13,14	Consensus guidelines based on systematic reviews
A bolus of 100–150 mL of hypertonic 3% saline can be given to correct severe hyponatremia	C	13,14	Consensus guidelines based on small studies
Vaptans appear to be safe for the treatment of severe hypervolemic and euvolemic hyponatremia but should not be used routinely	C	14	Consensus guidelines based on observational studies
Chronic hypernatremia should be corrected at a rate of 0.5 mEq/L/h, with a maximum change of 8–10 mEq/L in a 24-hour period	C	33	Expert opinion

Notes: Evidence rating key
- *A*: Consistent, good-quality patient-oriented evidence;
- *B*: Inconsistent or limited-quality patient-oriented evidence;
- *C*: Consensus, disease-oriented evidence, usual practice, expert opinion, or case series.

continuous infusion (0.5–2 mL/kg/h) or repeated 100–150 mL boluses. The goal is to raise sodium by 4–6 mEq/L to alleviate symptoms, but not >10–12 mEq/L in 24 hours or 18 mEq/L in 48 hours, to avoid osmotic demyelination. Adjunctive desmopressin may be used to control overcorrection. Clinical studies have demonstrated that combined desmopressin and hypertonic saline therapy allows safer, more predictable correction. Guidelines from European societies recommend a single bolus of 150 mL of 3% saline with frequent sodium checks. On reviewing specific clinical studies: one involving 25 patients with sodium <120 mEq/L showed that combining 3% saline with scheduled desmopressin prevented dangerous overcorrection while raising sodium safely by 3–7 mEq/L. Another trial in marathon runners used a 100 mL bolus of 3% saline to correct exercise-associated hyponatremia with encephalopathy, achieving rapid symptom relief without excessive correction. Importantly, the guideline-recommended correction targets are based on avoiding osmotic demyelination, which has historically been devastating and often irreversible (**Flowchart 2**).

ROLE OF VAPTANS

Vaptans (vasopressin receptor antagonists such as conivaptan and tolvaptan) selectively block ADH activity and increase free water excretion. Clinical trials (e.g., SALT, SALTWATER) demonstrated that tolvaptan significantly raises sodium levels in patients with SIADH, cirrhosis, and heart failure. However, long-term benefits on survival remain unclear. Adverse effects include thirst, polyuria, and hepatotoxicity, with tolvaptan being contraindicated in liver disease. Their high

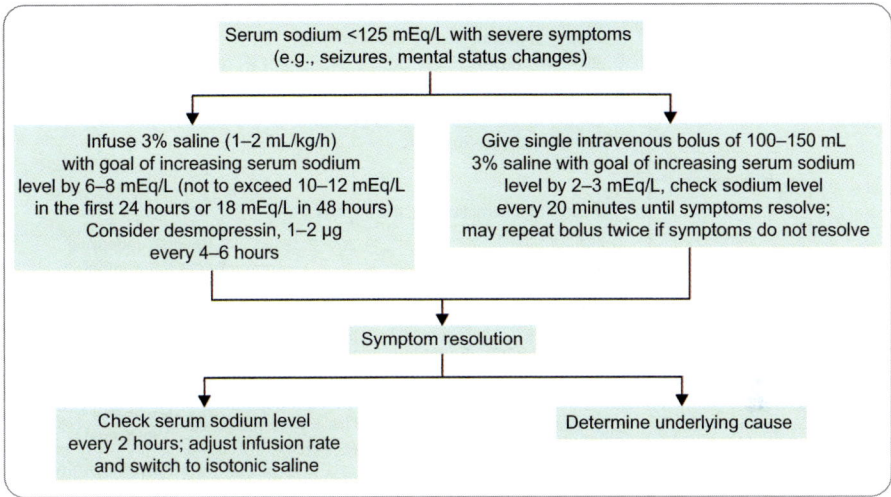

FLOWCHART 2: Algorithm for the treatment of severe symptomatic hyponatremia.

cost and potential for rapid overcorrection limit routine use. Current guidelines recommend against routine vaptan use, suggesting they be reserved for selected refractory cases.

HYPERNATREMIA: CAUSES, SYMPTOMS, AND DIAGNOSIS

Hypernatremia arises primarily from water deficit rather than sodium gain. Causes include gastrointestinal loss, diuretic therapy, osmotic diuresis (e.g., hyperglycemia, mannitol use), renal failure, fever, mechanical ventilation, and diabetes insipidus (central or nephrogenic). In rare cases, excessive sodium administration via hypertonic saline, sodium bicarbonate, or salt ingestion is responsible. Symptoms vary by age and acuity. Adults often have anorexia, weakness, irritability, nausea, and confusion. Severe acute hypernatremia can cause brain shrinkage, vascular rupture, and intracranial hemorrhage. Diagnosis is guided by history and physical examination, supplemented with urine osmolality and sodium measurements. In diabetes insipidus, urine remains inappropriately diluted (<300 mOsm/kg) despite hypernatremia. A desmopressin challenge test distinguishes central from nephrogenic diabetes insipidus **(Flowchart 3)**.

TREATMENT OF HYPERNATREMIA

The cornerstone of treatment is correction of water deficit while addressing the underlying cause. Oral or enteral free water is preferred; when intravenous fluids are required, hypotonic solutions such as 5% dextrose or 0.45% saline are used. Correction must be cautious: rapid reduction of sodium risks cerebral edema, especially in chronic cases. Recommended correction rates are ≤0.5 mEq/L/h, not exceeding 8–10 mEq/L in 24 hours. In acute hypernatremia, faster correction up to 1 mEq/L/h may be tolerated safely. Special considerations include calculating

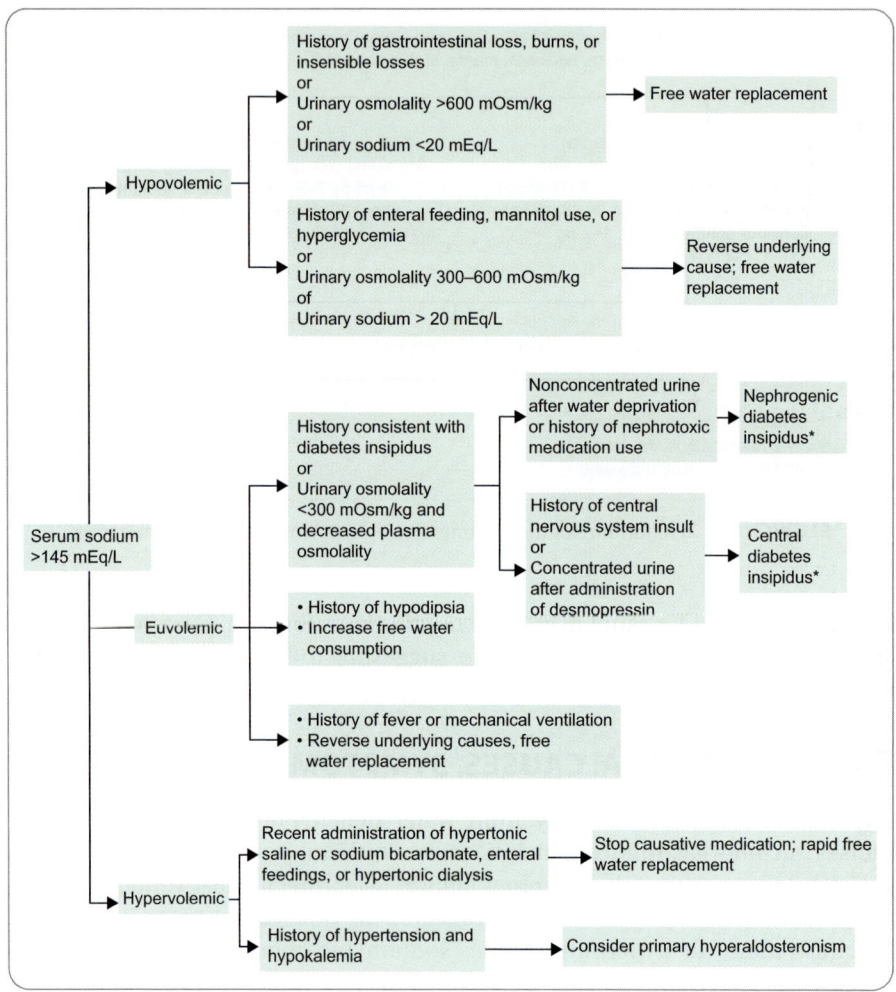

*The diagnosis of diabetes insipidus usually requires a combination of water deprivation and a trial of desmopressin. With water deprivation, patients with diabetes insipidus will have increased plasma osmolality but not urinary osmolality. In patients with central diabetes insipidus, urinary osmolality will increase by approximately 200 mOsm/kg after receiving desmopressin.

FLOWCHART 3: Evaluation of hypernatremia.

total body water deficit and monitoring serum electrolytes every 2–4 hours during therapy. The literature highlights that treatment strategies must be individualized depending on whether hypernatremia is acute or chronic and whether it is associated with hypovolemia, euvolemia, or hypervolemia. For hypovolemic hypernatremia, volume resuscitation with isotonic fluids may precede free water replacement. For euvolemic hypernatremia caused by diabetes insipidus, desmopressin is indicated in central forms, while nephrogenic forms may respond to thiazide diuretics or amiloride if lithium-induced. In hypervolemic hypernatremia due to iatrogenic sodium gain, discontinuation of sodium sources and administration of hypotonic fluids are essential. Frequent monitoring is emphasized, as overly aggressive treatment risks seizures from cerebral edema, while undercorrection prolongs morbidity and mortality risk.

CONCLUSION

This chapter emphasizes that sodium disorders are frequent, clinically significant, and potentially life-threatening. Hyponatremia and hypernatremia must be classified by volume status, with careful attention to an underlying disease processes. Diagnostic algorithms integrating urine studies, osmolality, and clinical context are essential for appropriate classification. Management strategies differ by etiology, but the guiding principles are gradual correction and prevention of iatrogenic complications. Ultimately, optimal outcomes depend on individualized therapy, close monitoring, and addressing the root cause of sodium imbalance.

FURTHER READINGS

1. Hoorn EJ, Zietse R. Hyponatremia and mortality: moving beyond associations. Am J Kidney Dis. 2013;62(1):139-49.
2. Mannesse CK, Vondeling AM, van Marum RJ, van Solinge WW, Egberts TC, Jansen PA. Prevalence of hyponatremia on geriatric wards compared to other settings over four decades: a systematic review. Ageing Res Rev. 2013;12(1):165-73.
3. Gankam-Kengne F, Ayers C, Khera A, de Lemos J, Maalouf NM. Mild hyponatremia is associated with an increased risk of death in an ambulatory setting. Kidney Int. 2013;83(4):700-6.
4. Hawkins RC. Age and gender as risk factors for hyponatremia and hypernatremia. Clin Chim Acta. 2003;337(1-2):169-72.
5. Pfennig CL, Slovis CM. Sodium disorders in the emergency department: a review of hyponatremia and hypernatremia. Emerg Med Pract. 2012; 14(10):1-26.
6. Verbalis JG, Goldsmith SR, Greenberg A, Korzelius C, Schrier RW, Sterns RH, et al. Diagnosis, evaluation, and treatment of hyponatremia: expert panel recommendations. Am J Med. 2013;126(10 suppl 1):S1-S42.

SECTION 12

Neurology

CHAPTER 33

Guillain–Barré Syndrome: Expanding Clinical Spectrum

Gurinder Mohan, Kapeesh Khanna, Asra Brar, Sehajnoor Singh

■ CASE SCENARIO

A 32-year-old previously healthy man presented with rapidly progressive, symmetric limb weakness evolving from mild fatigue to quadriplegia within days, eventually requiring mechanical ventilation. Examination revealed preserved cranial nerves, intact sensation, global areflexia, and severe motor weakness (proximal > distal, neck flexors also weak). Initial cerebrospinal fluid (CSF) was normal, but repeat CSF after 2 weeks showed albuminocytologic dissociation. Nerve conduction studies demonstrated absent compound muscle action potential (CMAPs) with preserved sensory nerve action potential (SNAPs), consistent with motor axonal involvement. Serum *Campylobacter jejuni* immunoglobulin G (IgG) was positive.

Question
Based on the above clinical presentation, examination findings, and investigations, what is the most likely diagnosis?

This case highlights some important aspects of Guillain–Barré syndrome (GBS). While typically GBS symptoms reach a clinical nadir by 2 weeks, occasionally weakness can progress at an alarming speed requiring intubation and mechanical ventilation within a few days of onset. Once extensive axonal degeneration was documented and evaluation for other causes was unrevealing, the diagnosis of acute motor axonal neuropathy (AMAN) was established. In this setting, early supportive interventions and multidisciplinary rehabilitation are recommended rather than combining or repeating immunotherapies. This case also highlights the presence of subclinical infection in GBS, which, in a recent study, was found to be present in 28% of patients. Although antecedent infection testing does not alter care, it may offer valuable prognostic information.

■ INTRODUCTION

Guillain–Barré syndrome is an acute, immune-mediated polyneuropathy representing one of the most common neuromuscular emergencies encountered in clinical practice. With an incidence of 0.81–1.91 cases per 100,000 person-years,

GBS affects patients across all age groups but shows a slight male predominance and increased incidence with advancing age. This condition demands immediate recognition and prompt intervention due to its potential for rapid progression and life-threatening complications.

PATHOPHYSIOLOGY

Guillain–Barré syndrome develops as a consequence of an aberrant immune response, most often triggered by antecedent infections such as *Campylobacter jejuni*, *Cytomegalovirus*, Epstein–Barr virus, or *Mycoplasma pneumoniae*. Through the process of molecular mimicry, antibodies generated against microbial antigens cross-react with peripheral nerve components, particularly gangliosides present on axonal membranes or Schwann cells. This autoimmune attack leads to inflammatory injury manifested either as segmental demyelination, which slows or blocks nerve conduction, or as direct axonal degeneration, which produces more severe deficits and delayed recovery. The pathological pattern varies between subtypes, with acute inflammatory demyelinating polyradiculoneuropathy (AIDP) predominating in Western countries and AMAN or acute motor–sensory axonal neuropathy (AMSAN) being more frequent in certain Asian and Latin American regions. Understanding these mechanisms not only helps explain the heterogeneity in clinical presentation but also provides insights into prognosis, as axonal variants are often associated with slower or incomplete recovery compared to demyelinating forms **(Fig. 1)**.

Key Pathogenic Mechanisms

- *Demyelinating forms (AIDP):* Attack on myelin proteins leading to conduction block
- *Axonal forms (AMAN/AMSAN):* Attack on gangliosides (GM1, GD1a) at nodes of Ranvier
- *Miller Fisher syndrome*: Anti-GQ1b antibodies targeting cranial nerves

CLINICAL PRESENTATION

The clinical presentation of GBS follows a characteristic temporal pattern that helps distinguish it from other acute neuropathies and guides management decisions.

Classic Four-phase Clinical Course

1. *Prodromal phase*: This phase follows an antecedent event such as an infection, surgery, or vaccination. Patients may also report vague symptoms like malaise, fatigue, or body aches before neurological features appear.
2. *Progressive phase*: Neurological symptoms such as weakness, paresthesias, or autonomic changes develop and progress over days to weeks. By definition, worsening occurs within 4 weeks, and in severe cases, patients may rapidly lose the ability to walk or breathe independently.

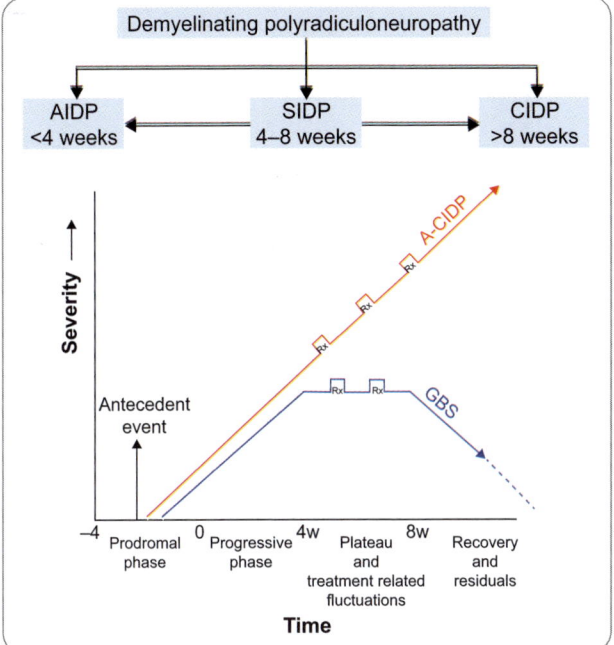

FIG. 1: GBS and its variants form a continuum: Symptom progression under 4 weeks suggests AIDP, 4–8 weeks points to SIDP, and over 8 weeks or multiple relapses indicates CIDP, while up to 10% of GBS cases may show treatment-related fluctuations.

(AIDP: acute inflammatory demyelinating polyradiculoneuropathy; CIDP: chronic inflammatory demyelinating polyradiculoneuropathy; GBS: Guillain–Barré syndrome; SIDP: subacute inflammatory demyelinating polyradiculoneuropathy)

3. *Plateau phase*: The rapid deterioration stops, and symptoms remain stable without further worsening. This stage usually lasts 1–4 weeks, during which patients often require supportive care for weakness, pain, or autonomic instability.
4. *Recovery phase*: Gradual improvement in strength and function begins, often over weeks to months. While most patients regain independence, some may be left with mild residual deficits **(Fig. 2)**.

Core Clinical Features

The clinical manifestations of GBS involve multiple systems, with motor symptoms typically dominating the presentation.

Motor symptoms:
- Symmetric ascending weakness (legs → arms)
- Proximal and distal muscle involvement
- Hyporeflexia or areflexia (may be delayed up to 1 week)
- Cranial nerve involvement (facial weakness in 50% and bulbar dysfunction in 40%)

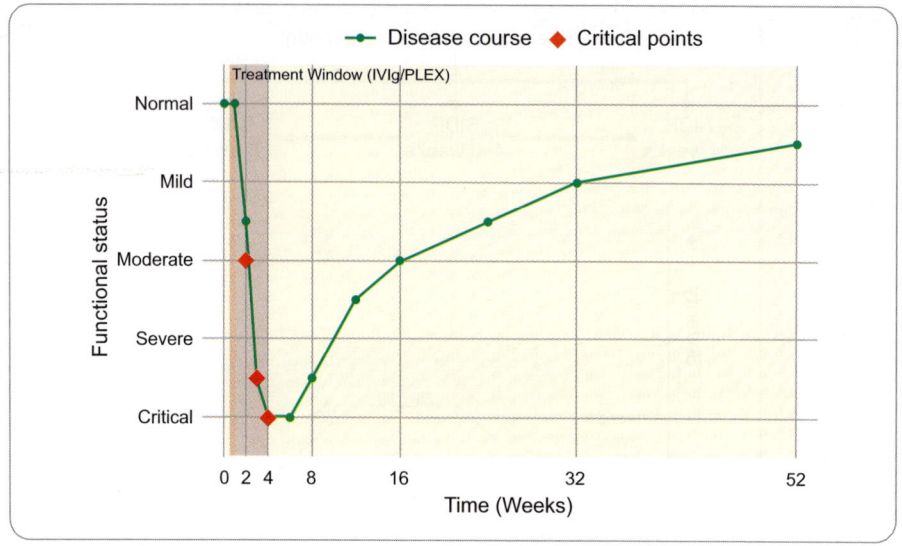

FIG. 2: GBS clinical timeline.
(GBS: Guillain–Barré syndrome)

Sensory symptoms:
- Distal paresthesias (acroparesthesia)—early symptom
- Mild objective sensory loss (often delayed)
- Neuropathic pain (common, often severe)

Autonomic features (66% of patients):
- Cardiac arrhythmias
- Blood pressure lability
- Orthostatic hypotension
- Gastrointestinal dysmotility
- Urinary retention

Respiratory involvement: This represents the most life-threatening complication of GBS.
- Required in 10–30% of patients
- Can progress rapidly, requiring emergency intubation

DIAGNOSTIC CRITERIA

The diagnosis of GBS is primarily clinical, relying on a detailed history and careful neurological examination. It is supported by characteristic laboratory findings, such as albuminocytological dissociation in CSF, and electrodiagnostic studies showing demyelination or axonal involvement. Standardized diagnostic criteria help establish the diagnosis with greater accuracy while also highlighting atypical features that may suggest alternative conditions or mimics, such as myelopathies, neuromuscular junction disorders, or metabolic neuropathies **(Box 1)**.

> **BOX 1: Core diagnostic criteria for GBS.**
>
> *Required features:*
> - Progressive weakness in more than one limb
> - Areflexia or hyporeflexia
>
> *Supporting features:*
> - Progression over days to 4 weeks
> - Relative symmetry
> - Mild sensory symptoms/signs
> - Cranial nerve involvement
> - Autonomic dysfunction
> - Pain
> - Elevated CSF protein
> - Characteristic electrodiagnostic features
>
> (CSF: cerebrospinal fluid; GBS: Guillain–Barré syndrome)

Red Flags Suggesting Alternative Diagnosis

The following clinical features should prompt consideration of other conditions:
- Severe respiratory dysfunction with limited limb weakness at onset
- Slow progression >4 weeks without cranial/autonomic involvement
- Severe sensory signs with limited weakness
- Bladder/bowel dysfunction at onset
- Sharp sensory level
- Marked persistent asymmetric weakness
- Fever at onset
- CSF pleocytosis > 50 cells/µL

CLASSIFICATION OF GUILLAIN–BARRÉ SYNDROME SUBTYPES

Recognition of different GBS subtypes is important for prognosis and management planning. Each subtype has distinct clinical features and recovery patterns **(Table 1 and Flowchart 1)**.

Localized Variants

Several localized variants present with restricted anatomical involvement:
- *Pharyngeal–cervical–brachial*: Mimics botulism
- *Paraparetic*: Mimics spinal cord lesion
- *Bifacial palsy with paresthesias*: Isolated cranial involvement
- *Acute pandysautonomia*: Pure autonomic involvement

DIAGNOSTIC INVESTIGATIONS

A systematic approach to laboratory and ancillary investigations is essential to support the diagnosis of GBS and to rule out other possible causes of acute

SECTION 12: Neurology

TABLE 1: GBS subtypes and clinical features.

Subtype	Frequency	Key features	Electrophysiology
AIDP	85–90% (Western countries)	Classic sensorimotor GBS	Demyelinating features
AMAN	More common in Asia	Pure motor, rapid recovery possible	Axonal motor involvement
AMSAN	Less common	Severe motor–sensory, poor prognosis	Axonal motor–sensory
Miller Fisher	5%	Ophthalmoplegia, ataxia, and areflexia	Anti-GQ1b positive (85–90%)

(AIDP: acute inflammatory demyelinating polyradiculoneuropathy; AMAN: acute motor axonal neuropathy; AMSAN: acute motor–sensory axonal neuropathy; GBS: Guillain–Barré syndrome)

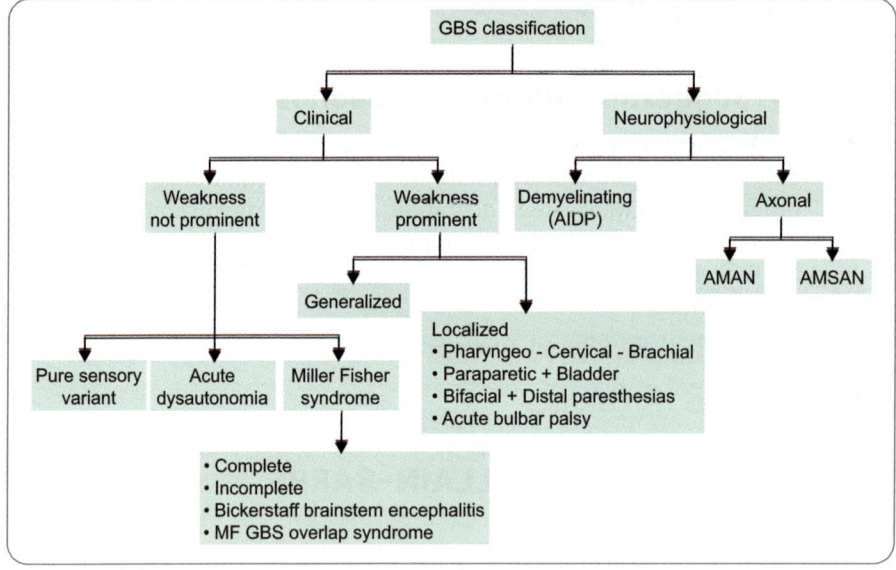

FLOWCHART 1: GBS classification.

(AIDP: acute inflammatory demyelinating polyradiculoneuropathy; AMAN: acute motor axonal neuropathy; AMSAN: acute motor–sensory axonal neuropathy; GBS: Guillain–Barré syndrome; MF: Miller Fisher)

neuropathy. The CSF analysis often shows albuminocytological dissociation, while nerve conduction studies and electromyography (EMG) provide objective evidence of demyelination or axonal damage. Additional tests, such as basic blood work, infectious serologies, and imaging studies, may be required to exclude alternative neurological or systemic conditions that can mimic GBS.

Cerebrospinal Fluid Analysis

Lumbar puncture remains a key diagnostic test in suspected GBS.
- *Classic finding*: Albuminocytologic dissociation
- *Protein*: Often normal in the first week, elevated >90% by week 2

- *Cell count*: Usually <10 cells/μL (up to 20 acceptable)
- *Red flag*: >50 cells/μL suggests an alternative diagnosis

Electrodiagnostic Studies

Nerve conduction studies and EMG provide crucial diagnostic and prognostic information, though findings evolve over time.

Early findings (first week):
- Prolonged or absent F-waves
- Absent H-reflexes
- May be normal initially

Later findings:
- *AIDP*: Conduction block, temporal dispersion, and prolonged distal latencies
- *AMAN*: Reduced CMAP amplitudes and preserved conduction velocities
- *"Sural sparing":* Preserved sural SNAP with abnormal upper limb sensory responses

Antiganglioside Antibodies

While helpful in specific subtypes, antiganglioside antibody tests have limited routine clinical utility.
- *Anti-GQ1b*: Positive in 85–90% of Miller Fisher syndrome
- *Anti-GM1*: Associated with AMAN, especially post-*C. jejuni*
- *Limited routine utility*: Negative results do not exclude GBS.

TREATMENT

The management of GBS requires a combination of disease-specific immunotherapy and meticulous supportive care. Early recognition and timely initiation of therapy significantly improve patient outcomes by reducing complications and speeding recovery. Intravenous immunoglobulin (IVIG) and plasma exchange (PLEX) are the mainstay treatments, both shown to shorten the disease course and enhance functional recovery. Equally important is supportive care, which includes close monitoring of respiratory function, prevention of complications such as deep vein thrombosis or infections, and multidisciplinary rehabilitation to aid in long-term recovery.

Supportive Care Priorities

Vigilant monitoring for complications is essential in all GBS patients (**Flowchart 2**).

Respiratory Monitoring
- *20/30/40 rule*: Vital capacity < 20 mL/kg, maximum inspiratory pressure (MIP) < 30 cmH$_2$O, and maximum expiratory pressure (MEP) < 40 cmH$_2$O
- *Erasmus GBS Respiratory Insufficiency Score (EGRIS)*: Score > 4 indicates high risk.
- Monitor every 2–4 hours in the acute phase.

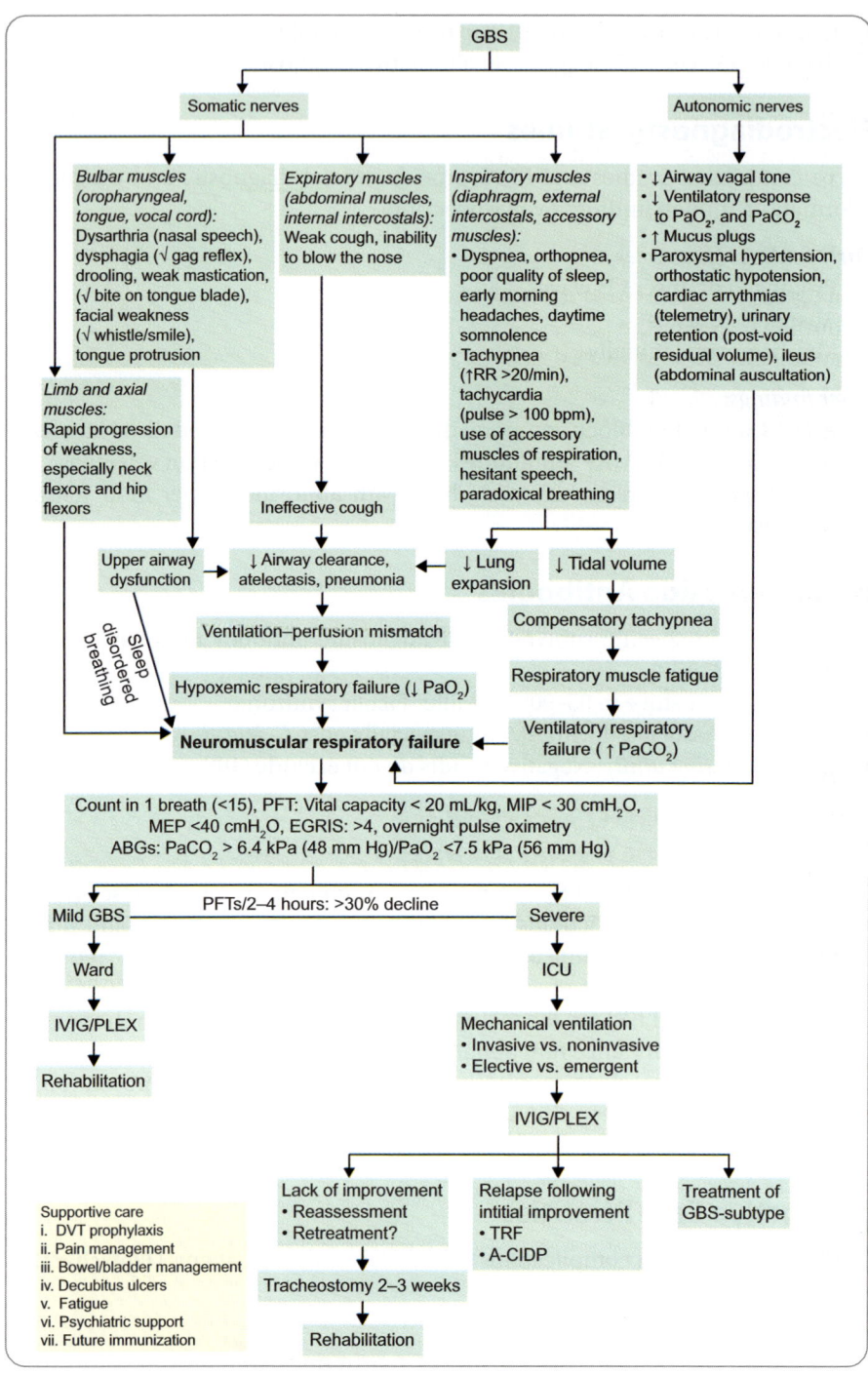

FLOWCHART 2: Treatment strategy for respiratory involvement.

(ABG: arterial blood gas; DVT: deep vein thrombosis; EGRIS: Erasmus GBS Respiratory Insufficiency Score; GBS: Guillain–Barré syndrome; ICU: intensive care unit; IVIG: intravenous immunoglobulin; MEP: maximum expiratory pressure; MIP: maximum inspiratory pressure; PFT: pulmonary function test; PLEX: plasma exchange; RR: respiratory rate; TRF: treatment-related fluctuations)

Intensive Care Unit Indications
- Dysautonomia
- Bulbar dysfunction
- Severe/Rapidly worsening weakness
- Respiratory distress

Immunotherapy
Two equally effective treatments are available for GBS, with choice depending on institutional factors and patient characteristics **(Table 2)**.

Treatment Indications
- Inability to walk 10 meters independently
- Should be started within 2 weeks (IVIg) or 4 weeks (PLEX) of symptom onset
- Consider for ambulatory patients with rapid progression or bulbar/respiratory involvement

Treatment Failures
- Up to 40% show no improvement after initial therapy.
- *Avoid*: Combination therapy or repeat courses (no proven benefit)
- Focus on aggressive supportive care and rehabilitation.

Contraindicated Treatments
Certain treatments have been proven harmful and must be avoided.
- *Corticosteroids*: Detrimental effect proven in multiple trials
- *Depolarizing neuromuscular blockers*: Risk of hyperkalemia

PROGNOSIS

Understanding prognostic factors helps guide treatment decisions and patient counseling.

OUTCOME PREDICTORS

Several clinical and laboratory factors influence long-term outcomes.

TABLE 2: Immunotherapy options.				
Treatment	**Dosing**	**Duration**	**Efficacy**	**Considerations**
IVIg	0.4 g/kg/day	5 days	Equal to PLEX	Easier administration, better tolerated
IVIg	1 g/kg/day	2 days	Equal efficacy	Higher treatment-related fluctuations in children
Plasma exchange	200–250 mL/kg	5 sessions over 10 days	Equal to IVIg	Requires vascular access, more complications
(IVIg: intravenous immunoglobulin; PLEX: plasma exchange)				

Favorable Prognosis Indicators
- Younger age
- Rapid onset and early plateau
- Preserved CMAP amplitudes
- Demyelinating subtype

Poor Prognosis Indicators
- Advanced age (>60 years)
- Rapid progression to severe weakness
- Need for mechanical ventilation
- Low CMAP amplitudes (axonal loss)
- Preceding diarrheal illness

RECOVERY EXPECTATIONS

Most patients with GBS achieve good functional recovery, though the timeline can be prolonged.
- *80% can walk independently at 1 year.*
- *>50% recover completely.*
- *20% have significant residual deficits.*
- Recovery may continue beyond 1 year, especially in axonal forms.

MORTALITY

While overall mortality is low, certain complications carry a significant risk.
- *Overall mortality:* 3–7%
- *Ventilated patients:* ~20% (higher in resource-limited settings)
- *Common causes of death*: ARDS, infections, pulmonary embolism, and sudden cardiac arrest

DIFFERENTIAL DIAGNOSIS

A systematic approach to differential diagnosis prevents misdiagnosis and inappropriate treatment **(Tables 3 and 4)**.

TABLE 3: Key differential diagnoses.

Presentation	Consider
Pure motor weakness	Motor neuron disease, myopathy, myasthenia gravis, and botulism
Paraparesis with sensory level	Spinal cord compression and transverse myelitis
Asymmetric weakness	Vasculitic neuropathy and multiple mononeuropathies
Cranial neuropathies	Brainstem stroke, myasthenia gravis, and botulism
CSF pleocytosis	CNS infections and inflammatory disorders

(CNS: central nervous system; CSF: cerebrospinal fluid)

TABLE 4: GBS versus acute CIDP.

Feature	GBS	Acute-onset CIDP
Time to maximal deficit (Nadir)	<4 weeks	>8 weeks or repeated relapses
Clinical course	Monophasic, usually single episode	Multiphasic, ≥3 relapses or ongoing progression
Response to initial immunotherapy	Plateau after IVIg/PLEX, slow recovery	Temporary improvement, then relapse after initial immunotherapy
Motor or sensory involvement	Sensory symptoms present, often mild	Sensory deficits and ataxia more prominent, vibration/proprioception loss
Cranial nerve/autonomic features	Common (facial, bulbar, autonomic)	Rarely prominent in A-CIDP
Preceding infection	Typical (GI/respiratory illness)	Rare or absent
Need for ventilation	10–30%	Rare in A-CIDP
Long-term treatment	Not indicated after recovery	Maintenance immunosuppressive therapy may be required
Electrodiagnostic features	Demyelination/axonal on NCS/EMG	*Similar demyelinating features*: Serial studies show continued activity

(CIDP: chronic inflammatory demyelinating polyradiculoneuropathy; EMG: emectromyography; GBS: Guillain–Barré syndrome; GI: gastrointestinal; IVIg: intravenous immunoglobulin; NCS: nerve conduction studies; PLEX: plasma exchange)

SPECIAL CONSIDERATIONS

Treatment-related Fluctuations

This phenomenon occurs in a subset of patients and must be distinguished from other conditions.
- Occurs in ~10% of patients within 8 weeks of treatment
- Distinguished from acute-onset CIDP by:
  - Fewer relapses (<3)
  - Response to retreatment with the same therapy
  - More likely to have an antecedent infection and autonomic involvement

COVID-19 and Vaccination

Current evidence regarding the relationship between COVID-19 and GBS:
- *COVID-19*: No established causal relationship with GBS
- *mRNA vaccines*: No increased GBS risk
- *Ad.26.COV2.S vaccine*: Small increased risk (32.4 vs. 1–2 per 100,000 person-years)

CONCLUSION

The following practical points help optimize patient care and outcomes:
- *Early recognition is crucial*: Do not wait for classic ascending paralysis—GBS can present with cranial nerve involvement first.
- *Respiratory monitoring is paramount*: Clinical assessment is more important than absolute pulmonary function test (PFT) values.
- *CSF can be normal early*: Do not exclude GBS based on normal CSF in the first week.
- *Electrodiagnostic studies evolve*: Repeat testing may be needed for subtype classification.
- *Treatment timing matters*: Earlier treatment (within 2 weeks) provides maximum benefit.
- *Avoid corticosteroids*: Proven harmful in multiple studies
- *Recovery is often prolonged*: Set realistic expectations with patients and families.
- *Multidisciplinary care is essential*: Early involvement of PT, OT, and respiratory therapy.

FURTHER READINGS

1. Jankovic J, Mazziotta JC, Pomeroy SL, Newman NJ. Bradley's Neurology in Clinical Practice. Guillain-Barré syndrome and related disorders. 8th edition. 2021.
2. Willison HJ, Jacobs BC, van Doorn PA. Guillain-Barré syndrome. Lancet. 2016;388(10045): 717-27.
3. Hughes RAC, Raphaël JC, Swan AV, van Doorn PA. Intravenous immunoglobulin for Guillain-Barré syndrome. Cochrane Database Syst Rev. 2014;(9):CD002063.

CHAPTER 34

Approach to Myelopathy

Ashutosh Kumar Karn, Amit Aggarwal, MPS Chawla

INTRODUCTION

Myelopathy refers to dysfunction of the spinal cord, presenting with motor, sensory, and autonomic deficits. Prompt and structured evaluation is critical, as many causes are reversible. The term "transverse myelitis" is now discouraged, with preference for "inflammatory myelopathy" to reflect diverse immune-mediated mechanisms involving aquaporin 4 (AQP4) or myelin oligodendrocyte glycoprotein (MOG) antibodies, T/B cell infiltration, and innate immune activation. Common triggers include autoimmune, demyelinating, infectious, and paraneoplastic conditions. At the same time, recognition of noninflammatory mimics—such as vascular, structural, or metabolic disorders—has improved diagnostic accuracy and reduced unnecessary immunosuppression. After excluding compressive causes, the next step is identifying the underlying etiology.

SPINAL CORD ANATOMY AND CLINICAL SYNDROMES

The adult spinal cord spans from the cervicomedullary junction to the conus medullaris at the lower border of L1, measuring approximately 45 cm—shorter than the 70 cm vertebral column. Vertebral levels do not match spinal segments: Cervical levels align, upper thoracic lie two levels above, and lower thoracic three. T9–T11 vertebrae correspond to lumbar segments and T12–L1 to sacral segments. Nerve roots below L1 form the cauda equina, where lesions produce asymmetric lower motor neuron (LMN) signs as shown in **Figure 1**. This vertebra–segment mismatch is essential in lesion localization; for example, a T8 vertebral fracture may cause sensory loss at the T12 level. **Figure 2** depicts the spinal cord cross-section showing various tracts.

The spinal cord contains many tracts, but three key ones for localization are lateral corticospinal, posterior column, and spinothalamic as depicted in **Figure 3**.

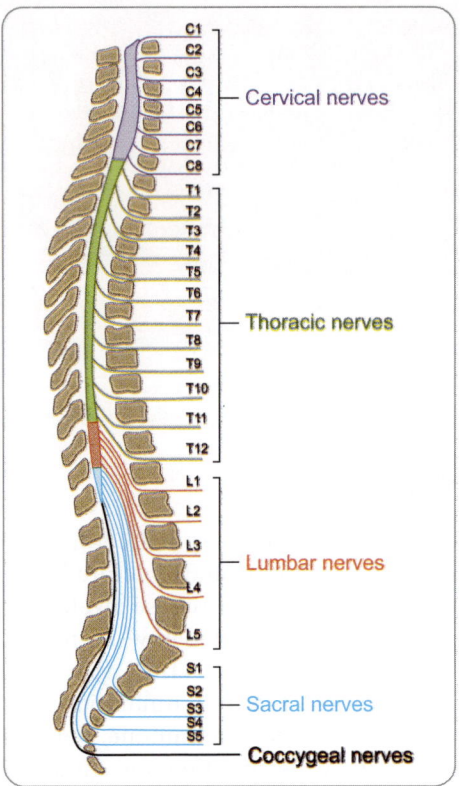

FIG. 1: Relationship between spinal cord segments, spinal nerves, and vertebral column.

Posterior Column

The posterior column transmits fine touch, vibration, and conscious joint position sense. The pathway ascends ipsilaterally, decussates in the medulla, and projects to the sensory cortex. Posterior column lesions produce ipsilateral loss of vibration and proprioception below the lesion, sensory ataxia with a positive Romberg's test, Lhermitte's sign, paresthesias (including glove-and-stocking and girdle sensations), and washbasin sign.

Lateral Spinothalamic Tract

The lateral spinothalamic tract conveys pain and temperature from the opposite side. First-order dorsal root ganglia (DRG) neurons enter the dorsal horn, ascend one to two segments, and synapse in the dorsal gray and second-order fibers cross via the anterior commissure and ascend as the lateral spinothalamic tract—sacral fibers lateral and cervical fibers medial—to the thalamus and then project to the cortex. Lesions cause contralateral analgesia and tract pain.

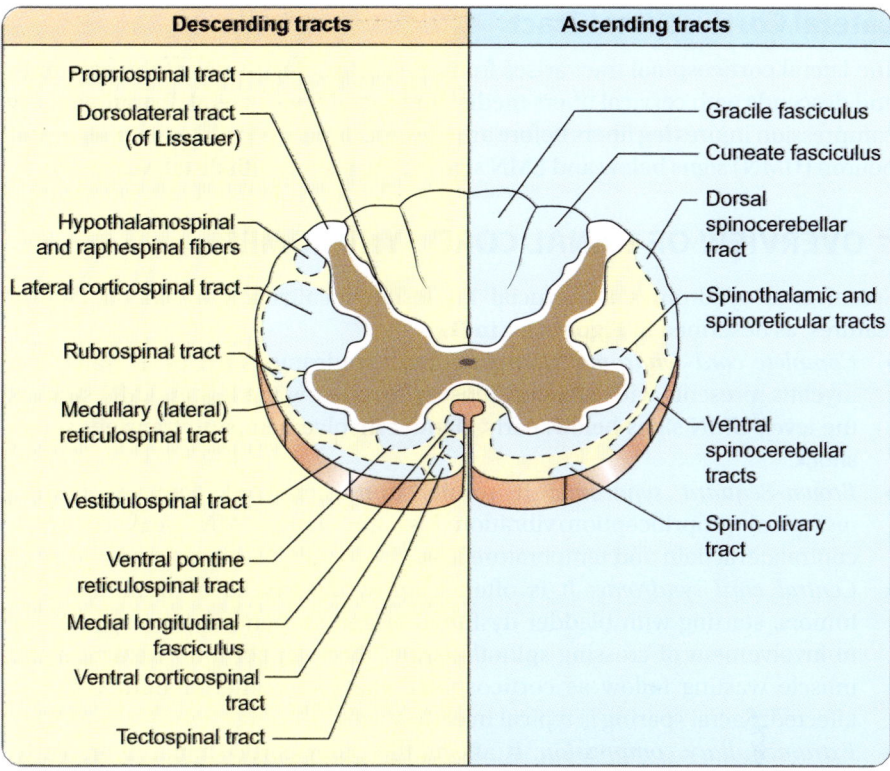

FIG. 2: Cross-section of the spinal cord showing central gray matter with ascending and descending tracts of the outer white matter.

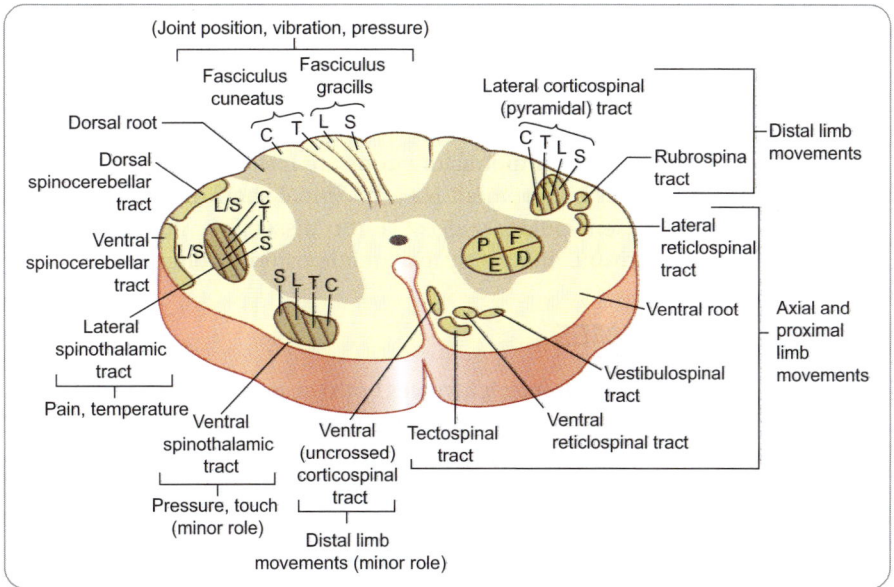

FIG. 3: Main tracts with the arrangement of fibers.

Lateral Corticospinal Tract

The lateral corticospinal tract arises from the cortex, decussates at the pyramids, and descends with cervical fibers medial and sacral fibers lateral. Extramedullary compression injures leg fibers before arm; lesions produce ipsilateral upper motor neuron (UMN) signs below and LMN signs at the lesion, with distal weakness.

■ OVERVIEW OF SPINAL CORD SYNDROMES

Spinal cord syndromes are crucial for lesion localization based on clinical features, as described in **Figures 4A to D**.

- *Complete cord syndrome*: Complete cord syndrome, such as in transverse myelitis, presents with bilateral sensory loss below the lesion, LMN signs at the level, UMN signs below, early bladder involvement, and transient spinal shock.
- *Brown–Séquard syndrome*: It results from hemicord damage, causing ipsilateral proprioception/vibration loss and LMN–UMN weakness, with contralateral pain and temperature loss.
- *Central cord syndrome*: It is often from syringomyelia or intramedullary tumors, starting with bladder dysfunction and suspended sensory loss due to involvement of crossing spinothalamic fibers. Upper limb weakness and muscle wasting follow as corticospinal tracts and anterior horn cells are affected. Sacral sparing is typical in early stages.
- *Extramedullary compression*: It affects the outer corticospinal fibers early, causing increased lower limb tone and plantar responses, with later bladder symptoms. Root pain aggravated by straining and vertebral signs help differentiate extradural (e.g., metastasis) from intradural (e.g., meningioma) causes.
- *Anterior spinal artery syndrome*: The anterior spinal artery supplies the anterior two thirds of the spinal cord, with key reinforcement from the artery of Adamkiewicz (T9–T12). Occlusion causes infarction sparing the posterior column, leading to bilateral UMN signs below and LMN signs at the lesion level. Pain, temperature, and motor functions are lost, while proprioception remains intact. Bladder involvement is early. Spinal shock may mimic LMN features initially. Absent pulses suggest aortic dissection. Posterior spinal artery infarcts are rare and affect only ipsilateral posterior columns.

■ OTHER SYNDROMES

- *Posterolateral column syndrome*: It involves both the posterior column and the lateral corticospinal tract, typically seen in subacute combined degeneration from vitamin B12 deficiency. Other causes include human immunodeficiency virus (HIV) myelopathy, copper deficiency, and zinc toxicity.
- *Posterior column syndrome*: It affects only the posterior column, with syphilitic myelopathy as the main cause, though idiopathic cases exist.
- *Anterior horn syndrome*: It results from damage to anterior horn cells, seen in spinal muscular atrophy (SMA), poliomyelitis, and Hirayama disease, producing LMN signs.

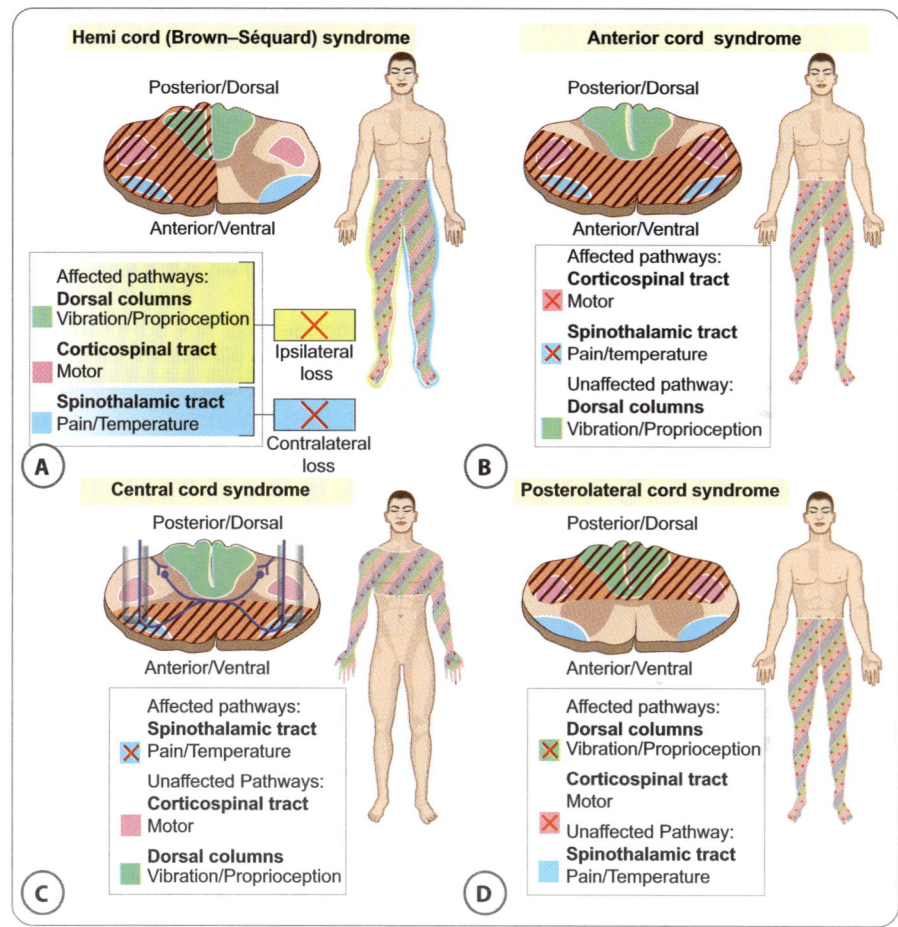

FIGS. 4A TO D: Spinal cord syndromes.

- *Anterior horn corticospinal tract syndrome*: As in amyotrophic lateral sclerosis (ALS), it involves both upper and lower motor neuron findings due to combined tract and cell damage.

CLINICAL APPROACH TO MYELOPATHY

When a patient presents with weakness or sensory symptoms suggesting a likely lesion in the spinal cord, we need to approach it in a stepwise manner, as elaborated in **Table 1**.

Clinical Localization of Spinal Cord Disorders

Spinal cord lesions are localized axially (intramedullary vs. extramedullary) and longitudinally (cervical, thoracic, lumbar, or sacral). Examples include transverse myelitis (intramedullary) and cervical spondylosis with myelopathy (extramedullary) as described in **Tables 2 and 3**. Longitudinal localization identifies the specific segmental level within each region, as explained in **Table 4**.

TABLE 1: Stepwise approach to myelopathy.

Steps	Question/Focus	Details
1	Do symptoms and signs suggest spinal cord involvement?	Suspect spinal cord disease if the patient has UMN-type weakness with/without tract-specific sensory loss *Caveats:* • UMN signs may be masked by LMN features (e.g., epiconus/conus lesions) • LMN syndromes (e.g., GBS) may mimic UMN lesions in the acute phase • Anterior horn cell pathologies (e.g., viral, ischemia) can mimic GBS • Spinal shock may mimic LMN weakness in early UMN lesions
2	Where is the lesion localized?	• Longitudinal localization (based on motor, sensory, reflex, and dermatomal levels)
3	What are the substrates involved?	*Identify affected anatomical structures based on transverse localization:* • Posterior columns • Spinothalamic tract • Corticospinal tract • Central gray matter
4	What is the syndromic diagnosis?	*Based on the pattern of signs/symptoms from step 2:* • Typical spinal cord syndrome • Syndrome-plus (if additional features exist)
5	What is the possible etiology?	*Consider based on clinical profile:* • Age/Gender • Onset (hyperacute/acute/subacute/chronic) • Progression (static/progressive/relapsing) • Symmetry • Associated systemic disease • Family history
6	What is the possible pathology?	*Examples:* • Demyelination (e.g., MS, NMO) • Infection (e.g., viral, bacterial, TB) • Neoplasm • Vascular (e.g., infarct, AVM)
7	What is the functional status?	*Assess mobility and independence:* • Ambulatory • Dependent • Bedbound • Important for rehabilitation planning

(AVM: arteriovenous malformation; GBS: Guillain–Barré syndrome; LMN: lower motor neuron; MS: multiple sclerosis; NMO: neuromyelitis optica; TB: tuberculosis; UMN: upper motor neuron)

TABLE 2: Comparison of intramedullary versus extramedullary spinal cord lesions.

Feature	Extramedullary spinal cord lesion	Intramedullary spinal cord lesion
Site of involvement	Outside the cord (intradural or extradural)	Within the cord
Symmetry	Asymmetrical	Symmetrical
Spontaneous pain	Radicular, localized distribution, early and important symptom	Funicular, burning type, poorly localized, usually bilateral, and often involves large areas of the body
Sensory changes	Contralateral loss of pain and temperature, ipsilateral loss of proprioception (Brown–Séquard type)	Dissociative sensory loss, spotty changes
Changes in saddle area pain and temperature	More marked than at level of lesion, sensory level below site of lesion	Less marked than at level of lesion, sensory loss suspended
Dissociative sensory loss (loss of spinothalamic senses and preservation of posterior column senses)	Rare	Characteristic feature
Location of sensory loss	May present with ascending sensory level	Can cause suspended sensory loss, most prominent at level of lesion
LMN involvement	Segmental	Marked and widespread with atrophy and fasciculation
UMN involvement	Prominent	Can be late and less prominent
Distribution of motor weakness	Cervical lesions cause ipsilateral arm weakness, followed by ipsilateral leg weakness before spreading to the contralateral side	Cervical lesions can cause unilateral or bilateral upper limb paresis and sparing of lower limbs in early stages (suspended weakness)
DTR (deep tendon reflexes)	Increased early	Late
Bladder and bowel	Late	Early
Trophic changes	Not marked	Can be marked
Spinal subarachnoid block and changes in spinal fluid	Early and marked	Late and less marked
Etiology	Intradural (meningioma, nerve sheath tumor), extradural (herniated disc, metastases, myeloma, osteoma)	Ependymoma, astrocytoma, syringomyelia/syrinx, hemangioblastoma, multiple sclerosis, myelitis

(LMN: lower motor neuron; UMN: upper motor neuron)

TABLE 3: Localization in the spinal cord.

Domain	Clinical feature	Localization insight
Sensory localization	Band-like radicular pain or segmental paresthesia	*Indicates lesion level*: • Cervical → radiates to arms • Thoracic → wraps around chest/abdomen • Lumbar/Sacral → radiates to legs
	Uppermost level of sensory loss	Useful in acute myelopathies (e.g., transverse myelitis, disc prolapse)
	Intramedullary lesion pattern	Initial "jacket-like" sensory loss due to crossing fibers; descending pain loss on the opposite side as the lesion progresses
	Extramedullary lesion pattern	Initial sacral sensory loss ascending upward due to the lateral spinothalamic fiber arrangement
	Variable sensory loss patterns	Especially common in progressive cervical myelopathies
Motor localization	LMN signs at the lesion level + UMN signs below	Segmental LMN signs help pinpoint the lesion site
	Example: Bilateral pyramidal signs + absent biceps reflex	Suggests C5–C6 cervical cord lesion
Reflex localization	Absent reflex above brisk reflexes	Indicates pyramidal tract involvement at a specific spinal segment
	Absent biceps/supinator + brisk lower limb reflexes	Localizes to C5–C6
	Absent triceps reflex	Suggests C7 involvement
	Paraplegia + absent lower abdominal reflex + intact upper	Localizes to T10 segment
	Absent both upper and lower abdominal reflexes	Suggests lesion above T6
Autonomic localization	Loss of bladder/bowel control, sweating, piloerection	Autonomic dysfunction below the lesion level
	Lower limb edema	Due to impaired vasomotor tone and temperature regulation
	Erectile dysfunction	*Lesion above L1 impairs voluntary erections*: • Psychogenic erections require intact descending pathways • Reflex erections arise from S2 to S4 segments
	Ejaculatory dysfunction	Often impaired; mediated by multiple spinal segments

(LMN: lower motor neuron; UMN: upper motor neuron)

CHAPTER 34: Approach to Myelopathy

TABLE 4: Longitudinal localization of spinal cord lesions.

Level/Syndrome	Motor signs	Reflex changes	Sensory findings	Other key features/Notes
Foramen magnum	UMN weakness, round-the-clock progression, or cruciate hemiplegia	Exaggerated reflexes	Onion skin facial sensory loss; C2 suboccipital pain	Downbeat nystagmus, papilledema, Lhermitte's sign
High cervical (C1–C4)	Quadriparesis, SCM and trapezius weakness, possible diaphragmatic palsy	Generalized hyperreflexia	Sensory loss from C2 downward	Involves the spinal accessory and phrenic nerves
C5–C6	LMN weakness in the deltoid, biceps	↓ Biceps, ↓ supinator; ↑ triceps, ↑ finger flexors	Inversion of the brachioradialis reflex; lateral arm sensory spared	Brachioradialis tap may cause finger flexion only
C7	Wrist flexor/extensor weakness	↓ Triceps; paradoxical triceps reflex	↓ Sensation over third/fourth digits	↑ Finger flexor reflex
C8–T1	Hand muscle wasting, spastic paraparesis	↓ Finger flexor reflex	↓ Sensation over the fifth digit, medial forearm/arm	± Horner's syndrome
Thoracic cord (T4–T12)	Spastic paraplegia	Reflexes vary: Absent at the lesion level; ↑ below	Reliable sensory level; nipple (T4), umbilicus (T10)	Root pain, bladder/bowel/sexual dysfunction, autonomic dysreflexia (>T6), Beevor's sign (T10)
L1	Spastic paraparesis	↑ Knee and ankle jerk	Sensory loss below the groin	Lower abdominal weakness is hard to detect
L2–L4	Weakness in the hip flexors, thigh muscles	↓ Knee jerk; ↑ ankle jerk	↓ Sensation over the anteromedial thigh	Absent cremasteric reflex in L2; spared anterior thigh in pure L4 lesion
L5	Weak EHL, foot dorsiflexion	↑ Ankle jerk; normal knee jerk	↓ Sensation in L5 distribution	Preserved hip/knee function
S1–S2	Weak plantarflexion, foot muscle weakness	↓ Ankle jerk; normal knee jerk	↓ Sensation in the sole, heel, outer foot, posterior thigh, saddle	Consider epiconus if L4–S2 involved
Conus medullaris	Pelvic floor weakness	Absent anal and bulbocavernosus reflexes	Saddle anesthesia (S3–S5)	Early bladder/bowel/sexual dysfunction; symmetric presentation
Cauda equina	LMN-type asymmetrical leg weakness	Variable knee/ankle reflexes	Asymmetric radicular sensory loss	Late bowel/bladder issues; severe radicular pain early

(EHL: extensor hallucis longus; LMN: lower motor neuron; SCM: sternocleidomastoid; UMN: upper motor neuron)

Localization in the Spinal Cord

Spinal cord localization relies on motor, sensory, reflex, and autonomic findings, primarily dermatomes. Identifying the most caudal intact neurological level helps determine the lesion level; this requires both root and segmental functions at that level.

Localization in the Upper Spinal Cord (Craniocervical Junction and High Cervical Cord) Syndromes

Upper spinal cord lesions (cervical/thoracic) show UMN signs and early bladder involvement. Sensory levels help localize thoracic lesions, but reflexes are more reliable. LMN signs indicate lesion level; UMN signs may originate above. Examining tracts and vascular zones aid in the diagnosis. Various clinical phenomena are seen in the lesion of high cervical cord/craniocervical junction, that is, jaw jerk, cruciate hemiplegia, downbeat nystagmus, Elsberg "U" phenomenon, reversed dissociated sensory loss, V1 sensory loss, neck tongue sign, lingual pseudoathetosis, myelopathy hand, scapulohumeral reflex, trapezius reflex, and glove and stocking sensory loss. The pathways and clinical significance of "jaw jerk reflex" are explained in detail in **Table 5**. The cruciate syndromes have been described in **Table 6** and craniocervical junction syndromes have been detailed in **Table 7**.

Myelopathy Mimics: Key Considerations

Several conditions can mimic progressive myelopathy. DOPA-responsive dystonia and stiff person syndrome may present with spasticity and normal spinal imaging. Brainstem vascular malformations and parafalcine meningiomas can cause long tract signs or spastic paraparesis. Brain imaging is essential when spinal imaging is negative. Superior sagittal sinus thrombosis and carotid stenosis

TABLE 5: Jaw jerk reflex.

Aspect	Details
Definition	A monosynaptic stretch reflex causing a subtle upward jerk of the jaw via the masseter, temporalis, and medial pterygoid muscles
Elicitation	Tap the relaxed chin with a reflex hammer while supporting with an index finger
Neural pathway	• *Afferent:* Masseter muscle spindles → mesencephalic nucleus of CN V • *Efferent:* Motor nucleus of CN V → pons
Clinical significance	• *Normal:* Often imperceptible • Exaggerated jaw jerk suggests bilateral UMN lesions above the trigeminal motor nucleus (e.g., suprabulbar pathology) • Craniocervical junction lesions may show limb hyperreflexia without exaggerated jaw jerk • Lesions at the foramen magnum may exaggerate the reflex due to brainstem dysfunction

(CN: cranial nerve; UMN: upper motor neuron)

TABLE 6: Cruciate syndromes.

Phenomenon	Details
Location	Lesions at pyramidal decussation (craniocervical junction; medulla to C2)
Cruciate hemiplegia	Ipsilateral upper limb UMN weakness + contralateral lower limb UMN weakness
Cruciate paralysis	Bilateral upper limb UMN weakness, lower limbs spared
Mechanism	Decussation pattern: Upper limb fibers cross rostrally, so midline or lateral lesions at the pyramids result in characteristic upper-limb-focused weakness
Differential diagnosis	Central cord syndrome may mimic cruciate paralysis due to anterior horn involvement at cervical levels

(UMN: upper motor neuron)

TABLE 7: Craniocervical junction syndromes.

Phenomenon	Description	Localization/Etiology
Elsberg "U" phenomenon	*Sequential limb weakness*: Ipsilateral arm → leg → contralateral leg → arm	Intradural compressive myelopathy at the cervicomedullary junction; vascular/pressure factors
Downbeat nystagmus	Downward fast component of vertical nystagmus on down gaze	Cervicomedullary junction; Chiari I, foramen magnum tumors, demyelination
Reversed dissociated sensory loss	Impaired vibration/position in upper limbs and torso; lower regions spared	Medial lemniscus decussation compression; basilar invagination, odontoid lesions
Trigeminal (V1) sensory changes	Loss of pain/temp in forehead/peripheral face; perioral area spared	High cervical cord lesion; spinal trigeminal nucleus (onion peel pattern)
Neck-tongue syndrome	Neck pain with ipsilateral tongue paresthesia, worsened by movement	Irritation of lingual afferents via ansa cervicalis; atlanto-occipital instability
Myelopathy hand	Finger escape; reduced grip-release cycle in ulnar fingers	Pyramidal tract lesion in the high cervical cord
Trapezius jerk	Shoulder elevation upon tapping the trapezius muscle	Reflex from C3–C4 segments; exaggerated in UMN lesions above C3
Scapulohumeral reflex	Abduction of the humerus or scapular elevation upon tapping the scapula/acromion	Indicates UMN lesion cranial to C3

(UMN: upper motor neuron)

may also present as paraparesis. Guillain–Barré syndrome may resemble or be mistaken for myelopathy.

False Localizing Signs in Spinal Lesions

False localizing signs occur when spinal cord lesions produce symptoms away from the actual lesion site. Due to somatotopic fiber arrangement, cervical compression may affect sacral fibers first, causing misleading sensory loss. High cervical or foramen magnum lesions can cause hand atrophy, dysesthesia, and limb UMN signs. The *"finger escape sign"* reflects ulnar finger weakness in high cervical myelopathy. Cervical stenosis may mimic ALS with mixed UMN/LMN signs. Mechanisms include ischemia, venous stasis, and mechanical distortion, often yielding misleading clinical presentations.

Cord-specific Clinical Phenomena

Spinal cord disorders often present with characteristic signs aiding lesion localization, severity assessment, and distinguishing degenerative from nondegenerative causes. Key features include Lhermitte's sign, flexor/extensor spasms, girdle sensation, spinal shock, and postural patterns of paraplegia.

Flexor spasms suggest severe UMN lesions with loss of supraspinal inhibition. They are uncommon in degenerative diseases and often lead to paraplegia in flexion due to unopposed flexor tone.

Lhermitte's sign is an electric shock-like sensation on neck flexion, indicating dorsal column dysfunction. It may also occur in neck extension (reverse sign) or with ascending paresthesia (inverse sign), seen in multiple sclerosis (MS), B12 deficiency, and cervical spondylosis.

Spinal shock is a temporary state following acute spinal cord injury, characterized by loss of motor, sensory, and reflex functions below the lesion. Initially, patients show flaccid paralysis, atonic bladder and bowel, and absent reflexes. The return of bulbocavernosus or anal reflexes signals the end of spinal shock, followed by UMN signs like spasticity and Babinski response. Recovery occurs in phases: Areflexia (0–24 hours), reflex return (1–3 days), early hyperreflexia (4 days–1 month), and spasticity (1–12 months). Reflex recovery follows a predictable order. Differentiation from conus/epiconus lesions relies on reflex. The presence of the bulbocavernosus reflex and a delayed plantar response supports a diagnosis of spinal shock due to a pyramidal (UMN) lesion, rather than an LMN lesion in the conus or epiconus region. Mechanisms include loss of descending input, elevated glycine, and synaptic changes.

Girdle sensation is a band-like pain or tightness from T3 to T11, often mimicking thoracic pathology. It may actually result from cervical cord compression, especially affecting the anterior spinal artery, especially around the T4 watershed zone, making it a false localizing sign.

A few diagnostic clues toward clinical localization of the lesion to the spinal cord are discussed in **Box 1**.

Etiologic Spectrum

The differential diagnosis of noncompressive myelopathy is extensive. A systematic classification based on the inflammatory versus noninflammatory framework is essential for a structured evaluation as defined in **Table 8**.

BOX 1: Clinical interpretation of neurological signs.

Signs strongly suggestive of spinal cord:
- Suspended band of sensory loss
- Sensory level on torso
- Spinal tract crossed findings (pyramidal on one side and contralateral spinothalamic)
- Dissociated sensory loss conforming to cord syndrome (syringomyelia, anterior spinal artery)
- Root plus long tract signs (sarcoidosis, spondylosis)
- Isolated tractopathy (anterior horn, posterior column, spinothalamic)
- Lhermitte's sign
- Urinary retention*

Signs consistent with, but not diagnostic of, spinal cord:
- Bilateral symmetric sensory loss with normal reflexes (consider polyneuropathy)
- Paraparesis without sensory signs (consider parasagittal location)
- Hyporeflexia (consider polyneuropathy)
- Unilateral or bilateral upper motor neuron signs (consider brain or brainstem)
- Ascending sensory loss (consider AIDP or CIDP)
- Exertional worsening of symptoms (consider vascular, MS, or lumbar stenosis)

Signs NOT suggestive of spinal cord:
- Monoparesis of the arm
- Cranial nerve deficits (other than V)
- Pure lower motor neuron signs
- Paratonia (frontal lobe), stiffness rather than spasticity (SPS, PD)
- Dysarthria, dysphagia, brisk jaw reflex (brainstem or ALS)
- Weakness with normal sensation and reflexes (MG)
- Proximal muscle weakness (watershed or myopathy)

*Isolated urinary retention would be an unusual initial spinal cord symptom and raises the possibility of bifrontal pathology or mechanical/pharmacological obstruction.

(AIDP: acute inflammatory demyelinating polyneuropathy; ALS: amyotrophic lateral sclerosis; CIDP: chronic inflammatory demyelinating polyneuropathy; MG: myasthenia gravis; MS: multiple sclerosis; PD: Parkinson's disease; SPS: stiff-person syndrome)

TABLE 8: Etiologic classification of noncompressive myelopathies.

Category	Subcategory	Specific etiologies	Typical temporal profile
Inflammatory (myelitis)	Demyelinating	Multiple sclerosis (MS), acute disseminated encephalomyelitis (ADEM)	• *Subacute*: Relapsing-remitting MS • *Acute*: ADEM
	Antibody-mediated	Neuromyelitis optica spectrum disorder (NMOSD), MOG antibody-associated disease (MOGAD)	Acute/Subacute, relapsing
	Systemic inflammatory	Neurosarcoidosis, systemic lupus erythematosus (SLE), Sjögren's syndrome	Subacute to chronic

Continued

Continued

Category	Subcategory	Specific etiologies	Typical temporal profile
	Infectious/ Postinfectious	Viral (VZV, HSV, Enterovirus), bacterial (TB, syphilis), parasitic (schistosomiasis)	Acute to chronic
	Paraneoplastic	Anti-Hu, anti-CRMP5, antiamphiphysin	Subacute, progressive
Noninflammatory	Vascular	Spinal cord infarction, dural arteriovenous fistula (dAVF), AVM, cavernoma	Hyperacute: Infarct; chronic: dAVF
	Metabolic/ Nutritional	Vitamin B12 deficiency, copper deficiency, nitrous oxide toxicity	Subacute to chronic
	Others	Radiation myelitis, drug-induced	Chronic

(AVM: arteriovenous malformation; CRMP5: collapsin response mediator protein 5; HSV: herpes simplex virus; MOG: myelin oligodendrocyte glycoprotein; TB: tuberculosis; VZV: varicella-zoster virus)

Temporal Profile: A Key Diagnostic Tool

The speed of symptom progression offers vital clues to spinal cord pathology. Hyperacute onset (≤6 hours) suggests vascular events like infarction. Acute progression (6–48 hours) points to infectious or postinfectious myelitis, such as acute flaccid myelitis. Subacute onset (2–21 days) is typical of inflammatory myelopathies like MS, neuromyelitis optica spectrum disorder (NMOSD), and MOG antibody-associated disease (MOGAD). Chronic evolution (>21 days) indicates compressive, metabolic, or vascular causes. A relapsing–remitting course strongly supports an autoimmune etiology, particularly MS, NMOSD, or MOGAD. Temporal patterns guide accurate and timely diagnosis **(Fig. 5)**.

Clinicoradiological Approach to Myelopathy

The initial step is identifying an intramedullary T2 hyperintensity and ruling out compression. Subsequent branching is determined by the temporal profile (acute vs. chronic) and key magnetic resonance imaging (MRI) features (lesion length and axial location), guiding the differential diagnosis toward specific etiologies as described in **Flowchart 1**. The various imaging signs of myelopathy have been enumerated in **Table 9**.

High-yield Serologic and Cerebrospinal Fluid Biomarkers

- *Aquaporin-4 immunoglobulin G (AQP4-IgG)*: The pathogenic antibody and specific diagnostic marker for NMOSD. Its detection confirms the diagnosis and mandates specific relapse-prevention therapies.
- *MOG-IgG*: The diagnostic marker for MOGAD, a distinct inflammatory demyelinating disease. Both AQP4-IgG and MOG-IgG should be tested using live cell-based assays for optimal sensitivity and specificity.

CHAPTER 34: Approach to Myelopathy

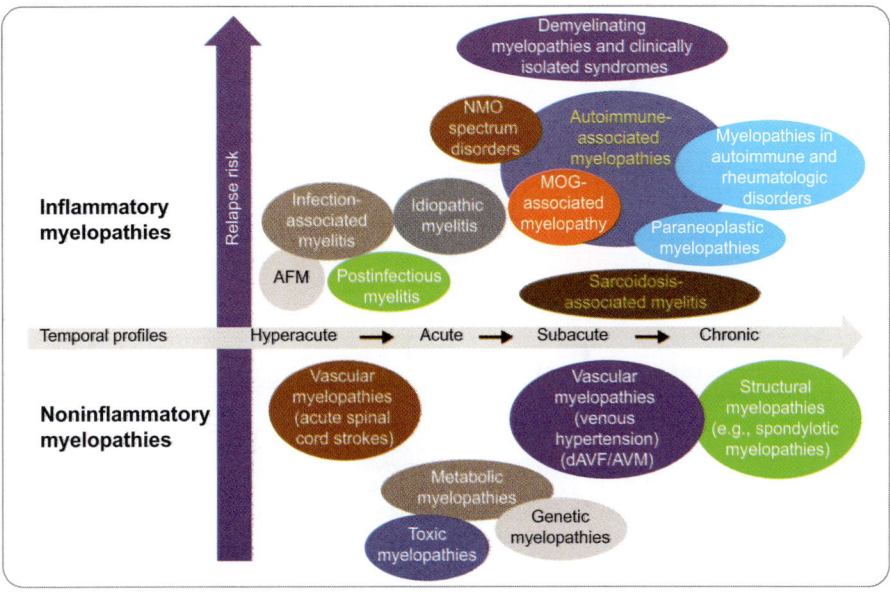

FIG. 5: Temporal profile of symptom evolution in myelopathies with diverse pathogenic mechanisms.

(AFM: acute flaccid myelitis; AVM: arteriovenous malformation; dAVF: dural arteriovenous fistula; MOG: myelin oligodendrocyte glycoprotein; NMO: neuromyelitis optica)

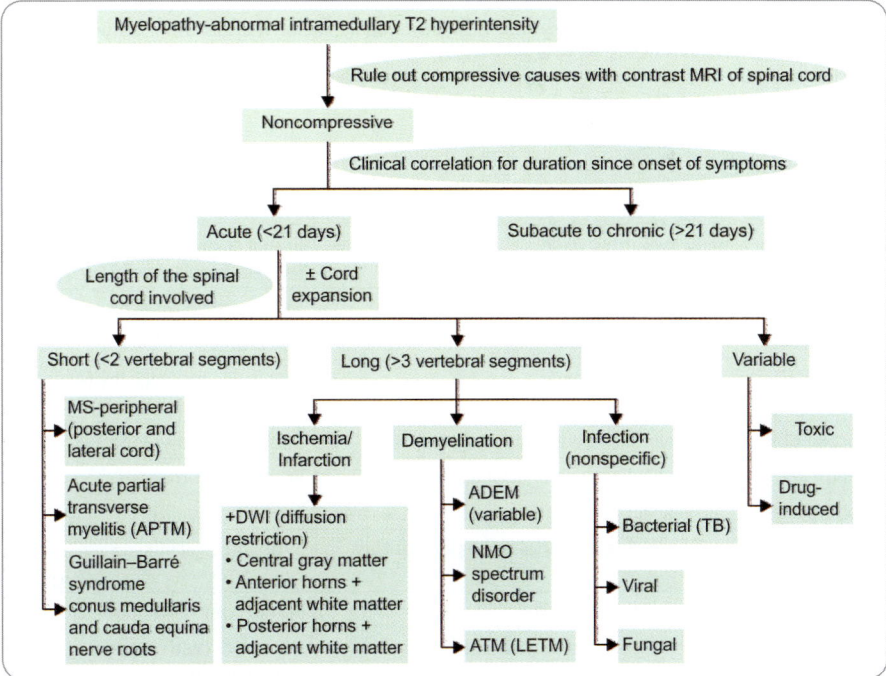

FLOWCHART 1: Continued

Continued

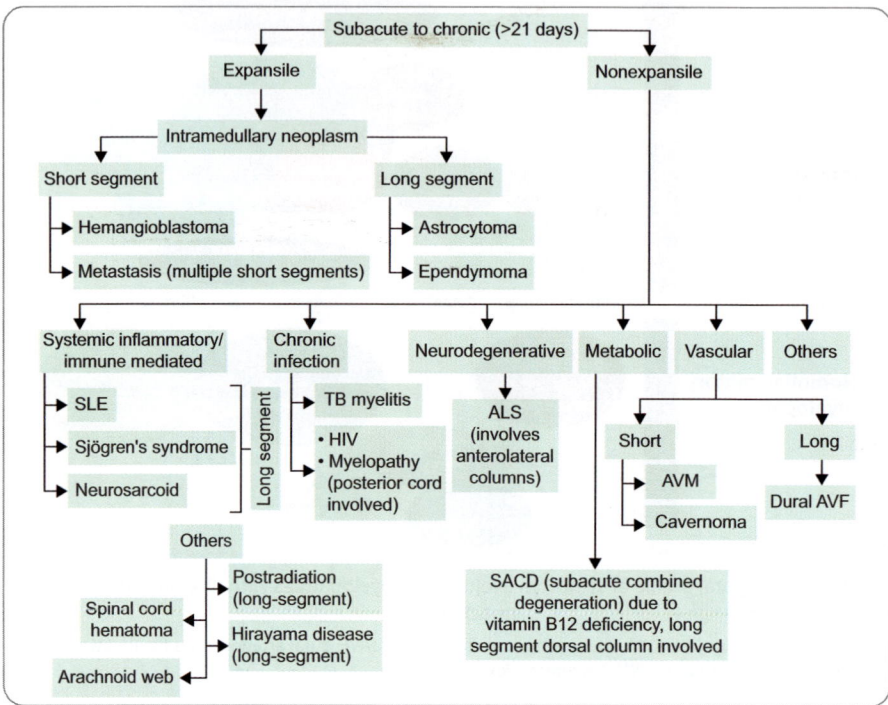

FLOWCHART 1: Clinicoradiological approach to myelopathy. (The initial step is identifying an intramedullary T2 hyperintensity and ruling out compression).

(ADEM: acute disseminated encephalomyelitis; ALS: amyotrophic lateral sclerosis; ATM: acute transverse myelitis; AVF: arteriovenous fistula; AVM: arteriovenous malformation; HIV: human immunodeficiency virus; LETM: longitudinally extensive transverse myelitis; MS: multiple sclerosis; MRI: magnetic resonance imaging; NMO: neuromyelitis optica; SLE: systemic lupus erythematosus; TB: tuberculosis)

TABLE 9: Myelopathy signs (T2-weighted, T1-weighted with gadolinium).		
Imaging sign	**MRI sequence**	**Associated condition(s)**
Owl or snake eyes sign	T2-weighted axial	Spinal cord ischemia, infection-related flaccid myelitis (WNV)
"H" sign	T2-weighted axial	MOG-related myelitis
Trident sign	T1-weighted with gadolinium (sagittal)	Sarcoidosis
Inverted "V" sign	T2-weighted axial	Metabolic myelopathy (e.g., vitamin B12 deficiency)
Pancake sign	T1-weighted with gadolinium (axial)	Spondylotic myelopathy
"Y" sign	T1-weighted with gadolinium (sagittal)	Epidural lipomatosis
Flip-flop sign	T2- and T1-weighted pre- and postcontrast	Syphilitic myelitis
Candle-guttering appearance	T2-weighted sagittal or T1-postcontrast	Syphilitic myelitis
Scalpel sign	T2-weighted sagittal	Spinal cord herniation
Missing-piece sign	T1-weighted with gadolinium (sagittal)	Dural AVF (with patchy enhancement)

(AVF: arteriovenous fistula; MOG: myelin oligodendrocyte glycoprotein; WNV: West Nile virus)

TABLE 10: Interpretation of oligoclonal band patterns.

Pattern	Description	Clinical interpretation
1	No bands in CSF or serum	Normal; no evidence of intrathecal IgG synthesis
2	Bands exclusively in CSF	Intrathecal IgG synthesis; highly suggestive of MS in the appropriate clinical and radiological context
3	Bands in CSF with additional identical bands in serum	Intrathecal IgG synthesis in the setting of a systemic immune response
4	Identical "mirror" bands in CSF and serum	Systemic immune response with passive transfer of IgG into CSF; nonspecific
5	Monoclonal band in CSF and serum	Suggests a systemic monoclonal gammopathy (e.g., MGUS, myeloma)

(CSF: cerebrospinal fluid; IgG: immunoglobulin G; MGUS: monoclonal gammopathy of undetermined significance; MS: multiple sclerosis)

- *CSF oligoclonal bands (OCBs)*: The interpretation of paired CSF and serum OCBs is critical for differential diagnosis, as described in **Table 10**.

SUMMARY OF STRATEGIC APPROACH FOR ETIOLOGICAL DIAGNOSIS OF MYELOPATHIES

The strategic approach for establishing a precise etiologic diagnosis of myelopathies includes a comprehensive clinical history and neurologic examination combined with laboratory analysis of blood and CSF along with neuroimaging studies, as depicted in **Figure 6**.

CONCLUSION

A precise diagnosis of myelopathy is essential, as treatment differs significantly between inflammatory and noninflammatory causes. Inflammatory myelopathies require immunotherapy—high-dose steroids initially, followed by plasma exchange or intravenous immunoglobulin (IVIg) for severe cases, and long-term, etiology-specific immunosuppression. Noninflammatory myelopathies demand targeted treatment: Surgical decompression for compressive lesions, embolization for vascular malformations, or nutritional repletion for deficiencies. Immunosuppressants are ineffective and potentially harmful in noninflammatory cases. Accurate diagnosis guides appropriate therapy, prevents harm, and optimizes neurological recovery and long-term functional outcomes.

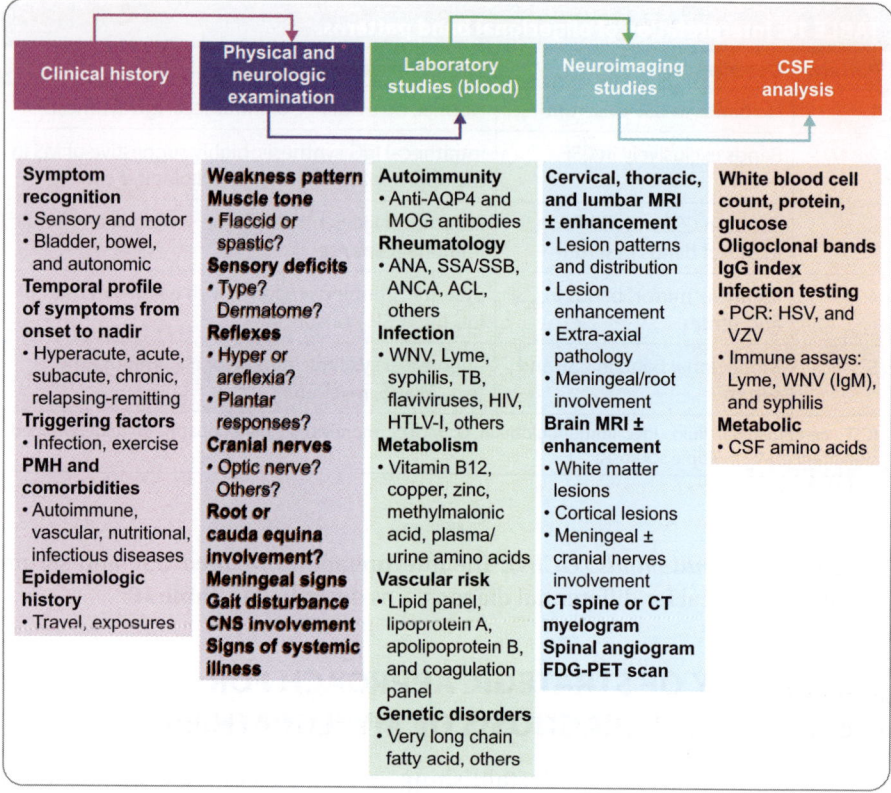

FIG. 6: Strategic approach for etiological diagnosis of myelopathies.

(ACL: anticardiolipin; ANA: antinuclear antibodies; ANCA: antineutrophil cytoplasmic autoantibody; AQP4: aquaporin 4; CNS: central nervous system; CSF: cerebrospinal fluid; FDG-PET: fluorodeoxyglucose positron emission tomography; HIV: human immunodeficiency virus; HSV: herpes simplex virus; HTLV-1: human T-cell lymphotropic virus type 1; IgG: immunoglobulin G; IgM: immunoglobulin M; MOG: myelin oligodendrocyte glycoprotein; PCR: polymerase chain reaction; PMH: past medical history; SSA/SSB: anti-Ro/Sjögren's syndrome A and anti-La/Sjögren's syndrome B; TB: tuberculosis; VZV: varicella zoster virus; WNV: West Nile virus)

FURTHER READINGS

1. Swarup MS, Chandola S, Batra R, Tiwari A, Bhargava R, Saini S, et al. Radiological approach to non-compressive myelopathies. Egypt J Radiol Nucl Med. 2022;53:65.
2. Pardo CA. Clinical approach to myelopathy diagnosis. Continuum (Minneap Minn). 2024;30(1):14-52.
3. Wingerchuk DM, Banwell B, Bennett JL, Cabre P, Carroll W, Kimbrough T, et al. International consensus diagnostic criteria for neuromyelitis optica spectrum disorders. Neurology. 2015;85(2):177-89.
4. Jurynczyk M, Jacob A, Fujihara K, Palace J. Myelin oligodendrocyte glycoprotein antibody-associated disease: practical considerations. Pract Neurol. 2022;22(6):458-67.
5. Kira J, Ochi H. Juvenile muscular atrophy of the distal upper limb (Hirayama disease). Neurol India. 2021;69(Suppl):S329-35.

CHAPTER 35

Autonomic Dysfunction in Diabetes Mellitus

Jugal Kishor Sharma

INTRODUCTION

Diabetes mellitus (DM) is a chronic metabolic disorder characterized by persistent hyperglycemia due to defects in insulin secretion, insulin action, or both. Chronic hyperglycemia leads to widespread microvascular and macrovascular complications, including neuropathy, nephropathy, and retinopathy. Among these, autonomic neuropathy is one of the most complex and debilitating complications, often indicating advanced and long-standing disease. Autonomic dysfunction in diabetes refers to damage to the sympathetic and parasympathetic nerves that regulate involuntary body functions such as heart rate, blood pressure, digestion, bladder control, and thermoregulation. It can occur in both type 1 and type 2 diabetes, with risk and severity increasing with longer disease duration and poor glycemic control. Notably, subclinical autonomic neuropathy may develop within a few years of onset – even earlier in type 2 diabetes where it can be present at diagnosis.

Autonomic dysfunction in diabetes is thus far from rare; various studies suggest anywhere from 20% to over 50% of diabetic individuals have some evidence of autonomic involvement, depending on the population studied, and the prevalence approaches 90% in type 1 diabetics with decades of disease. Despite this high prevalence, DAN often remains undiagnosed until clinically apparent. The condition carries a grave prognosis if unrecognized—cardiovascular autonomic neuropathy (CAN), in particular, is associated with increased mortality risk—underscoring the importance of early detection and intervention. Key risk factors for diabetic autonomic neuropathy include long duration of diabetes, chronic hyperglycemia, hypertension, dyslipidemia, and obesity, especially in the presence of other diabetic complications.

PATHOPHYSIOLOGY

The pathogenesis of diabetic autonomic neuropathy is multifactorial, involving chronic metabolic and vascular insults to nerve fibers. Sustained hyperglycemia triggers several biochemical and structural cascades:

- *Polyol pathway activation*: Excess intracellular glucose is shunted to sorbitol and fructose via aldose reductase. Accumulation of these polyols causes

osmotic stress, depletes nerve myo-inositol, and impairs Na^+/K^+-ATPase activity, ultimately leading to axonal swelling and degeneration.
- *Advanced glycation end-products (AGEs)*: Hyperglycemia drives non-enzymatic glycation of proteins and lipids, producing AGEs that disrupt neuronal cytoskeleton and damage the microvasculature supplying nerves.
- *Oxidative stress*: The diabetic state promotes overproduction of reactive oxygen species, which damage neuronal membranes, organelles, and DNA. Oxidative injury to mitochondria and Schwann cells impairs nerve fiber function.
- *Ischemia of vasa nervorum*: Diabetes-related microangiopathy leads to occlusive changes in the vasa nervorum (the small blood vessels that perfuse nerves). Resultant endoneurial ischemia and hypoxia cause fiber loss and demyelination.
- *Inflammation and immune mechanisms*: Chronic inflammation in diabetes, along with altered immune responses, can contribute to nerve injury through cytokine-mediated damage and autoimmune mechanisms targeting nerve components.

Together, these processes result in distal axonal degeneration and segmental demyelination of autonomic nerve fibers. Both sympathetic and parasympathetic neurons are affected. Early in the course, small unmyelinated fibers tend to lose function (often asymptomatically), while more extensive fiber loss produces the diverse clinical manifestations of autonomic failure.

■ CLINICAL SPECTRUM OF AUTONOMIC DYSFUNCTION

Autonomic dysfunction in diabetes can involve almost every organ system under autonomic control. The clinical spectrum is broad, and manifestations may appear in isolation or together. Major system-wise presentations of diabetic autonomic neuropathy include:

■ CARDIOVASCULAR AUTONOMIC NEUROPATHY

Damage to cardiac sympathetic and vagal fibers can lead to significant cardiovascular abnormalities. *CAN is the most studied and clinically significant form of DAN*, and it is an independent risk factor for cardiovascular mortality. Common features include:
- *Resting tachycardia*: Elevated resting heart rate (often >90–100 bpm) due to loss of vagal tone.
- *Exercise intolerance*: Diminished heart rate and blood pressure response to exercise, limiting exertional capacity.
- *Orthostatic hypotension*: A fall in blood pressure >20 mm Hg systolic (or >10 mm Hg diastolic) upon standing, due to impaired sympathetic vasoconstriction and heart rate response. Patients may experience dizziness, lightheadedness, or syncope on postural change.
- *Silent myocardial ischemia*: Painless myocardial infarctions or ischemia owing to blunted cardiac pain sensation. This can delay recognition of acute coronary syndromes.

- *Cardiac arrhythmias and sudden death*: Autonomic denervation of the heart increases the risk of atrial arrhythmias and lethal ventricular arrhythmias.

Cardiovascular autonomic neuropathy is a powerful predictor of mortality in diabetes, conferring up to a five-fold higher risk of cardiac death. It may initially be asymptomatic (detected only by decreased heart rate variability), but progression leads to the above clinical signs. Given its prognostic importance, routine screening for CAN is advised in long-standing diabetes.

GASTROINTESTINAL AUTONOMIC NEUROPATHY

Autonomic damage to the enteric nervous system can affect any part of the gastrointestinal tract, leading to disordered motility from esophagus to colon. *Diabetic gastroparesis*—delayed gastric emptying due to vagal neuropathy of the stomach—is a hallmark of GI involvement and often underdiagnosed. It can cause erratic glycemic control as food absorption becomes unpredictable.
Symptoms of gastrointestinal autonomic neuropathy include:
- *Esophageal dysmotility*: Dysphagia and odynophagia from impaired esophageal peristalsis and sphincter function.
- *Gastroparesis*: Early satiety, postprandial fullness, nausea, vomiting, and bloating due to delayed gastric emptying. This can lead to poor appetite, weight changes, and extreme glucose fluctuations.
- *Enteropathy*: Alternating constipation and diarrhea. Constipation is especially common (due to prolonged colonic transit), but patients may also experience nocturnal diarrhea or fecal incontinence in severe cases.

In advanced cases, malnutrition and dehydration can result from chronic vomiting or severe diarrhea. Diabetic gastroparesis is particularly challenging to manage and significantly impacts quality of life. It should be suspected in diabetics with upper GI symptoms and erratic glucose control after meals.

GENITOURINARY AUTONOMIC NEUROPATHY

Autonomic neuropathy frequently involves the genitourinary system, with substantial effects on bladder function and sexual health. Typical manifestations include:
- *Bladder dysfunction (diabetic cystopathy)*: A neurogenic bladder characterized by decreased sensation of bladder filling, loss of detrusor contractility, incomplete emptying, and urinary retention. This leads to hesitancy, dribbling, and elevated post-void residual volumes.
- *Recurrent urinary tract infections*: Due to urinary stasis and retention, diabetics with autonomic bladder involvement have an increased risk of UTIs.
- *Erectile dysfunction (ED)*: Up to 50–75% of men with longstanding diabetes develop ED. Autonomic neuropathy impairs penile vasodilation and engorgement. It is often an early presenting symptom of DAN in men.
- *Female sexual dysfunction*: Women may experience reduced vaginal lubrication, dyspareunia (painful intercourse), and anorgasmia as a result of autonomic nerve damage affecting genital blood flow and lubrication reflexes.

These genitourinary issues carry significant psychosocial burden. Erectile dysfunction in particular may prompt evaluation for autonomic neuropathy and often coexist with cardiovascular disease. Early recognition allows for interventions (medical or mechanical) to improve urinary and sexual function and prevent complications such as upper urinary tract damage from chronic retention.

SUDOMOTOR AND THERMOREGULATORY DYSFUNCTION

Sympathetic denervation in diabetes can disrupt normal sweat gland function and thermoregulation:
- *Distal anhidrosis*: Loss of sweating in the feet and distal lower extremities is common, resulting in dry, cracked skin that is prone to ulceration and infection. Impaired sweating in the feet contributes to the pathogenesis of diabetic foot ulcers.
- *Compensatory hyperhidrosis*: Patients may exhibit excessive sweating of the upper body (head, neck, and trunk) especially after meals or at night, as proximal sweat glands overcompensate for peripheral anhidrosis.
- *Heat intolerance*: Diminished overall sweating capacity and blood flow adjustments can lead to poor heat tolerance and difficulty with temperature regulation in hot environments.

This characteristic pattern of sudomotor dysfunction (anhidrosis in the feet with gustatory or upper-body hyperhidrosis) is highly suggestive of diabetic autonomic neuropathy. Regular skin care and monitoring are needed to prevent dryness-related complications.

PUPILLOMOTOR AND OTHER NEUROLOGIC MANIFESTATIONS

Autonomic neuropathy can also involve the pupils and various neuroendocrine reflexes:
- *Impaired pupillary light reflex*: Diabetic autonomic neuropathy may cause pupils to constrict poorly in response to light (due to parasympathetic damage), leading to symptoms of night vision difficulty and glare.
- *Hypoglycemia unawareness*: Perhaps one of the most dangerous manifestations, longstanding diabetes with autonomic failure can blunt the sympathetic adrenergic response to hypoglycemia. Patients may lose the typical warning symptoms (tremors, palpitations, and anxiety) of low blood sugar, putting them at risk for severe hypoglycemic episodes without awareness.
- *Altered circadian blood pressure variation*: Healthy individuals exhibit a "dipping" of blood pressure at night. Autonomic neuropathy can abolish this nocturnal dip (a non-dipping pattern), which is associated with higher cardiovascular risk.

These miscellaneous manifestations underscore that diabetic autonomic neuropathy is truly systemic. Patients should be specifically queried about symptoms such as abnormal sweating, vision changes, or loss of hypoglycemia symptoms, as these may otherwise go unreported.

DIAGNOSTIC APPROACHES

Early detection of autonomic dysfunction is critical, as timely interventions may slow progression and improve outcomes. The diagnosis of diabetic autonomic neuropathy involves a combination of careful clinical evaluation, simple bedside tests, and specialized autonomic function testing where available. A detailed history and physical should seek clues of autonomic impairment (orthostatic vital signs, pupillary responses, skin changes, etc.), followed by objective testing.

Cardiovascular autonomic function tests (AFTs): Standardized cardiovascular reflex tests are the cornerstone for assessing CAN and are recommended for routine screening of diabetic patients with peripheral neuropathy or long-standing disease. These tests evaluate heart rate and blood pressure responses to various maneuvers, primarily reflecting cardiac vagal and sympathetic integrity. The battery of five classic tests and their interpretations are summarized in **Table 1**.

Each individual test result can be informative, but a *definite diagnosis of CAN* usually requires at least two abnormal heart rate tests (deep breathing, standing, or Valsalva) or one abnormal heart rate test plus abnormal blood pressure response. These bedside autonomic function tests are noninvasive, reproducible, and easy to perform. They remain highly useful for early detection and can even uncover subclinical autonomic dysfunction before symptoms arise.

In addition to these reflex tests, other tools are utilized to evaluate autonomic function in different organ systems or more severe cases:

- *Heart rate variability analysis*: 24-hour Holter monitoring and spectral analysis of heart rate variability can quantify cardiac autonomic regulation and often reveal early CAN (loss of high-frequency variability).

TABLE 1: Cardiovascular autonomic reflex tests commonly used to diagnose cardiovascular autonomic neuropathy (CAN) in diabetes.

Test	Predominant autonomic function	Abnormal response (interpretation)
Heart rate response to deep breathing (E:I ratio)	Parasympathetic (vagal)	Reduced HR variability with respiration (e.g., <10 bpm difference or E:I ratio <1.2) indicates vagal dysfunction
Valsalva maneuver (Valsalva ratio)	Parasympathetic and sympathetic	Blunted heart rate/blood pressure response (Valsalva ratio <1.1) suggests autonomic failure. Avoid if proliferative retinopathy is present
Heart rate response to standing (30:15 ratio)	Parasympathetic (vagal)	30:15 R-R interval ratio <1.03 upon immediate standing is abnormal, indicating vagal impairment
Blood pressure response to standing	Sympathetic (adrenergic)	Orthostatic drop ≥20 mm Hg systolic or ≥10 mm Hg diastolic is diagnostic of orthostatic hypotension
Blood pressure response to sustained handgrip	Sympathetic (adrenergic)	Increase in diastolic BP <16 mm Hg during sustained handgrip exercise indicates impaired sympathetic vasomotor function

- *Head-up tilt-table testing*: Formal tilt testing can confirm orthostatic hypotension and evaluate baroreflex sensitivity, useful if bedside orthostatic vitals are equivocal and to assess syncope etiologies.
- *Gastric emptying studies*: Scintigraphic gastric emptying tests or breath tests (using radiolabeled meal) help diagnose diabetic gastroparesis in patients with upper GI symptoms.
- *Quantitative sudomotor axon reflex test (QSART)*: A specialized sweat test measuring autonomic axon reflex-mediated sweating, helpful to document sudomotor dysfunction objectively. Simple bedside alternatives include the thermoregulatory sweat test or skin conductance measurements.
- *Urodynamic studies*: In diabetics with significant bladder dysfunction, urodynamic testing can characterize the neurogenic bladder (e.g., impaired detrusor contractility, increased post-void residuals) and guide management.

Notably, advanced autonomic testing methods are available in research or specialized centers. For example, *cardiac sympathetic imaging* with radiotracers {such as [^{123}I]-metaiodobenzylguanidine scintigraphy} can directly assess cardiac sympathetic innervation and has been used to detect early cardiac autonomic neuropathy. While not routine, such tests underscore the systemic nature of DAN and may help in research settings or complex cases.

CLINICAL STAGING OF AUTONOMIC NEUROPATHY

Diabetic autonomic neuropathy typically progresses through recognizable stages, from subclinical involvement to advanced widespread failure. The staging can be defined as:

- *Early (subclinical) stage*: Abnormal autonomic function test results are present (e.g., reduced heart rate variability or borderline postural BP drop) without obvious symptoms. Patients are generally unaware of any autonomic dysfunction at this stage.
- *Clinical stage*: The patient exhibits clear symptoms and signs of autonomic failure in one or more organ systems—for example, symptomatic orthostatic hypotension, gastrointestinal dysmotility, or bladder dysfunction. This stage often indicates more significant nerve damage.
- *Advanced stage*: Severe, multisystem involvement is present, with disabling symptoms across several domains (cardiovascular, GI, GU, etc.). For instance, a patient may have persistent orthostatic hypotension, gastroparesis requiring nutritional support, and neurogenic bladder with retention.

Importantly, patients may not progress linearly through these stages in all systems—for example, they might have clinical CAN but only subclinical GI neuropathy. *Early identification at the subclinical stage offers the best opportunity for intervention.* If autonomic dysfunction is detected through testing before symptoms develop, aggressive management of risk factors (especially hyperglycemia) may delay progression to symptomatic disease. This underlines the value of routine screening in at-risk diabetic patients.

MANAGEMENT

There is currently *no definitive cure* for diabetic autonomic neuropathy; management focuses on optimizing glycemic control, alleviating symptoms, reducing risks of complications, and improving quality of life. A multifaceted, individualized approach is required, often involving multiple specialties (endocrinology, cardiology, neurology, gastroenterology, and urology). Key components of management include:

Glycemic control: Tight and sustained glycemic control remains the cornerstone for preventing or slowing progression of neuropathy. Landmark trials have demonstrated that intensive diabetes management can delay the onset of autonomic neuropathy. In type 1 diabetes, the DCCT showed significant reduction in neuropathy with strict blood glucose control, and similarly, the UKPDS showed reduced neuropathic complications in type 2 diabetes with improved A1c. Therefore, early and intensive glycemic control (while avoiding severe hypoglycemia) is recommended to all patients to mitigate further nerve damage. Newer technologies such as continuous glucose monitoring and insulin pumps can aid in achieving stable glycemia.

Lifestyle modification: Lifestyle interventions are important adjuncts to both prevent and manage autonomic neuropathy. Recommended measures include:
- *Regular physical activity*: Engaging in aerobic exercise can improve cardiovascular fitness, blood pressure stability, and insulin sensitivity. Exercise training has been shown to enhance heart rate variability and may modestly improve autonomic function over time.
- *Dietary adjustments and weight management*: A balanced diet focusing on glycemic control (with adequate fiber and hydration) and achieving a healthy body weight can reduce metabolic stress on nerves. Small, frequent meals may help symptoms of gastroparesis or orthostatic hypotension (by minimizing postprandial BP drops).
- *Smoking cessation and reduced alcohol intake*: Tobacco and excessive alcohol are neurotoxic and can exacerbate neuropathy. Avoiding these can slow progression and improve symptoms (e.g., orthostatic tolerance).
- *Adequate hydration and salt intake*: For those with orthostatic hypotension, ensuring good hydration and modest salt supplementation (if not contraindicated) can expand intravascular volume and mitigate blood pressure drops. Compression stockings and elevation of the head end of the bed at night are additional non-pharmacological strategies for orthostatic symptoms.

Pharmacological management: Targeted pharmacotherapy is used to manage specific manifestations of autonomic dysfunction. While these treatments are symptomatic and do not cure neuropathy, they can substantially improve patient comfort and function:
- *Cardiovascular manifestations*:
  - *Orthostatic hypotension*: Midodrine (an alpha-agonist) is often first-line to raise standing blood pressure. Other options include fludrocortisone (to expand plasma volume), droxidopa, or octreotide. Wearing compression stockings and using vasoconstrictor agents before arising can help.

- *Resting tachycardia*: Low-dose beta-blockers (such as bisoprolol or metoprolol) can be used carefully to reduce excessive resting heart rate and improve exercise tolerance.
- *Silent ischemia*: It requires increased vigilance—although no direct treatment exists for the neuropathy component, these patients warrant regular cardiac screening (stress tests) and aggressive management of cardiovascular risk factors, given their higher risk of silent coronary events.

- *Gastrointestinal symptoms*:
  - *Gastroparesis*: Prokinetic agents such as metoclopramide (with careful use due to side effects), domperidone (where available), or low-dose erythromycin (a motilin agonist) can enhance gastric emptying. Dietary modifications are crucial—patients benefit from small, frequent meals that are low in fat and fiber (to speed gastric transit). In refractory cases, gastric electrical stimulation or jejunal feeding tubes may be considered.
  - *Diabetic diarrhea*: Empirical antibiotics (e.g., tetracycline or metronidazole) can treat small intestinal bacterial overgrowth; loperamide or diphenoxylate can reduce stool frequency; clonidine has been used for its inhibitory effects on intestinal secretions. Episodes of nocturnal diarrhea might respond to an alpha-2 agonist at bedtime.
  - *Constipation*: A high-fiber diet (if tolerated), adequate fluid intake, and exercise form the foundation. Osmotic laxatives (like polyethylene glycol) or stimulant laxatives can be added as needed for symptom relief.

- *Genitourinary and sexual dysfunction*:
  - *Bladder dysfunction*: Emphasize timed voiding schedules and double-voiding techniques to aid bladder emptying. Bethanechol (a cholinergic agonist) may help in some cases. For persistent urinary retention, intermittent self-catheterization is often necessary to protect renal function.
  - *Erectile dysfunction*: Phosphodiesterase-5 inhibitors (sildenafil and tadalafil) are effective in many diabetic men with ED, improving ability to achieve and maintain erections. Vacuum erection devices or intracavernosal injection therapy are options if PDE-5 inhibitors fail. Psychosexual counseling should be offered, since ED can have psychological interplay as well.
  - *Female sexual dysfunction*: Local vaginal estrogen therapy (for postmenopausal women), lubricants to alleviate dryness, and targeted counseling can improve sexual comfort. There is no specific pharmacotherapy for female autonomic sexual dysfunction, so a multidisciplinary approach (gynecologist and counselor) is often needed.

- *Sudomotor dysfunction*:
  - *Anhidrosis (dry skin)*: Regular skin care with emollient creams to moisturize dry areas is recommended. Avoiding extreme temperatures and frequent skin checks (especially on feet) help prevent cracking and ulceration.
  - *Hyperhidrosis*: Focal hyperhidrosis (such as gustatory sweating on the face or upper body) can be managed with strong topical antiperspirants (aluminum chloride). In severe cases, botulinum toxin injections in the affected area provide relief by blocking sympathetic cholinergic

nerves. Systemic anticholinergic medications (such as glycopyrrolate or oxybutynin) can reduce sweating but are often limited by side effects.

It is important to individualize therapy and start with conservative measures before escalating to medications, given the potential side effects (for example, midodrine can cause supine hypertension, and metoclopramide can cause tardive dyskinesia). Patient education is central—patients should understand their condition and the strategies to manage it (such as rising slowly to avoid orthostatic dizziness, or dietary measures for gastroparesis).

Emerging therapies: A number of disease-modifying treatments are under investigation aiming to slow or reverse diabetic neuropathy. These include *antioxidants* (such as α-lipoic acid and acetyl-L-carnitine), which have shown some efficacy in improving neuropathic symptoms and nerve conduction in trials, presumably by reducing oxidative stress. Aldose reductase inhibitors (to block the polyol pathway) were explored in the past and newer agents in this class continue to be evaluated. ACE inhibitors and ARBs—besides their cardiovascular benefits—may have microvascular protective effects that could slow neuropathy progression. Novel approaches such as *autonomic neuromodulation* (through devices or nerve stimulation techniques) are also being studied for therapeutic potential. While none of these emerging treatments have become standard care yet, they offer hope that future interventions might more directly address the underlying nerve damage in DAN.

A comprehensive *multidisciplinary management* is recommended for patients with established autonomic neuropathy. This means not only treating individual symptoms, but also rigorously controlling cardiovascular risk factors (blood pressure and lipids), providing psychosocial support, and coordinating care among specialists. For example, a patient with diabetic autonomic neuropathy might benefit from an endocrinologist to optimize glycemia, a cardiologist for arrhythmia or blood pressure management, a gastroenterologist for refractory GI symptoms, and a neurologist for autonomic testing and guidance. Such coordinated care can substantially improve patient outcomes and safety.

PROGNOSIS AND COMPLICATIONS

Diabetic autonomic neuropathy, especially cardiovascular autonomic neuropathy, portends a serious prognosis. CAN is strongly linked to increased mortality—studies indicate a 2–5 fold higher risk of death in diabetics with CAN compared to those without. The excess mortality is largely due to silent myocardial infarctions, fatal arrhythmias, and cardiogenic sudden death. Additionally, autonomic neuropathy contributes to a range of morbid complications—gastrointestinal autonomic neuropathy can lead to malnutrition, dehydration, and poor glycemic control (from erratic absorption); bladder dysfunction predisposes to chronic urinary infections and renal impairment; and patients with hypoglycemia unawareness are at risk for life-threatening hypoglycemic episodes. The impact on quality of life is also profound—for instance, erectile dysfunction and gastrointestinal issues can cause significant psychological distress and disability.

Despite these challenges, *early identification and proactive management* of autonomic neuropathy can markedly improve the outlook. Patients diagnosed in subclinical stages who receive intensified therapy (for diabetes and comorbid conditions) may experience slower progression. Even in clinical stages, aggressive treatment of symptoms (e.g., using midodrine for orthostasis or prokinetics for gastroparesis) and complication prevention (foot care, hydration, etc.) can reduce hospitalizations and improve day-to-day functioning. The presence of autonomic neuropathy should also prompt clinicians to redouble efforts in controlling cardiovascular risk factors, as this will mitigate some of the mortality risk. With vigilant care, many patients with DAN can stabilize their symptoms and avoid the most severe complications, though ongoing monitoring is essential.

PREVENTION AND SCREENING

Preventing diabetic autonomic neuropathy revolves around optimum diabetes management and regular screening to catch early signs of dysfunction. The American Diabetes Association (ADA) and other expert bodies emphasize tight glycemic control from the outset of diabetes as the primary preventive strategy. In addition, *routine screening for autonomic neuropathy* in high-risk patients is recommended. Current guidelines advise:

- *Type 2 diabetes*: Begin screening for autonomic dysfunction at the time of diagnosis of diabetes and repeat annually thereafter. (Many type 2 patients have had years of undetected hyperglycemia prior to diagnosis, so autonomic neuropathy may already be present.)
- *Type 1 diabetes*: Start screening 5 years after diagnosis (once the patient has had several years of chronic hyperglycemia), and then annually. Youth with type 1 diabetes should be monitored especially as they transition to longer disease duration in adulthood.
- Pay particular attention to patients who already exhibit peripheral neuropathy or have persistently poor glycemic control, as they are at elevated risk for autonomic involvement. In such individuals, more frequent or earlier screening may be justified.

Screening can be performed in the outpatient clinic using the simple bedside tests described earlier (heart rate variability with deep breathing, orthostatic BP measurement, etc.). Incorporating a structured autonomic assessment into routine diabetes visits—even a short battery of bedside tests—greatly aids early detection. Importantly, patients should also be educated to report subtle symptoms (like reduced exercise tolerance or abnormal sweating) which might prompt further evaluation. By implementing regular screening protocols, clinicians can identify autonomic dysfunction in its subclinical phase and intervene early with stricter metabolic control and symptom-specific measures, potentially altering the trajectory of this complication. In summary, prevention of DAN is best achieved by strict glycemic management and risk factor modification from day one of diabetes, and screening is the safety net to ensure it is recognized before irreversible damage occurs.

CONCLUSION

Autonomic dysfunction in diabetes mellitus represents a complex, multisystem disorder with significant clinical and prognostic implications. Despite its relatively high prevalence, diabetic autonomic neuropathy often remains under-recognized until it has progressed to a moderate or advanced stage. Clinicians must maintain a high index of suspicion for autonomic involvement in any longstanding diabetic patient, especially those with other complications or poor glycemic control.

Early detection through focused history, examination, and simple autonomic function tests is essential. Once diagnosed, a *comprehensive management plan* should be instituted—addressing glycemic control, symptomatic treatments, and prevention of secondary complications—ideally through a multidisciplinary team approach. Regular follow-up is important to adjust therapies and to monitor for progression or new autonomic issues in other organ systems. Patient education is equally vital, empowering individuals to manage their condition (for example, teaching measures to avoid orthostatic dizziness or to treat hypoglycemia promptly despite blunted symptoms).

In the evolving landscape of diabetes care, attention to autonomic dysfunction has become an integral component of holistic management. By combining early screening, intensive therapy, and coordinated care, healthcare providers can significantly mitigate the impact of autonomic neuropathy—improving not only survival, but also the day-to-day well-being and functional status of people living with diabetes.

FURTHER READINGS

1. Spallone V. Update on the Impact, Diagnosis and Management of Cardiovascular Autonomic Neuropathy in Diabetes: What Is Defined, What Is New, and What Is Unmet. Diabetes Metab J. 2019;43(1):3-30.
2. Vinik AI, Maser RE, Mitchell BD, Freeman R. Diabetic autonomic neuropathy. Diabetes Care. 2003;26(5):1553-79.
3. Vinik AI, Ziegler D. Diabetic cardiovascular autonomic neuropathy. Circulation. 2007;115(3):387-97.
4. Verrotti A, Prezioso G, Scattoni R, Chiarelli F. Autonomic neuropathy in diabetes mellitus. Front Endocrinol (Lausanne). 2014;5:205.
5. Sharma JK, Rohatgi A, Sharma D. Diabetic autonomic neuropathy: a clinical update. J R Coll Physicians Edinb. 2020;50(3):269-73.
6. The DCCT Research Group. The effect of intensive treatment of diabetes on the development and progression of long-term complications in insulin-dependent diabetes mellitus. N Engl J Med. 1993;329(14):977-86.
7. UK Prospective Diabetes Study (UKPDS) Group. Intensive blood-glucose control with sulphonylureas or insulin compared with conventional treatment and risk of complications in type 2 diabetes (UKPDS 33). Lancet. 1998;352(9131):837-53.
8. Serhiyenko VA, Serhiyenko AA. Cardiac autonomic neuropathy: risk factors, diagnosis and treatment. World J Diabetes. 2018;9(1):1-24.
9. American Diabetes Association. Diabetic Neuropathy: Standards of Medical Care in Diabetes—2016. Diabetes Care. 2016;39(Suppl 1):S72-S80.
10. de Azevedo Vieira ARS, Porto-Dantas LB, do Prado Romani FA, Carvalho PS, Pop-Busui R, Pedrosa HC. Autonomic neuropathic symptoms in patients with diabetes: practical tools for screening in daily routine. Diabetol Metab Syndr. 2023;15(1):83.

CHAPTER 36

Neuromyelitis Optica Spectrum Disorder

Prabhjit Kaur, Aastha Takkar

INTRODUCTION

Neuromyelitis optica spectrum disorder (NMOSD), earlier termed *Devic's disease*, is a severe inflammatory demyelinating disease of the central nervous system (CNS) that primarily targets the optic nerves and spinal cord. The disorder is characterized by recurrent relapses, often resulting in significant morbidity and disability. The central pathophysiological event involves autoimmunity against aquaporin-4 (AQP4), a water channel protein expressed on astrocytic end-feet that maintains the integrity of the blood–brain barrier. The presence of AQP4-IgG (also known as NMO-IgG) serves as a specific and pathogenic biomarker of NMOSD.

The disease was first described by Allbutt in 1870, and later detailed by Devic and Gault in 1894, who provided a systematic description of optic neuritis and myelitis occurring in the same patient. For several decades, controversy persisted over whether NMOSD represented a variant of multiple sclerosis (MS) or a distinct disease. Subsequent advances in clinical, radiological, immunological, and pathological understanding have clearly established NMOSD as a separate entity.

EPIDEMIOLOGY

Neuromyelitis optica spectrum disorder is a rare disorder, but its prevalence and incidence vary considerably across ethnic and geographic populations. The prevalence of NMOSD ranges from 0.3 to 4.4 per 100,000 people. It predominantly affects women (66–88%) and typically presents between 30 and 40 years of age. Pediatric-onset disease is uncommon, accounting for <5% of cases. Although NMOSD occurs worldwide, most epidemiological data come from developed countries, reflecting greater access to magnetic resonance imaging (MRI) and antibody testing. Its proportion among demyelinating disorders varies geographically 1–2% in the United States and Italy, 13.7% in India, and over 30% in Thailand. Indian data are limited; a southern Indian study estimated a prevalence of 2.7 per 100,000.

IMMUNOPATHOLOGY AND PATHOGENESIS

The hallmark lesion of NMOSD is necrosis of both gray and white matter in the spinal cord, associated with perivascular deposition of immunoglobulins and complement components in a rosette-like pattern. These findings support a humoral, antibody-mediated mechanism of injury.

The proposed pathogenesis involves an unidentified antigenic stimulus that triggers peripheral production of AQP4-IgG antibodies. These antibodies cross a disrupted or permeable blood-brain barrier and bind to AQP4 on astrocytic membranes. The antibody-antigen interaction results in internalization of AQP4, complement activation, cytokine release, and recruitment of inflammatory cells such as neutrophils and eosinophils. The ensuing astrocyte loss leads to secondary demyelination and neuronal injury.

Unlike MS, where intrathecal synthesis of oligoclonal bands (OCBs) is a characteristic finding, AQP4-IgG in NMOSD is produced peripherally. Consequently, CSF OCBs are absent in most cases. The peripheral antibody source also explains the marked responsiveness of NMOSD to plasma exchange therapy.

CLINICAL FEATURES

The classical manifestations include longitudinally extensive transverse myelitis (LETM) and optic neuritis (ON), which may occur sequentially or simultaneously. ON is typically severe, often unilateral but occasionally bilateral, and may cause profound, sometimes irreversible, visual loss. Bilateral or rapidly sequential ON is more suggestive of NMOSD than MS.

Spinal cord lesions commonly involve the cervical region and extend across three or more vertebral segments. Attacks often cause severe paraparesis or tetraparesis with sensory level, sphincter dysfunction, and pain. Paroxysmal tonic spasms, dysesthesias, and Lhermitte's sign are frequently reported. Extension of spinal lesions into the medulla can result in intractable hiccups, nausea, vomiting, or respiratory compromise.

Although initially believed to involve only the optic nerves and spinal cord, brain lesions are now recognized in the majority of patients during the disease course. These lesions preferentially occur in regions of high AQP4 expression, such as the periependymal area, hypothalamus, and brainstem. Brainstem involvement may produce hearing loss, vertigo, diplopia, facial weakness, or trigeminal neuralgia. The disease course may be monophasic or relapsing; the latter is much more common (80–90% of cases). Female sex, late onset, coexisting autoimmune disorders, and longer inter-attack intervals predict relapsing disease.

DIFFERENTIATION FROM MULTIPLE SCLEROSIS

Neuromyelitis optica spectrum disorder differs from MS in its epidemiological profile, immunopathogenesis, radiological appearance, CSF characteristics, and ophthalmologic findings. Recognition of these differences is crucial, as several MS-specific immunomodulatory drugs can exacerbate NMOSD.

DIFFERENTIAL DIAGNOSIS

While MS remains the closest mimic, autoimmune diseases such as systemic lupus erythematosus (SLE) and Sjögren's syndrome (SS) can produce overlapping clinical and radiological features. Autoantibodies such as ANA or SSA may be present even in the absence of systemic manifestations. NMOSD has also been described as a paraneoplastic phenomenon, particularly in association with solid tumors, where patients demonstrate typical NMOSD features with AQP4-IgG positivity.

DIAGNOSIS

The discovery of AQP4-IgG in 2004 revolutionized NMOSD diagnosis. AQP4-IgG is present in approximately 70% of patients, with 73% sensitivity and 91% specificity for distinguishing NMOSD from MS.

The Wingerchuk et al. criteria (1999, revised in 2006) formed the basis of diagnostic classification. The 2006 revision required optic neuritis and myelitis as essential features plus at least two of three supportive criteria: (1) contiguous spinal cord lesion extending ≥3 vertebral segments, (2) brain MRI not meeting MS criteria, and (3) serum AQP4-IgG positivity.

In 2014, the International Panel for NMO Diagnosis (IPND) introduced unified diagnostic criteria under the term *NMOSD*. The criteria incorporate six core clinical features-optic neuritis, acute myelitis, area postrema syndrome, brainstem, diencephalic, or cerebral presentations-and stratify patients by AQP4-IgG status.

For AQP4-IgG-positive NMOSD, at least one core clinical feature is sufficient after excluding alternative diagnoses. For seronegative cases, two or more core features (including optic neuritis, LETM, or area postrema syndrome) plus characteristic MRI findings are required.

INVESTIGATIONS

Neuroimaging

Magnetic resonance imaging of the spinal cord typically demonstrates longitudinally extensive T2-hyperintense lesions spanning three or more vertebral segments, often involving the central gray matter. Lesions may enhance with gadolinium and evolve to atrophy or cavitation. In contrast, MS lesions are usually short, asymmetric, and peripherally located.

Optic nerve MRI reveals T2-hyperintensity or gadolinium enhancement extending over more than half the nerve length or involving the optic chiasm. Brain MRI may be normal initially but later shows lesions in AQP4-rich regions such as the periventricular area, hypothalamus, and brainstem. Callosal lesions tend to be large and heterogeneous, unlike the small, well-defined lesions typical of MS.

Cerebrospinal Fluid

Cerebrospinal fluid (CSF) abnormalities are frequent during relapses. Elevated protein and pleocytosis (>50 cells/μL, often neutrophilic) are common, whereas

OCBs are absent or transient. This contrasts sharply with MS, where persistent OCBs and intrathecal IgG synthesis are characteristic.

Antibody Assays

Cell-based assays (microscopy or flow cytometry) provide the highest sensitivity and specificity for AQP4-IgG detection. ELISA and indirect immunofluorescence are less reliable and prone to false results. Some AQP4-negative patients are positive for myelin oligodendrocyte glycoprotein (MOG) antibodies; these cases are usually younger, more often male, and follow a monophasic course with better recovery.

Ophthalmic Evaluation

Fundus examination often shows optic disc edema. Optical coherence tomography (OCT) demonstrates greater thinning of the retinal nerve fiber layer compared to MS, indicating more severe axonal loss. Visual field testing may reveal altitudinal defects, sometimes mimicking ischemic optic neuropathy, reflecting antibody-mediated ischemic injury.

MANAGEMENT

Treatment of Acute Relapses

High-dose intravenous methylprednisolone (1 g/day for 3–5 days) is the preferred first-line therapy, followed by a tapering course of oral prednisone over several months. Most patients respond within 2 weeks.

Plasma exchange (five to seven sessions over 2 weeks) is recommended for steroid-refractory relapses and is most effective when initiated within 5–10 days of symptom onset. In cases where plasma exchange is contraindicated, repeat steroid therapy at higher doses can be considered.

Relapse Prevention

Long-term immunosuppressive therapy is indicated for relapsing NMOSD or AQP4-IgG-positive patients even after a single severe attack. Commonly used agents include azathioprine, mycophenolate mofetil (MMF), rituximab, cyclophosphamide, and mitoxantrone.

- *Azathioprine* (2.5–3 mg/kg/day) combined with prednisone is widely used, especially in Asian populations. Regular hematologic and hepatic monitoring is mandatory.
- *Mycophenolate mofetil (MMF)* (1–3 g/day) inhibits lymphocyte proliferation and antibody synthesis, offering sustained remission even in azathioprine-resistant cases.
- *Rituximab*, an anti-CD20 monoclonal antibody, is highly effective in reducing relapses. The standard regimen is 375 mg/m^2 weekly for 4 weeks or 1 g twice at a 2-week interval, with re-dosing guided by B-cell counts.
- *Mitoxantrone* (12 mg/m^2 every 3 months) is reserved for refractory cases because of cardiotoxicity and leukemia risk.

- *Methotrexate* may be used when cost or tolerability limits other therapies.

Multiple sclerosis-specific agents such as interferon-β, natalizumab, and fingolimod are contraindicated, as they may exacerbate NMOSD.

Symptomatic Therapy

Management of residual symptoms is crucial for quality of life. Pain is often resistant to standard neuropathic agents and may require carbamazepine or lamotrigine. Spasticity can be managed with physiotherapy, baclofen, or localized injections. Fatigue and weakness benefit from graded exercise programs and energy-conservation strategies. Bladder dysfunction may necessitate clean intermittent catheterization, and psychological distress should be addressed with counseling and pharmacotherapy.

EMERGING AND INVESTIGATIONAL THERAPIES

Newer treatments target specific immune pathways implicated in NMOSD. Eculizumab, a monoclonal antibody against complement C5, significantly reduces relapse rates and disability. Anti-IL-6 receptor agents such as tocilizumab and satralizumab (SA-237) have also demonstrated efficacy in reducing relapses. Other investigational approaches include neutrophil elastase inhibition (sivelestat) and eosinophil stabilization with antihistamines such as cetirizine or ketotifen. Although promising, these biologics are expensive and may not be widely accessible.

CONCLUSION

Neuromyelitis optica spectrum disorder is a distinct autoimmune astrocytopathy characterized by AQP4-IgG-mediated injury, predominantly affecting the optic nerves and spinal cord. Early recognition, differentiation from MS, and prompt initiation of immunosuppressive therapy are critical to preventing irreversible disability. Advances in antibody testing and targeted biological therapies continue to refine both diagnostic precision and long-term management of this debilitating disorder.

FURTHER READINGS

1. Lucchineti CF, Mandler RN, Mc Gavern D, Bruck W, Gleich G, Ransohoff RM, et al. A role for humoral mechanisms in the pathogenesis of Devic's neuromyelitis optica. Brain 2002;125:1450-61.
2. Jacob A, Matiello M, Wingerchuk DM, Lucchinetti CF, Pittock SJ, Weinshenker BG. Neuromyelitis optica: changing concepts. J Neuroimmunol. 2007;187(1):126-38.
3. Wingerchuk DM, Lennon VA, Lucchinetti CF, Pittock SJ, Weinshenker BG. The spectrum of neuromyelitis optica. Lancet Neurol. 2007;6(9):805-15.
4. Graber DJ, Levy M, Kerr D, Wade WF. Neuromyelitis optica pathogenesis and aquaporin 4. J Neuroinflammation. 2008;5(1):1.
5. Papadopoulos MC, Verkman AS. Aquaporin 4 and neuromyelitis optica. Lancet Neurol. 2012;11(6):535-44.

6. Allbutt TC. On the ophthalmoscopic signs of spinal disease. Lancet. 1870;95(2420):76-8.
7. Devic E. Myélite subaiguë compliquée de névrite optique. Bull Med. 1894;8(1):1033-4.
8. Papadopoulos MC, Verkman AS. Aquaporin 4 and neuromyelitis optica. Lancet Neurol. 2012;11(6):535-44.
9. Ransohoff RM. Illuminating neuromyelitis optica pathogenesis. Proc Natl Acad Sci USA. 2012;109(4):1001-2.
10. Kitley J, Leite MI, Nakashima I, Waters P, McNeillis B, Brown R, et al. Prognostic factors and disease course in aquaporin-4 antibody-positive patients with neuromyelitis optica spectrum disorder from the United Kingdom and Japan. Brain. 2012;135(Pt 6):1834-49.
11. Asgari N, Lillevang ST, Skejoe HP, Falah M, Stenager E, Kyvik KO. A population-based study of neuromyelitis optica in Caucasians. Neurology. 2011;76(18):1589-95.
12. Pandit L. Neuromyelitis optica spectrum disorders: An update. Ann Indian Acad Neurol. 2015;18(Suppl 1):S1.
13. Pandit L, Kundapur R. Prevalence and patterns of demyelinating central nervous system disorders in urban Mangalore, South India. Mult Scler. 2014;20(12):1651-3.
14. Papais-Alvarenga RM, Carellos SC, Alvarenga MP, Holander C, Bichara RP, Thuler LC. Clinical course of optic neuritis in patients with relapsing neuromyelitis optica. Arch Ophthalmol. 2008;126(1):12-6.
15. Wingerchuk DM, Lennon VA, Pittock SJ, Lucchinetti CF, Weinshenker BG. Revised diagnostic criteria for neuromyelitis optica. Neurology. 2006;66(10):1485-9.
16. Wingerchuk DM, Hogancamp WF, O'Brien PC, Weinshenker BG. The clinical course of neuromyelitis optica (Devic's syndrome). Neurology. 1999;53(5):1107-14.
17. Jacob A, McKeon A, Nakashima I, Sato DK, Elsone L, Fujihara K, et al. Current concept of neuromyelitis optica (NMO) and NMO spectrum disorders. J Neurol Neurosurg Psychiatry. 2013;84(8):922-30.
18. Trebst C, Jarius S, Berthele A, Paul F, Schippling S, Wildemann B, et al. Update on the diagnosis and treatment of neuromyelitis optica: recommendations of the Neuromyelitis Optica Study Group (NEMOS). J Neurol. 2014;261(1):1-6.
19. Jacob A. Neuromyelitis optica-an update: 2007–2009. Ann Indian Acad Neurol. 2009;12(4):231.
20. Pittock SJ, Lennon VA, de Seze J, Vermersch P, Homburger HA, Wingerchuk DM, et al. The Prevalence of Non-organ-specific Autoantibodies and NMO-IgG in Neuromyelitis Optica (NMO) and Related Disorders. Neurology. 2006;66(5):A307.
21. Pittock SJ, Lennon VA. Aquaporin-4 autoantibodies in a paraneoplastic context. Arch Neurol. 2008;65(5):629-32.
22. Wingerchuk DM, Banwell B, Bennett JL, Cabre P, Carroll W, Chitnis T, et al. International consensus diagnostic criteria for neuromyelitis optica spectrum disorders. Neurology. 2015;85(2):177-89.
23. Pandit L. Transverse myelitis spectrum disorders. Neurol India. 2009;57(2):126.
24. Kim W, Kim SH, Huh SY, Kim HJ. Brain abnormalities in neuromyelitis optica spectrum disorder. Mult Scler Int. 2012;2012:735486.
25. Jarius S, Paul F, Franciotta D, Ruprecht K, Ringelstein M, Bergamaschi R, et al. Cerebrospinal fluid findings in aquaporin-4 antibody positive neuromyelitis optica: results from 211 lumbar punctures. J Neurol Sci. 2011;306(1):82-90.
26. Cabre P, Gonzalez-Quevedo A, Bonnan M, Saiz A, Olindo S, Graus F, et al. Relapsing neuromyelitis optica: long term history and clinical predictors of death. J Neurol, Neurosurg Psychiatry. 2009 ;80(10):1162-4.
27. Jacob A, Weinshenker BG, Violich I, McLinskey N, Krupp L, Fox RJ, et al. Treatment of neuromyelitis optica with rituximab: retrospective analysis of 25 patients. Arch Neurol. 2008;65(11):1443-8.
28. Pittock SJ, Lennon VA, McKeon A, Mandrekar J, Weinshenker BG, Lucchinetti CF, et al. Eculizumab in AQP4-IgG-positive relapsing neuromyelitis optica spectrum disorders: an open-label pilot study. Lancet Neurol. 2013;12(6):554-62.

SECTION 13

Oncology

SECTION
13

INTRODUCTION

Oncology

CHAPTER 37
Chronic Lymphocytic Leukemia

Madhuchanda Kar, Suman Meyur

INTRODUCTION

Chronic lymphocytic leukemia (CLL) is a clonal malignancy of mature B lymphocytes characterized by their progressive accumulation in peripheral blood, bone marrow, lymph nodes, and spleen. It is the most common adult leukemia in Western populations, accounting for nearly 30% of all leukemias in these regions, but is less frequent in Asia and India ($\approx$5–10%). The median age at diagnosis is 65–70 years, and a slight male predominance is seen.

Chronic lymphocytic leukemia and its tissue equivalent, small lymphocytic lymphoma (SLL), represent different manifestations of the same disease entity, distinguished primarily by the degree of lymphocytosis versus tissue involvement.

EPIDEMIOLOGY

Global incidence varies widely, with the highest rates reported in Europe and North America (4–6 per 100,000/year) and the lowest in East Asia (<1 per 100,000/year). The reasons for this disparity are not fully understood but may include genetic predisposition, environmental factors, and underdiagnosis in low-resource settings. In India, hospital-based cancer registries show a rising trend due to increased use of routine health check-ups and flow cytometry facilities.

PATHOGENESIS AND MOLECULAR BIOLOGY

Chronic lymphocytic leukemia originates from a mature, antigen-experienced B cell arrested at various stages of differentiation. Key pathogenetic mechanisms include:
- *B-cell receptor (BCR) signaling*: Aberrant BCR signaling is central to CLL survival and proliferation. Constitutive activation of BTK (Bruton's tyrosine kinase) and PI3K pathways promotes anti-apoptotic signaling via NF-κB, AKT, and ERK pathways.
- *Genetic alterations:* Recurrent cytogenetic lesions are detectable in >80% of patients by FISH or next-generation sequencing (NGS):

- *del(13q14):* Loss of miR-15a/16-1 leading to increased BCL2 expression (favorable prognosis).
- *trisomy 12:* Associated with atypical morphology and intermediate prognosis.
- *del(11q22-23):* ATM loss, bulky nodes, and aggressive course
- *del(17p13):* TP53 loss, resistance to chemotherapy (poor prognosis)
- *NOTCH1, SF3B1, BIRC3 mutations*—predict early relapse and Richter transformation.
- *Microenvironmental influence:* Chronic lymphocytic leukemia cells depend on the tumor microenvironment within bone marrow and lymph nodes. Stromal cells, nurse-like cells, and cytokines such as CXCL12/CXCR4 and IL-4 support CLL survival and resistance to therapy.

CLINICAL FEATURES

Many patients are asymptomatic at diagnosis, detected incidentally on CBC showing lymphocytosis.
When symptomatic, features include:
- Fatigue, weight loss, night sweats (B symptoms)
- Lymphadenopathy (most common sign)
- Splenomegaly ± hepatomegaly
- Recurrent infections due to hypogammaglobulinemia
- Autoimmune complications—autoimmune hemolytic anemia (AIHA) or immune thrombocytopenia (ITP) occur in 10–20%.
In the **Box 1** below, a real life case has been presented.

Box 1: Case presentation
- BK—65 years, M, pursued health screening by employer
- Asymptomatic—but feels more tired for past few months
- Not on any particular medicine
- No family history of cancer
- Physical examination—unremarkable

DIAGNOSTIC WORK-UP

- *Blood counts and smear:*
  - Absolute lymphocytosis $> 5 \times 10^9$/L for ≥3 months is required.
  - *Morphology*: Small mature lymphocytes with clumped chromatin, scant cytoplasm, and characteristic smudge cells due to lymphocyte fragility
- *Flow cytometry immunophenotyping:* Diagnostic immunophenotype (Matutes scoring system ≥4):
  - CD19, CD20 (dim), CD5, CD23, weak surface Ig (κ or λ)
  - Negative for CD10 and FMC7

  This confirms monoclonal B-cell nature.
- *Bone marrow examination:* Not required for diagnosis but useful before therapy or if cytopenias are present. It typically shows diffuse or interstitial infiltration by mature lymphocytes.

- *Cytogenetic and molecular studies*:
  - *FISH:* To detect del(13q), del(11q), del(17p), and trisomy 12
  - *Immunoglobulin heavy chain variable (IGHV) mutation analysis*:
    - Mutated IGHV → indolent disease
    - Unmutated IGHV → aggressive course
  - *TP53 sequencing* recommended before starting therapy, as TP53 mutation or del(17p) predicts *chemo-refractoriness*.
- *Serum markers:*
  - β_2-microglobulin, lactate dehydrogenase (LDH), and thymidine kinase are prognostic indicators **(Tables 1 and 2)**.
  - Hypogammaglobulinemia common in advanced stages

STAGING AND PROGNOSTIC SYSTEMS

The *CLL-International Prognostic Index (CLL-IPI)* **(Table 3)** integrates clinical and molecular factors:
Total score classifies patients into low, intermediate, high, or very high risk.

TABLE 1: Rai staging (US).

Stage	Clinical features	Risk
0	Lymphocytosis only	Low
I	+ Lymphadenopathy	Intermediate
II	+ Organomegaly	Intermediate
III	+ Anemia	High
IV	+ Thrombocytopenia	High

TABLE 2: Binet staging (Europe).

Stage	Criteria	Risk
A	<3 involved areas	Low
B	≥3 areas	Intermediate
C	Anemia and/or thrombocytopenia	High

TABLE 3: Risk stratification.

Factor	Points
Age >65 years	1
Clinical stage (Rai I-IV/Binet B-C)	1
β_2-microglobulin >3.5 mg/L	2
Unmutated IGHV	2
del(17p)/TP53 mutation	4
(IGHV: immunoglobulin heavy chain variable)	

DISEASE COURSE AND COMPLICATIONS

The CLL typically follows a *waxing and waning* course. Transformation into Richter syndrome (aggressive DLBCL or Hodgkin variant) occurs in 5–10% of cases. Other complications include:
- *Infectious risk*: Bacterial, viral (HSV, VZV), fungal
- *Secondary malignancies*: Melanoma, lung, GI cancers
- *Autoimmune cytopenias*: Coombs-positive AIHA, ITP

MANAGEMENT PRINCIPLES

- *Watchful waiting:* Asymptomatic early stage patients (Rai 0–I, Binet A) benefit from observation only, as early therapy offers no survival advantage.
- *Indications for treatment (iwCLL 2018 criteria):*
  - Progressive marrow failure (Hb <10 g/dL or platelets <100 × 10^9/L)
  - Massive/progressive lymphadenopathy (>10 cm) or splenomegaly
  - Rapid lymphocyte doubling (<6 months)
  - Disease-related symptoms (B symptoms)
  - Autoimmune complications unresponsive to corticosteroids

Therapeutic Options

- *Chemo-immunotherapy (historical standard):*
  - *FCR regimen (fludarabine, cyclophosphamide, rituximab)*: Standard for fit, young, TP53-wild-type patients
  - *BR regimen (bendamustine + rituximab)*: Alternative for elderly or frail patients.

  However, these regimens are now largely replaced by targeted therapies.
- *Targeted therapies*:
  - BTK inhibitors:
    - *Ibrutinib*, *acalabrutinib*, and *zanubrutinib*: Oral agents that inhibit B-cell receptor signaling and induce apoptosis
    - *Side effects*: Atrial fibrillation, bleeding, and hypertension
  - BCL2 inhibitor:
    - *Venetoclax*: Induces apoptosis by inhibiting BCL2
    - Given with *obinutuzumab* (CLL14 regimen) or *rituximab* for fixed-duration therapy
    - Risk of tumor lysis syndrome (TLS) during initiation—requires slow dose ramp-up
  - PI3K inhibitors:
    - *Idelalisib* and *duvelisib*: Used in relapsed CLL; limited by immune-mediated toxicities (colitis, hepatitis)
- *Monoclonal antibodies*: Rituximab, obinutuzumab, ofatumumab improve response rates when combined with chemo or venetoclax.
- *Cellular and novel immunotherapies:*
  - *CAR-T cell therapy (anti-CD19)*: Achieves durable remissions in relapsed/refractory CLL
  - *Bispecific antibodies* (e.g., epcoritamab, mosunetuzumab) are in advanced trials

○ *Allogeneic stem cell transplantation* is reserved for young, high-risk relapsed patients

Supportive and Preventive Care
- *Infection prophylaxis:*
  ○ Vaccinate against pneumococcus, influenza, and COVID-19
  ○ Avoid live vaccines
  ○ Consider IV immunoglobulin in recurrent infections with hypogammaglobulinemia
- *Autoimmune cytopenia management:* Corticosteroids, rituximab, or splenectomy if refractory
- *Avoid immunosuppressive therapy* unless clinically indicated
- *Regular follow-up* every 3–6 months with CBC and physical examination

Chronic lymphocytic leukemia in India—Key differences:
- Lower overall incidence but rising detection due to expanded flow cytometry access.
- Patients often present younger (median ≈ 58–60 years) and with more advanced disease.
- *Cytogenetic profile*: higher frequency of trisomy 12 and del(13q), lower of del(17p).
- Resource limitations influence treatment—bendamustine-rituximab or ibrutinib remain practical first-line options in many centers.

CONCLUSION
- CLL is a heterogeneous B-cell malignancy with variable course—from indolent to aggressive.
- *Flow cytometry* remains diagnostic cornerstone.
- *Cytogenetic and molecular profiling* are essential for prognosis and therapy selection.
- Modern therapy emphasizes *targeted agents* over chemotherapy.
- *Observation* is appropriate for asymptomatic early disease.
- *Richter transformation and autoimmune cytopenias* remain important complications.

"In the **Box 2** below, the management and outcome of the afore-mentioned case have been discussed."

BOX 2: The outline of management of the case

Our patient:
- Asymptomatic
- RAI stage 0
- BINET stage A
- FISH 13q del, mutated 1GVH
- *Decision*: low risk-watchful waiting
- No surveillance with CT Scan.

BK lived happily ever after!

FURTHER READINGS

1. Hallek M, Shanafelt TD, Eichhorst B. Chronic lymphocytic leukaemia. Lancet. 2018;391(10129):1524-37.
2. Gupta S, Singh PK, Jain M. Epidemiology of chronic lymphocytic leukaemia in India. Indian J Cancer. 2020;57(4):427-33.
3. Swerdlow SH, Campo E, Arber DA, Cazzola M, Cook JR, Döhner H, Dreyling M, Hasserjian RP, Jaffe ES, Orazi A, Quintanilla-Martinez L. Response to "The WHO classification of haematolymphoid tumours". Leukemia. 2022;36(11):2748-9.
4. Nabhan C, Rosen ST. CLL epidemiology and etiology. Curr Opin Hematol. 2014;21(4):281-7.
5. Sarma S, Mehta J. Spectrum of lymphomas in India. International journal of molecular and immuno oncology. 2024;19;9(1):16-24.
6. Stevenson, F.K., Krysov, S., Davies, A.J., Steele, A.J. and Packham, G., 2011. B-cell receptor signaling in chronic lymphocytic leukemia. Blood, The Journal of the American Society of Hematology, 118(16), pp.4313-4320.
7. Burger JA. BCR signaling in CLL. Blood. 2014;123(21):3277-86.
8. Döhner H, Stilgenbauer S, Benner A, Leupolt E, Kröber A, Bullinger L, et al. Genomic aberrations and survival in CLL. N Engl J Med. 2000;343(26):1910-6.
9. Rossi D, Gaidano G. Molecular pathogenesis of CLL. Blood Rev. 2016;30(4):233-43.
10. Herishanu Y, Pérez-Galán P, Liu D, Biancotto A, Pittaluga S, Vire B, et al. The lymph node microenvironment in CLL. Blood. 2011;117(2):563-74.
11. Zent CS, Kay NE. Autoimmune complications in CLL. Blood Rev. 2011;25(4):181-6.
12. Mauro FR, Foa R, Cerretti R, Giannarelli D, Coluzzi S, Mandelli F, et al. Autoimmune haemolytic anaemia in CLL. Blood. 2000;95(9):2786-92.
13. Bain BJ. Blood Cells: A Practical Guide, 6th edition. Hoboken: Wiley-Blackwell; 2015.
14. Matutes E, Owusu-Ankomah K, Morilla R, Garcia Marco J, Houlihan A, Que TH, et al. Immunophenotyping score in CLL. Leukemia. 1994;8(10):1640-5.
15. Stilgenbauer, S., Schnaiter, A., Paschka, P., Zenz, T., Rossi, M., Döhner, K., Bühler, A., Böttcher, S., Ritgen, M., Kneba, M. and Winkler, D., 2014. Gene mutations and treatment outcome in chronic lymphocytic leukemia: results from the CLL8 trial. Blood, The Journal of the American Society of Hematology, 123(21), pp.3247-3254.
16. International CLL-IPI Working Group. Development of the CLL-IPI. Lancet Oncol. 2016;17(6):779-90.
17. Tsimberidou AM, Keating MJ. Richter transformation. J Clin Oncol. 2005;23(24):4441-52.
18. Shanafelt, T. D., & Kay, N. E. (2014). Early therapy vs watchful waiting in CLL. Blood, 123(24), 3660-3668.
19. Hallek M, Cheson BD, Catovsky D, Caligaris-Cappio F, Dighiero G, Döhner H, et al. iwCLL guidelines for diagnosis and treatment. Blood. 2018;131(25):2745-60.
20. Fischer, K., Bahlo, J., Fink, A.M., Goede, V., Herling, C.D., Cramer, P., Langerbeins, P., Von Tresckow, J., Engelke, A., Maurer, C. and Kovacs, G., 2016. Long-term remissions after FCR chemoimmunotherapy in previously untreated patients with CLL: updated results of the CLL8 trial. Blood, the Journal of the American Society of Hematology, 127(2), pp.208-215.

CHAPTER 38

Multiple Myeloma: From Incurable to Potentially Curable

Pankaj Malhotra

INTRODUCTION

Multiple myeloma (MM) is a malignant disorder of plasma cells and ranks as the second most common hematological cancer worldwide, following non-Hodgkin lymphoma. Despite being less common than certain solid organ malignancies, its clinical significance is immense due to its complex biology, varied presentation, and historically poor outcomes. Over the past two decades, however, the outlook for patients with myeloma has transformed remarkably, largely because of major advances in diagnosis, monitoring, and treatment strategies. Once viewed as an incurable disease with dismal survival rates, myeloma is now increasingly considered a potentially curable malignancy for a subset of patients.

PRECURSOR CONDITION: MONOCLONAL GAMMOPATHY OF UNDETERMINED SIGNIFICANCE

Almost every case of MM is preceded by a clinically silent precursor state known as *monoclonal gammopathy of undetermined significance (MGUS)*. This premalignant condition is characterized by the presence of a monoclonal immunoglobulin protein (M-protein) in the blood without evidence of end-organ damage.

The prevalence of MGUS rises with age. It is estimated that about *3% of individuals above the age of 50 years* and *5-6% of individuals above 70 years* harbor this condition. While the annual risk of progression from MGUS to overt myeloma is relatively low (about 1% per year), the sheer prevalence of MGUS means that a substantial proportion of elderly populations remains at risk of developing symptomatic disease. Identifying and monitoring such individuals is therefore an important component of early detection and intervention strategies.

HISTORICAL PERSPECTIVE AND CHANGING PROGNOSIS

Multiple myeloma historically carried a very poor prognosis. Before the year 2000, the *median overall survival* of patients diagnosed with myeloma was barely *2-3 years*. Conventional chemotherapy regimens, most notably combinations involving melphalan and corticosteroids, were the mainstay of therapy. While these agents induced remission in some patients, relapses were inevitable, and durable long-term survival was rare.

The past two decades, however, have witnessed a paradigm shift. With the introduction of *novel therapeutic classes*, improvement in supportive care, and better risk stratification tools, the outlook for patients has dramatically improved. A patient diagnosed with MM today can expect a *median survival exceeding 10 years*, and approximately *30–40% of patients are now considered potentially curable*. This transformation is one of the most remarkable success stories in modern hematology.

ADVANCES IN THERAPEUTICS

The improvement in outcomes can be attributed to the development and availability of *targeted and immune-based therapies*. The most important classes of novel drugs include:

Immunomodulatory Drugs

Agents such as thalidomide, lenalidomide, and pomalidomide have become integral to myeloma management. They exert their effect by modulating the tumor microenvironment, enhancing immune surveillance, and directly inducing tumor cell apoptosis.

Proteasome Inhibitors

Drugs such as bortezomib, carfilzomib, and ixazomib target the proteasome pathway, which is crucial for protein degradation in plasma cells. By disrupting this pathway, they induce cellular stress and apoptosis in malignant cells.

Monoclonal Antibodies

The advent of monoclonal antibodies, particularly *daratumumab* and *isatuximab*, has been a game-changer. By targeting surface markers such as CD38, these antibodies enhance immune-mediated killing of myeloma cells.

Bispecific Antibodies

These agents simultaneously bind to a myeloma-specific antigen [e.g., B-cell maturation antigen (BCMA)] and to CD3 on T cells, thereby redirecting T cells to kill myeloma cells. Early clinical results have shown impressive efficacy, even in heavily pretreated patients.

Chimeric Antigen Receptor T-cell Therapy

Chimeric antigen receptor (CAR) T-cell therapy represents the forefront of personalized medicine. By engineering a patient's T cells to specifically target BCMA or other myeloma antigens, this therapy offers unprecedented remission rates in relapsed/refractory myeloma.

Other Novel Approaches

Histone deacetylase inhibitors, antibody–drug conjugates, and next-generation targeted therapies continue to expand the therapeutic arsenal.

Interestingly, traditional *chemotherapy agents* that once dominated treatment regimens are now rarely used, except in resource-limited settings. However, *high dose melphalan followed by autologous stem cell transplantation (ASCT)* remains a cornerstone of therapy. Despite the availability of several novel agents, ASCT continues to provide durable disease control and remains standard of care for eligible patients.

ADVANCES IN DISEASE MONITORING

Alongside therapeutic innovations, improvements in disease monitoring have contributed significantly to better outcomes. The most notable development is the use of *minimal residual disease (MRD) assessment*.

- *MRD negativity* has emerged as one of the strongest predictors of long-term survival and potential cure.
- It is now considered a surrogate marker for durable remission and has been incorporated into clinical trials as an endpoint.
- Techniques such as *next-generation flow cytometry* and *next-generation sequencing* allow for sensitive detection of even a single malignant plasma cell among a million normal cells.

This ability to measure disease at a molecular level enables physicians to tailor therapy more precisely, avoid overtreatment, and identify patients who may benefit from treatment intensification or novel approaches.

MULTIPLE MYELOMA IN THE INDIAN CONTEXT

In India, the management of MM has seen substantial progress in recent years. The *Ayushman Bharat* scheme has played an important role in improving accessibility by covering several antimyeloma drugs, thereby enabling patients to live longer and healthier lives.

However, significant challenges remain. Advanced therapies such as monoclonal antibodies, bispecific antibodies, and CAR T-cell therapies are still prohibitively expensive for most Indian patients. The cost of these therapies in Western countries is extremely high, often running into 1,000,000 or even crores of rupees. Encouragingly, several Indian companies and research institutes have started developing indigenous CAR T-cell therapies. These are available at *approximately one-tenth of the cost* of their Western counterparts, thereby bringing hope for greater affordability and accessibility in the near future.

ROLE OF THE INDIAN MYELOMA ACADEMIC GROUP

A landmark development in the Indian context has been the establishment of the *Indian Myeloma Academic Group (IMAGe)* in 2018. This society (www.imagesociety.co.in) has emerged as a unifying platform for clinicians, researchers, and patients.

The Indian Myeloma Academic Group organizes annual conferences and workshops that focus on:
- Creating awareness about plasma cell dyscrasias
- Promoting collaborative research
- Developing consensus guidelines tailored to the Indian healthcare setting
- Facilitating uniformity in clinical practice across the country

Through its efforts, IMAGe has significantly improved the standardization of care, ensuring that patients across India have access to evidence-based treatment protocols. It has also fostered collaborations with international groups, thereby contributing to global advancements in myeloma research.

FUTURE OF MYELOMA THERAPY

The trajectory of myeloma management strongly suggests that the future is bright. With rapid advancements in immunotherapy, cellular therapy, and precision medicine, the dream of curing myeloma appears increasingly realistic.

Key areas of ongoing development include:
- *Next-generation CAR T-cell therapies* with improved efficacy and reduced toxicity
- *Allogeneic cellular therapies* that may provide off-the-shelf solutions.
- *Combination immunotherapy regimens* that leverage synergistic effects of antibodies, bispecifics, and IMiDs
- *Personalized medicine approaches* based on genomic profiling of individual tumors
- *Improved supportive care measures*, including infection prophylaxis, bone health management, and rehabilitation strategies that enhance quality of life during prolonged survival.

CONCLUSION

Multiple myeloma has undergone a remarkable transformation over the past two decades. From being an almost uniformly fatal disease with survival measured in just a few years, it has evolved into a condition where *long-term remission and even cure are tangible possibilities.* Advances in therapeutics—ranging from IMiDs and proteasome inhibitors to CAR T-cell therapy—along with sensitive monitoring tools like MRD assessment, have driven this progress.

In India, schemes such as Ayushman Bharat and the efforts of organizations like IMAGe have ensured that patients are increasingly able to access modern therapies and benefit from the global advances in care. While challenges remain—particularly in terms of cost and accessibility of cutting-edge treatments—the overall direction is optimistic.

The journey of MM exemplifies how sustained research, global collaboration, and local initiatives can transform a once-incurable disease into one that may soon be considered *curable for a significant proportion of patients.*

FURTHER READINGS

1. Rajkumar, SV. Multiple myeloma: 2024 update on diagnosis, risk-stratification, and management. Am J Hematol. 2024;99(9):1802-24.
2. Simeone C, et al. Practice-changing updates on multiple myeloma: highlights from the 2024 ASH annual meeting. J Exp Clin Cancer Res. 2025;44:59.
3. Hsin-Ti Lin C, Tariq MJ, Ullah F, et al. Current Novel Targeted Therapeutic Strategies in Multiple Myeloma. Int J Mol Sci. 2024;25(11):6192.
4. Paikray E, Rout A, Tripathy R. Recent Advances in Multiple Myeloma. Biomed Pharmacol J. 2024;17(1).
5. Raza S, Shaughnessy, JD. A New Era In Multiple Myeloma Treatment: Advances and Future Directions. OncLive. 2024.
6. Bensinger WI. Recent advances in the treatment of multiple myeloma: a brief review. Acta Haematol. 2022;145(6):534-46.

SECTION 14

Pregnancy

Diabetes in Pregnancy

Preetkanwal Sibia, Vikas Sharma, Ajay Bhaskar

INTRODUCTION

The critical subject of diabetes in pregnancy, focusing on the identification and therapeutic management of both gestational diabetes mellitus (GDM) and preexisting diabetes. Timely and universal screening, particularly at 24–28 weeks, is crucial for early diagnosis and intervention. The goal of management is to achieve strict glycemic targets through lifestyle modification and, if needed, pharmacotherapy like insulin or oral agents.

TERMINOLOGIES

Gestational diabetes mellitus (GDM): Impaired glucose tolerance diagnosed at 24–28 weeks of pregnancy (2–10% of pregnancies) **(Fig. 1)**

Overt diabetes: Diabetes diagnosed early in pregnancy and is assumed to be previously undiagnosed type 2 diabetes (complicates 1–2% of pregnancies).

Preexisting diabetes accounts for 13–21% of diabetes in pregnancy, with remainder due to GDM.

Pregnancy is a state of enhanced beta cell function and insulin resistance.

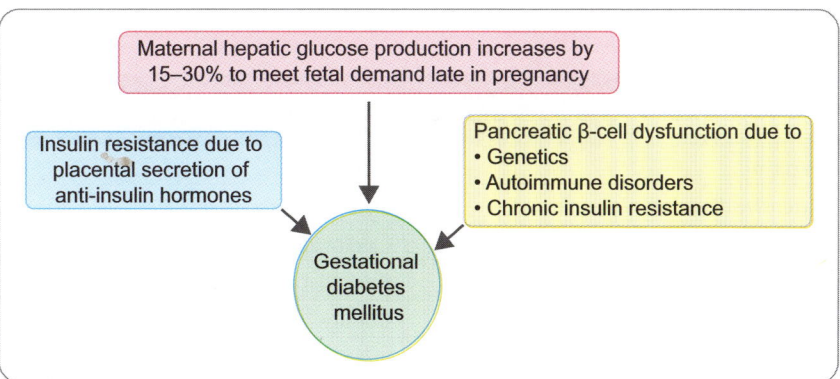

FIG. 1: The key factors in the pathophysiology of gestational diabetes mellitus (GDM).

Insulin resistance is due to placental secretion of diabetogenic hormones like GH, CRH, hPL, Prolactin, and progesterone.

Gestational diabetes mellitus develops if beta cell function is insufficient to overcome insulin resistance.

Most prominent in *third trimester*.

Prevalence is 25% in South Asia.

SCREENING FOR DIABETES

All pregnant women are screened at *first antenatal visit*.

If negative, repeat testing is done at *24–28 weeks* to rule out GDM in *high-risk groups* (ADA).

However, national DIPSI guidelines recommend screening of all pregnant women at 24 weeks.

High Risk Groups
- GDM in previous pregnancy
- Impaired glucose tolerance
- HbA1c > 5.7
- Elevated fasting glucose
- Family history of diabetes
- Pre-pregnancy BMI> 30 kg/m^2
- Older maternal age> 35 years
- Polycystic ovary syndrome (PCOS)

Why Screening Important?

Potential risks associated with gestational diabetes mellitus **(Table 1)**:

(Hypoglycemia, hypoCa, hypoMg, polycythemia hyperbilirubinemia, and hyperviscosity syndrome)

Gestational diabetes mellitus is not associated with increased risks of congenital anomalies.

Patients with GDM are at *10-fold* higher risk of developing subsequent diabetes mellitus **(Table 2)**.

TABLE 1: Short-term and long-term consequences associated with a specific medical condition (implied).

Short term	Long term
Hypertensive disorders of pregnancy	Maternal: Diabetes mellitus
Macrosomia	Cardiovascular disease
Polyhydramnios	Fetal: Diabetes
Operative delivery	Obesity
Fetal cardiomyopathy	Hypertension
Neonatal respiratory disorders	Metabolic syndrome
Neonatal metabolic problems	

TABLE 2: Absolute risk of type 2 diabetes mellitus.

1–5 years	9%
>5–10 years	12%
>10 years	16%

TABLE 3: American Diabetes Association criteria for diagnosis of diabetes.

Number	Criteria for diagnosis of diabetes (American Diabetes Association)	Threshold	Notes
1	HbA1c	≥6.5%	Test should be performed in a laboratory using a method that is NGSP certified and standardized to the DCCT assay
2	Fasting plasma glucose (FPG)	≥126 mg/dL (7 mmol/L)	Fasting is defined as no caloric intake for at least 8 hours
3	2-hour plasma glucose during an oral glucose tolerance test (OGTT)	≥200 mg/dL (11.1 mmol/L)	Test should be performed as described by the WHO, using a glucose load containing the equivalent of 75 g anhydrous glucose dissolved in water
4	Random plasma glucose	≥200 mg/dL (11.1 mmol/L)	Applicable in a patient with classic symptoms of hyperglycemia or hyperglycemic crisis

(DCCT: Diabetes Control and Complications Trial; NGSP: National Glycohemoglobin Standardization Program)

TABLE 4: IADPSG and ADA criteria for a positive 2-hour 75-g oral glucose tolerance test for the diagnosis of gestational diabetes.

Time point	Threshold (mg/dL)	Threshold (mmol/L)	Condition for diagnosis
Fasting	92	5.1	OR
1 hour	180	10	OR
2 hours	153	8.5	

Screening of Overt Diagnosis in Early Pregnancy

- Increasing proportion due to increased obesity and lack of routine screening.
- Associated with miscarriage and *congenital anomalies*.
- *Approach: Universal screening by HbA1c (ADA)*
- *75 g oral glucose 2-hour blood glucose level >140 (DIPSI)*
- Although choice of screening test varies from institution and clinician preference.

Screening for Gestational Diabetes Mellitus at 24–28 Weeks

- Done for high risk groups, however, universal screening appears to be most practical approach according to DIPSI.
- Screening is done with *one step approach* and *two step approach* (**Table 3**).
- Two step approach is better but one step approach is more feasible and economical to identify GDM in pregnant women (**Table 4**).

ACOG Two-step Approach for Screening and Diagnosis of Gestational Diabetes Mellitus

The American College of Obstetricians and Gynecologists (ACOG) recommends a two-step approach for identifying gestational diabetes mellitus (GDM).

Step one: Screening—
1. *Procedure:* Give a *50 g oral glucose solution* without regard to the time of day.
2. *Measurement:* Measure venous plasma or serum glucose concentration at *1 hour* after administration.
3. *Threshold for progression:* A glucose concentration of ≥135$ mg/dL (7.5 mmol/L) or greater than equal ≥140 mg/dL (7.8 mmol/L) is considered elevated and requires administration of a 100 g oral glucose tolerance test (step two).
   - *Note*: The ≥135 mg/dL threshold provides greater sensitivity, but results in more false positives and requires the full tolerance test for more patients than the ≥140 mg/dL threshold. The lower threshold should be considered in populations with higher prevalence of gestational diabetes.

Step two: Diagnosis (100-g oral glucose tolerance test)—
1. *Preparation:* Measure *fasting* venous plasma or serum glucose concentration.
2. *Procedure:* Give a *100-g oral glucose solution*.
3. *Measurement:* Measure venous plasma or serum glucose concentration at *1, 2, and 3 hours* after administration.
4. *Criteria for positive test*: A positive test is generally defined by *elevated glucose concentrations at two or more time points* (**Table 5**).

A 100 g oral glucose load is given in the morning to a patient who has fasted overnight for at least 8 hours. A positive test is generally defined as greater than equal glucose values at or above these thresholds.

Post-Delivery Screening

Individuals with GDM should be screened at *4–12 weeks* postpartum and periodically *every 3 years*.

Increased risk of developing type 2 diabetes mellitus.

TABLE 5: Diagnostic criteria for the 3 hour 100 g oral GTT for gestational diabetes mellitus.

Time point	Carpenter/Coustan thresholds	National Diabetes Data Group Thresholds
	Plasma or serum: mg/dL (mmol/L)	Plasma: mg/dL (mmol/L)
Fasting	95 (5.3)	105 (5.8)
1 hour	180 (10)	190 (10.6)
2 hours	155 (8.6)	165 (9.2)
3 hours	140 (7.8)	145 (8)

TREATMENT OF DIABETES IN PREGNANCY

Treatment of gestational diabetes mellitus can improve patient's outcome.

Many patients can achieve target glucose levels with nutritional therapy and moderate exercise alone, but up to *30% will require pharmacotherapy.*

Medical nutrition therapy: Refers to the dietary plan tailored for patients with diabetes based on medical, lifestyle, and personal factors.

The goals are:
- Achieve normoglycemia
- Prevent ketosis
- Prevent adequate nutrition
- Contribute to fetal well-being

The specific diet that achieves optimum maternal and newborn outcomes in GDM is unclear. In a systematic review of randomized trials comparing a variety of dietary interventions with conventional dietary recommendations for patients with GDM. When analyzed by diet subtype, low glycemic index, DASH, low carbohydrate, and ethnicity-based diets had beneficial effects on maternal glucose levels.

Meal plan: A typical meal plan for patients with GDM includes three small to moderate sized meals and two to four snacks.

Close follow-up is necessary to ensure nutritional adequacy. If insulin therapy is added to nutritional therapy, a primary goal is to maintain carbohydrate consistency at meals and snacks to facilitate insulin adjustments.

Calories: The caloric requirements of patients with GDM are the same as those for pregnant patients without GDM. For individuals with a prepregnancy BMI in the healthy range, caloric requirements in the first trimester are the same as before pregnancy and generally increase by 340 calories per day in the second trimester and 452 calories per day in the third trimester. Individuals who are underweight, overweight, or obese should work with a registered dietician to determine their specific caloric requirements.

Protein and fat intake: The remaining calories come from protein (20% of total calories or approximately 71 g/day and fats (40% of total calories; saturated fat intake should be <7% of total calories). Protein intake should be distributed throughout the day and included in all meals and snacks to promote satiety, slow the absorption of carbohydrates into the bloodstream, and provide adequate calories **(Table 6)**.

A bedtime high-protein snack is recommended to prevent accelerated (i.e., starvation) ketosis overnight and maintain fasting glucose levels within the target range.

Exercise

Adults with diabetes are encouraged to perform 30–60 minutes of moderate-intensity aerobic activity (40–60% maximal oxygen uptake) on most days of the week (at least 150 minutes of moderate-intensity aerobic exercise per week).

TABLE 6: Recommended total gestational weight gain ranges according to pre-pregnancy body mass index (BMI).

Pregnancy BMI	Total weight gain	
	Range in kg	Range in lb
Underweight (<18.5 kg/m^2)	12.5–18	28–40
Normal weight (18.5–24.9 kg/m^2)	11.5–16	25–35
Overweight (25–29.9 kg/m^2)	7–11.5	15–25
Obese (≥30 kg/m^2)	5–9	11–20

TABLE 7: Target glucose level.

	Venous blood glucose	Capillary blood glucose
FBS	<95	80–110
1 hour postprandial	<140	
2 hours postprandial	<120	<155
HbA1c	<6.5	

Exercise that increases muscle mass, including aerobic, resistance, and circuit training, appears to improve glucose management, primarily from increased tissue sensitivity to insulin.

As a result, exercise can reduce both fasting and postprandial blood glucose concentrations and, in some patients with GDM, the need for insulin may be obviated.

Glucose Monitoring

Patients should monitor their glucose levels. Glucose meters measure capillary blood glucose, almost all available glucose meters provide plasma equivalent values rather than whole-blood glucose values. Thus, results from most available glucose meters and venous plasma glucose measured in a laboratory should be comparable. Intermittent home blood glucose monitoring. It is suggested that patients monitor their blood glucose levels at the following times:
- Before breakfast (i.e., fasting glucose level)
- At one or at two hours after the beginning of each meal

Glucose Target

Glucose targets vary among international guidelines and the precise target for optimum maternal, fetal, and newborn outcome is not well-established. In the United States, the American Diabetes Association (ADA) **(Table 7)** and the American College of Obstetricians and Gynecologists (ACOG) recommend the following upper limits for glucose levels, with insulin therapy initiated if they are exceeded, but acknowledge that these thresholds have been extrapolated from recommendations proposed for pregnant patients with preexisting diabetes:
- *Fasting and preprandial blood glucose concentration*: <95 mg/dL (5.3 mmol/L)
- *1-hour postprandial blood glucose concentration*: <140 mg/dL (7.8 mmol/L)
- *2-hour postprandial glucose concentration*: <120 mg/dL (6.7 mmol/L)

Pharmacotherapy

Goal: The goal of pharmacotherapy is to manage glucose levels so that the majority are no higher than the upper limit of the target range, without inducing any episodes of hypoglycemia. Overly tight metabolic control [average blood glucose levels <86 mg/dL (4.8 mmol/L)] has no additional benefits and increases the risk for iatrogenic growth restriction.

Indications for pharmacotherapy:
- Glucose levels above the target range.
- If glucose targets cannot be maintained by medical nutritional therapy, then pharmacotherapy should be initiated, but the degree of hyperglycemia at which the disadvantages of initiating insulin therapy are clearly outweighed by the benefits has not been definitively determined and varies among providers.

The patients diagnosed with GDM after screening at 24–28 weeks and who have mostly postprandial hyperglycemia, fetal abdominal circumference >75th percentile, or estimated fetal weight (EFW) ≥90th percentile are managed with lifestyle interventions, glucose monitoring, and pharmacotherapy **(Flowchart 1)**.

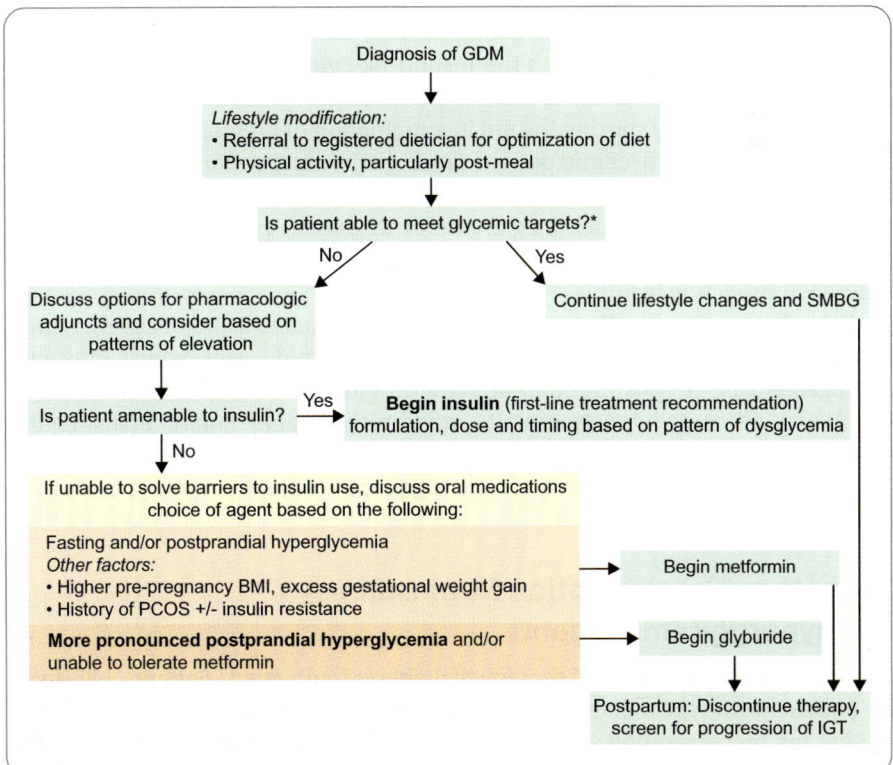

*Glycemic target (mg/dL): Fasting <95; 1 hour postprandial <140; 2 hours postprandial <120.
FLOWCHART 1: Step-wise management of gestational diabetes mellitus (GDM), from lifestyle changes to pharmacologic therapy.
(SMBG: self-monitoring of blood glucose)

Choice of pharmacotherapy: The options for pregnant patients who require pharmacotherapy are insulin (and some insulin analogs) or selected oral antihyperglycemic medications (metformin or glyburide).

Insulin is preferred because it is effective, easily adjusted based on glucose levels, and safe for the fetus, whereas data are lacking regarding long-term outcomes of offspring exposed to oral antihyperglycemic medications in utero.

In patients with type 1 or type 2 diabetes (preexisting diabetes), insulin remains the standard drug for glucose management during pregnancy. In patients with type 2 diabetes taking noninsulin antihyperglycemic agents, insulin is often started preconception to attain the optimal degree of glycemic management while allowing discontinuation of noninsulin agents without safety data in early pregnancy.

It is believed that oral antihyperglycemic medications are a reasonable alternative to insulin for patients in whom pharmacotherapy is indicated but who decline to take, or are unable to comply with, insulin therapy. Some guidelines consider oral antihyperglycemic medications an acceptable first-line approach in selected patients, such as those with normal fasting blood glucose levels and modest postprandial hyperglycemia.

In the preconception period, it is preferred to use insulins with a good fetal safety profile, such as neutral protamine hagedorn *(NPH), lispro, and aspart* insulins. Insulin glargine, a long-acting insulin, has greater mitogenic potential and higher affinity in binding to the insulin-like growth factor 1 receptor than other insulins, which could lead to increased fetal growth and macrosomia.

For patients newly starting insulin in anticipation of pregnancy, a long-acting insulin based on the glycemic pattern, dosing schedule, patient preference, and insurance coverage is initiated. For patients who are already on a stable long-acting insulin regimen (such as glargine or degludec) prior to pregnancy and meeting glucose targets, it is generally not recommended to switch them to a different long-acting insulin.

For a short-acting insulin, a rapid-acting insulin, such as lispro or aspart, is used instead of regular insulin. These insulins have a rapid onset, which improves management of the postprandial increase in glucose, and have a rapid offset, which may decrease hypoglycemia. A randomized trial of aspart versus regular insulin in pregnancy demonstrated less of a glucose rise postprandially with aspart than regular insulin, but there was no significant difference in hypoglycemia rates.

Patients on Preconception Noninsulin Antihyperglycemic Agents

Insulin remains the preferred therapy of diabetes in pregnant patients. However, for patients with type 2 diabetes on metformin monotherapy with glucose levels at goal for preconception, we suggest continuing metformin through the first trimester and adding insulin to achieve pregnancy glycemic goals once pregnancy is confirmed. Studies of metformin use in the first trimester suggest that it is not teratogenic and use of metformin may help maintain glycemic management during the period of organogenesis.

For patients on other noninsulin antihyperglycemic agents, it is suggested to switch to metformin and/or insulin therapy prior to conception. While glyburide has been studied in gestational diabetes and was previously the most frequently prescribed agent for this indication, its use is declining because of evidence of transplacental transfer and a possible increase in the risk of adverse outcomes in comparison with insulin.

There are limited data for other commonly used non-insulin antihyperglycemic medications such as glucagon like peptide 1 (GLP-1) agonists, sodium-glucose cotransporter-2 (SGLT-2) inhibitors, and dipeptidyl peptidase 4 (DPP-4) inhibitors. Patients should use contraception while taking these medications and stop using them before conceiving.

It is important to review signs and symptoms of hypoglycemia (e.g., tremor, palpitations, anxiety/arousal, sweating, hunger, dizziness, weakness, drowsiness, confusion) with the patient, as well as actions the patient (and close contacts) should take if hypoglycemia develops.

Patients should be instructed to carry a snack at all times.

If patients have a history of hypoglycemia or begin to experience hypoglycemia when tightening glucose management they should be given a prescription for glucagon and taught how to administer.

Reinforcement of hypoglycemia management is particularly important prepregnancy so that the patient is prepared in early pregnancy, when the frequency of hypoglycemia may increase due to tightened glucose management, changes in hormone levels, nausea and vomiting of pregnancy, and reduction in physical activity. Hypoglycemia is more likely to occur in patients with type 1 diabetes due to autoimmune destruction of the alpha cells that produce glucagon.

Meta-analyses comparing use of oral antihyperglycemic medications with insulin therapy have generally found that both approaches can improve some pregnancy outcomes in patients with GDM or type 2 diabetes.

There is a trend toward more frequent maternal hypoglycemia with use of insulin, and some patients on oral medications need supplemental insulin to achieve and maintain glucose levels in the target range.

However, it is difficult to draw firm conclusions about the optimal approach because of inconsistencies in criteria for GDM, glucose targets, patient adherence to treatment, clinical outcome measures across studies, and lack of long-term safety data.

Insulin

Dose: The insulin dose required to achieve target glucose levels varies among individuals, but the majority of studies have reported a total dose ranging from 0.7 to 2 units/kg (current pregnant weight). Dose titration to blood glucose levels is based upon frequent monitoring. At least four daily glucose measurements are required (fasting and one or two hours postprandial with the addition of pre-lunch and pre-dinner measurements as needed) to optimize therapy and ensure timely dose increases because insulin requirements increase with pregnancy progression. Indeed, the insulin requirement in twin gestations complicated by GDM may double with pregnancy progression.

Insulin pumps are not used in patients with GDM because there are no data to suggest that they are necessary or more effective than conventional therapy, and the cost of an insulin pump is not justified over the relatively short duration of a pregnancy.

If postprandial glucose levels throughout the day remain high, adjustments in the rapid-acting insulin dose are typically in the range of 10–20%. The upper end of this range is not likely to lead to hypoglycemia in patients with both obesity and GDM unless a meal is omitted after insulin is given.

If only the post-dinner glucose level remains elevated, then we add an injection of 6–10 units of rapid-acting insulin immediately before dinner.

If only the post-lunch glucose level remains elevated, we add an injection of 6–10 units of rapid-acting insulin immediately before lunch. If both post-breakfast and post-lunch glucose levels are elevated, increasing the morning NPH may be sufficient.

If the fasting glucose level is elevated after postprandial levels in the target range, we add an intermediate-acting basal insulin, preferably at bedtime but with dinner is another option on an individualized basis. The initial dose is 0.2 units/kg body weight.

Oral Antihyperglycemic Medications

Metformin and glyburide are the only noninsulin antihyperglycemic medications used in pregnancy. Both offer the advantage of significantly decreased cost compared with insulin and metformin is not associated with hypoglycemia.

Clinically important pregnancy outcomes are generally similar for metformin and glyburide, with only limited evidence of benefit of one oral medication over the other.

Need for supplemental insulin: The frequency of treatment failure (inability to maintain glucose levels in the target range) is similar for glyburide and metformin and ranges from approximately 15–30% in most trials directly comparing the two medications.

Placentar Transfer

Both medications cross the placenta (in contrast to insulin). Fetal metformin levels are 200% of the maternal level and glyburide levels are 70% of the maternal level, which has unknown long-term consequences.

Although metformin and glyburide have not been associated with an increased risk of congenital anomalies, when either medication is prescribed, patients should be made aware that information regarding the long-term effects of transplacental passage, including possible fetal programming effects, are largely unknown, so caution is required.

Metformin

A typical dosing regimen is to start metformin extended release (XR) 500 mg orally once daily (with dinner) and, if tolerated, increase by 500 mg (e.g., 1,000 mg with dinner or 500 mg with dinner plus 500 mg with breakfast) based on the degree of glucose elevations. The dose can then be increased by 500–1,000 mg orally per week until reaching the usual effective dose of 1,500–2,000 mg orally per day divided into two doses (maximum daily dose is 2,500 mg). An immediate release preparation is also available, but the XR is preferred as it may cause fewer gastrointestinal side effects and fewer daily doses may be needed.

The most common side effects of metformin are gastrointestinal, including a metallic taste in the mouth, mild anorexia, nausea, abdominal discomfort, and soft bowel movements or diarrhea. These symptoms are usually mild, transient, and reversible after dose reduction or discontinuation of the drug. Symptoms can be mitigated by starting at a low dose with slow-dose escalation as needed. In a clinical trial, only 2% of study subjects discontinued.

The ADA recommends avoiding metformin in patients with hypertension, preeclampsia, or at risk for fetal growth restriction due to the potential for impaired growth or acidosis in the setting of placental insufficiency.

Glyburide

Starting doses of 2.5–5 mg once daily are commonly used, increased as needed to a maximum of 20 mg per day. Twice-daily dosing is often necessary to maintain glucose levels in the target range. One group that investigated glyburide pharmacokinetics in pregnancy suggested pregnant patients take the drug 30–60 minutes before a meal, rather than with the meal, to improve efficacy. In this study, plasma glyburide concentrations in pregnant patients with GDM did not increase until 1 hour after drug ingestion, peaked at 2–3 hours, and returned to baseline by 8–10 hours. Thus, the drug took longer to reach peak concentration and was metabolized more rapidly than in nonpregnant females.

Maternal hypoglycemia is the most common side effect.

Patients who fail to achieve glycemic control with oral pharmacotherapy: If oral pharmacotherapy alone does not adequately manage glucose levels, supplemental insulin can be prescribed and may be easier for the patient than switching to a multidose insulin only regimen. In contrast to nonpregnant patients, dual use of oral agents (e.g., metformin plus glyburide) is not recommended in pregnancy because of minimal safety and efficacy data and concerns about adverse fetal effects since both drugs cross the placenta.

MATERNAL PROGNOSIS

Most patients with GDM are normoglycemic after giving birth. However, they are at high risk for recurrent GDM and developing prediabetes (impaired glucose tolerance or impaired fasting glucose) or overt diabetes over the subsequent 5 years and beyond.

Recurrence-GDM in one pregnancy is a strong predictor of recurrence in a subsequent pregnancy. In a study including over 65,000 pregnancies, the frequency of GDM in the second pregnancy among patients with and without previous GDM was 41 and 4%, respectively.

Long-term risk: A history of GDM is predictive of an increased risk of developing type 2 diabetes, metabolic syndrome, cardiovascular disease (CVD), and even type 1 diabetes. These risks appear to be particularly high in patients with both GDM and a hypertensive disorder of pregnancy. GDM has been called a "marker," "stress test," or "window" for future diabetes and CVD, but it is not considered causal.
- *Impaired glucose tolerance*: As many as 30% of patients with GDM have impaired glucose tolerance during the early postpartum period
- *Type 2 diabetes*: In a meta-analysis, patients with GDM were at an almost 10-fold higher risk of developing subsequent type 2 diabetes than patients with normoglycemic pregnancies

CONCLUSION

Successful management significantly improves maternal and fetal outcomes, preventing complications like macrosomia and neonatal metabolic issues. Following delivery, it's vital to discontinue GDM therapy and screen the mother for the progression to impaired glucose tolerance or type 2 diabetes mellitus, as a history of GDM is a strong predictor of her long-term risk for diabetes and cardiovascular disease.

FURTHER READINGS

1. American Diabetes Association (ADA). Standards of Medical Care in Diabetes—2025. Diabetes Care. 2025;48(Suppl 1):S1-S206.
2. American College of Obstetricians and Gynecologists (ACOG). Practice Bulletin No. 190: Gestational Diabetes Mellitus. Obstet Gynecol. 2018;131(2):e49-e64.
3. Ministry of Health and Family Welfare, Government of India. DIPSI Guidelines for Screening and Management of Gestational Diabetes Mellitus in India. New Delhi: Ministry of Health and Family Welfare; 2018.
4. UpToDate. Management of diabetes mellitus in pregnancy. UpToDate; 2024.
5. Loscalzo J, Fauci A, Kasper D, Hauser S, Longo D, Jameson JL. Harrison's Principles of Internal Medicine, 21st edition. Chapter 422: Diabetes Mellitus: Diagnosis, Classification, and Pathophysiology. New York: McGraw-Hill Education; 2022.
6. International Federation of Gynecology and Obstetrics (FIGO). FIGO Initiative on Gestational Diabetes Mellitus: A Pragmatic Guide for Diagnosis, Management and Care. Int J Gynecol Obstet. 2015;131(Suppl 3):S173-S211.
7. Metzger BE, Lowe LP, Dyer AR, Trimble ER, Chaovarindr U, Coustan DR, et al. Hyperglycemia and Adverse Pregnancy Outcomes (HAPO) Study. N Engl J Med. 2008;358:1991-2002.

SECTION 15

Pulmonology

SECTION

15

aulrenology

CHAPTER 40

Obstructive Sleep Apnea: What a Physician Needs to Know

Puneet Rijhwani, Vidita Kalra, Ram Kishan Jat, Shrikant Chaudhary

INTRODUCTION

Obstructive sleep apnea (OSA) is the most prevalent and clinically significant entity within the spectrum of sleep-disordered breathing—conditions marked by abnormal respiratory patterns during sleep that may coexist with cardiovascular, respiratory, neurological, or endocrine disorders.

Obstructive sleep apnea lies at the severe end of this spectrum, with primary snoring representing the mild end. It results from repetitive upper airway collapse during sleep, leading to intermittent airflow obstruction.

The hallmark features of OSA include obstructive apneas, hypopneas, and respiratory effort-related arousals (RERAs), which disrupt normal sleep architecture and impair gas exchange.

Clinically, OSA manifests as excessive daytime sleepiness and cognitive and behavioral disturbances (particularly in children) and has been independently linked to systemic hypertension, increased cardiovascular morbidity, and a heightened risk of occupational and motor vehicle accidents.

Recognizing and managing OSA are essential for physicians, given its high prevalence, multisystem impact, and significant implications for long-term health outcomes.

EPIDEMIOLOGY AND RISK FACTORS: WHAT A PHYSICIAN NEEDS TO KNOW

Obstructive sleep apnea is a common yet underdiagnosed disorder with a steadily increasing global burden, largely fueled by rising obesity rates. For physicians, understanding the epidemiological trends and associated risk factors is essential for early identification and risk stratification.

- *Global prevalence:* A comprehensive literature-based analysis estimated that nearly *one billion adults* aged 30–69 years are affected by OSA globally. Among all nations, *India ranks fourth* in terms of OSA burden, underscoring the need for increased awareness among Indian healthcare providers.

- *Sex differences: Male sex is a well-established risk factor,* with studies showing a prevalence of sleep-disordered breathing of *24% in men* and *9% in women* aged 30-60 years. Diagnostic criteria for sleep apnea syndrome are met by approximately *4% of men* and *2% of women*, with more recent data suggesting a possible increase to 9% and 4%, respectively. Indian data reflects similar trends, with a community-based study showing an OSA prevalence of *13.5% in men* and *5.5% in women*. However, the risk equalizes postmenopause, likely due to hormonal influences.
- *Obesity and body mass index (BMI): Obesity is the most significant modifiable risk factor*, with up to *60% of OSA patients* being overweight or obese. In younger adults, especially, a *higher BMI strongly correlates with increased OSA risk*. Notably, a *10% increase in weight* raises the risk of developing moderate-to-severe OSA by sixfold and increases the *apnea–hypopnea index (AHI)* by 32%. Additionally, *nearly 90% of patients* with obesity hypoventilation syndrome have coexisting OSA. Physicians must prioritize weight assessment and counseling as part of OSA risk reduction.
- *Age-related risk:* OSA prevalence rises steadily with *advancing age*, peaking in the *sixth to seventh decades* and then plateauing. Compared to individuals aged 20-29 years, those aged 60-80 years have a *34.5 times greater risk*, highlighting the importance of age as an independent risk factor.
- *Anatomical predispositions:* Structural abnormalities that narrow the upper airway—such as *enlarged tonsils or adenoids*, a *small nasal cavity*, or a *low-lying soft palate with a bulky uvula*—predispose individuals to airway collapse during sleep. *Craniofacial anomalies* like *micrognathia, retrognathia*, and a *broad craniofacial base* also elevate risk. Notably, studies among *Asian men with severe OSA* showed that many were *nonobese*, suggesting that *craniofacial architecture*, rather than BMI alone, plays a pivotal role in certain populations.
- *Genetic susceptibility:* Family history is clinically relevant. First-degree relatives of OSA patients have a two to four *times greater risk*, and *genetic influences* on fat distribution, craniofacial features, and neuromuscular tone may explain up to *40% of the variability in AHI*.
- *Other recognized risk factors*: Physicians should remain alert to additional contributors, such as:
  - Smoking
  - Menopause (due to hormonal changes; hormone replacement may be protective)
  - Chronic nasal congestion
  - Environmental pollutants (notably nitrogen dioxide and PM2.5 exposure)
- *Comorbid conditions:* While causality is still being explored, several *chronic diseases are strongly associated* with OSA, including:
  - Hypertension
  - Type 2 diabetes mellitus
  - Congestive heart failure
  - Coronary artery disease
  - Atrial fibrillation
  - Stroke

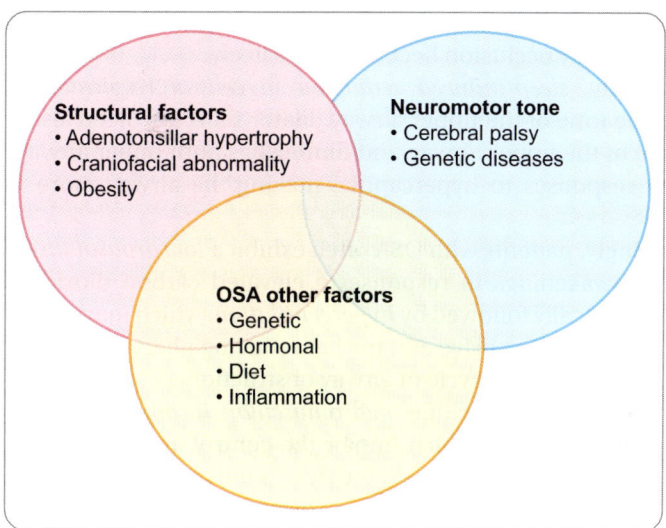

FIG. 1: Various factors.
(OSA: obstructive sleep apnea)

- Chronic lung disease
- Endocrine disorders (e.g., hypothyroidism, acromegaly)
- End-stage renal disease
- Gastroesophageal reflux disease (GERD)

As OSA often coexists with these conditions, physicians must maintain a *high index of suspicion* in patients presenting with these comorbidities—even in the absence of classic OSA symptoms **(Fig. 1)**.

PATHOPHYSIOLOGY

The pathogenesis of OSA involves a complex interplay of anatomical and neuromuscular factors that predispose the upper airway to collapse during sleep.

During inspiration, the pharyngeal airway—lacking rigid structural support from bone or cartilage—is subjected to increasingly negative intraluminal pressures. This creates a suction effect that pulls the airway walls inward. In healthy individuals, the patency of this airway is maintained by tonic and reflex activity of the pharyngeal dilator muscles.

In OSA patients, particularly those with anatomically narrow or collapsible airways, there is a sleep-related reduction in neuromuscular output. This results in transient episodes of airway obstruction, manifesting as *apneas* (complete collapse) or *hypopneas* (partial collapse). These episodes are typically interrupted by arousals triggered via chemoreceptor reflexes, which restore muscle tone and reestablish airflow. Common anatomical sites of collapse include the *soft palate* (most frequent), *tongue base, lateral pharyngeal walls,* and *epiglottis*.

Several structural factors increase the risk of airway collapse. These include *obesity* (with fat deposition around the airway), *age-related laxity, craniofacial abnormalities*, and genetically determined upper airway dimensions. When these structural predispositions encounter a collapsing transmural pressure during inspiration, airway occlusion becomes more likely.

Additionally, *sleep-induced reduction in central respiratory drive* further decreases the tone of the upper airway dilator muscles. Sleep also increases the compliance of the upper airway and diminishes both upper airway reflexes and ventilatory responses to hypercapnia, making the airway more vulnerable to collapse.

Interestingly, patients with OSA often exhibit a *low arousal threshold*, leading to frequent awakenings in response to elevated carbon dioxide levels. These arousals are typically followed by *hyperventilation*, which may cause *hypocapnia*, suppressing respiratory drive and further reducing pharyngeal muscle activity—thereby perpetuating the cycle of airway obstruction.

Other contributors include *neuromuscular incoordination* or underlying neuromuscular diseases, which impair the control and timing of upper airway muscles.

A reduction in *lung volume* during sleep, particularly in the setting of *aging* or *obesity*, removes the caudal traction normally exerted by inflated lungs on the upper airway. This further increases the propensity for collapse, particularly in the supine position **(Figs. 2A and B)**.

CLINICAL FEATURES

A physician must remain vigilant for the diverse and often subtle clinical manifestations of *OSA*, as early identification can significantly alter disease progression and complications.

Patients typically present with *daytime symptoms* that may impair functioning and quality of life:
- Difficulty maintaining full wakefulness or alertness
- Persistent fatigue, more frequently reported by women
- Generalized tiredness
- Impaired concentration and attention
- A sensation of unrefreshing or nonrestorative sleep despite adequate duration

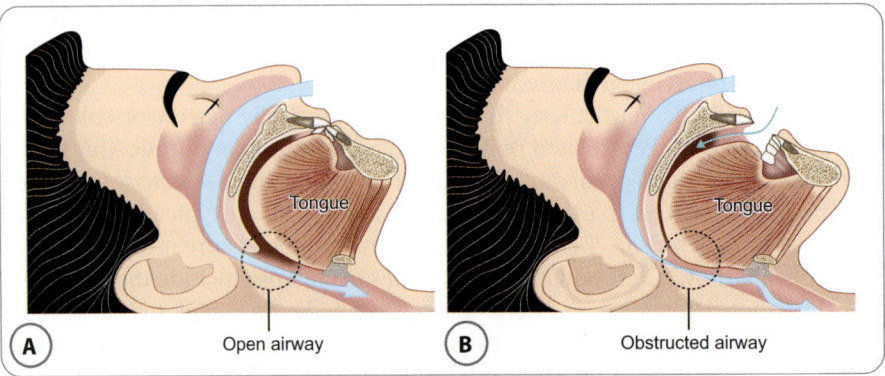

FIGS. 2A AND B: Airway specification.

The *Epworth Sleepiness Scale* is a useful tool to quantify subjective sleepiness and fatigue in clinical settings.

Nocturnal symptoms, often reported by bed partners, are key diagnostic clues and include:
- Loud, habitual snoring
- Gasping or choking episodes during sleep
- Snorting
- Observed breathing pauses

A systematic review encompassing 42 studies highlighted *nocturnal gasping or choking* as the most specific symptom for OSA (likelihood ratio 3.3), while *snoring*, although commonly reported, had limited specificity (likelihood ratio 1.1). Snoring showed a *high sensitivity (80%)* but *low specificity (50%)*, whereas gasping or choking had *moderate sensitivity (52%)* and *high specificity (84%)*. These figures underscore the importance of correlating symptoms rather than relying on any single complaint.

Additional *clinical symptoms* that should prompt evaluation for OSA include:
- *Morning headaches* (present in 12–18% of patients), which persist for several hours after awakening
- *Insomnia*, seen in up to 30% of OSA cases, with a higher prevalence in women
- *Nocturia*, affecting approximately 40% of patients and correlating with OSA severity in individuals under 50 years; continuous positive airway pressure (CPAP) therapy has been shown to significantly reduce nighttime urination frequency

Physical examination provides valuable insight into underlying risk factors and comorbidities. Physicians should specifically assess for:
- *Central obesity,* the most consistent clinical correlate
- *Increased waist and neck circumference* (neck > 17 inches in men, >16 inches in women)
- *Craniofacial abnormalities* and features of *upper airway crowding* on oropharyngeal examination

The *Mallampati classification* and *Friedman tongue position* serve as rapid screening tools to estimate the degree of airway narrowing, both showing a positive correlation with OSA severity **(Figs. 3 and 4)**.

DIAGNOSIS

The American Academy of Sleep Medicine (AASM) has outlined clear recommendations for the diagnostic evaluation of OSA, emphasizing the importance of objective testing in clinical decision-making.

Diagnostic assessment is warranted in individuals presenting with excessive daytime sleepiness in combination with at least two of the following features:
- Persistent loud snoring
- Witnessed apneas or episodes of choking during sleep
- Presence of systemic arterial hypertension

The AASM explicitly advises against relying solely on screening tools, symptom-based questionnaires, or predictive algorithms for diagnosing OSA

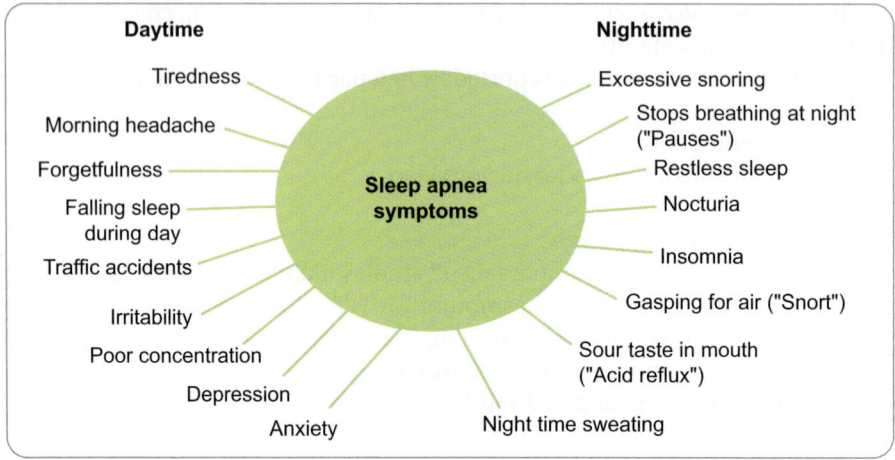

FIG. 3: Sleep apnea symptoms.

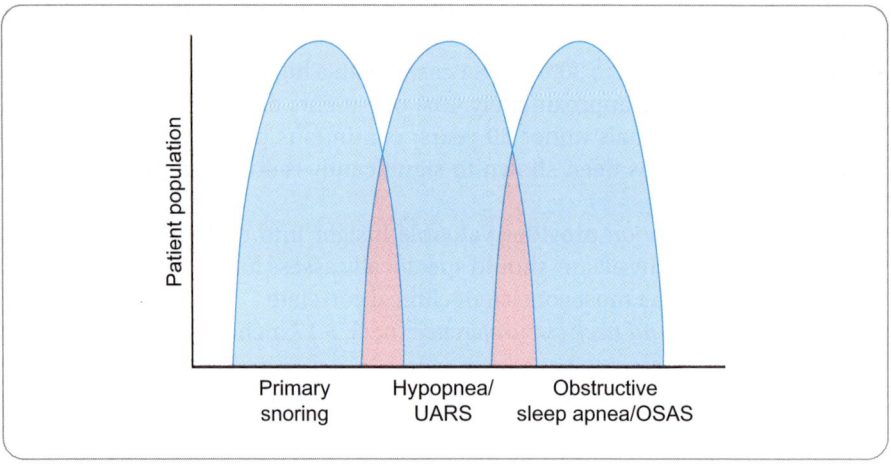

FIG. 4: Graphical representation of sleep differentiation with patient population.
(OSAS: obstructive sleep apnea syndrome; UARS: upper airway resistance syndrome)

in adults when polysomnography (PSG) or home-based sleep studies are not available. These tools, while useful for risk stratification, are not substitutes for definitive diagnostic testing. Common examples include:
- Berlin Questionnaire
- STOP-Bang Questionnaire
- NoSAS score (noted for better predictive performance)
- Multivariable Apnea Prediction (MVAP) instrument

For confirmatory diagnosis, physicians should utilize either home sleep apnea testing (HSAT), also referred to as out-of-center sleep testing (OCST), or in-laboratory PSG. While HSAT is appropriate in selected patients, PSG remains the gold standard, particularly in cases where HSAT is nondiagnostic, technically compromised, or equivocal.

As per the AASM and the International Classification of Sleep Disorders (ICSD), 3rd edition, the diagnostic criteria for OSA include the following:
- ≥15 *predominantly obstructive respiratory events per hour of sleep* (on PSG or HSAT), even in the absence of related symptoms or comorbid conditions
  OR
- ≥5 *obstructive respiratory events per hour of sleep*, accompanied by one or more of the following:
  - Complaints of excessive sleepiness, fatigue, nonrestorative sleep, or insomnia
  - Nocturnal gasping, choking, or breath-holding episodes
  - Observed breathing interruptions or habitual snoring, as reported by a bed partner or caregiver
  - Comorbidities such as systemic hypertension, type 2 diabetes mellitus (T2DM), coronary artery disease, atrial fibrillation, heart failure, stroke, cognitive decline, or mood disturbances

Definitions of respiratory events:
- *Apnea:* ≥90% reduction in airflow for ≥10 seconds, with continued respiratory effort
- *Hypopnea:* ≥30% reduction in airflow lasting ≥10 seconds, associated with either arousal or ≥3% oxygen desaturation
- *Respiratory effort-related arousal (RERA):* Arousal caused by increased respiratory effort and reduced airflow lasting ≥10 seconds, which does not meet the criteria for apnea or hypopnea

Physicians should interpret diagnostic data using two key indices:
1. *AHI:* Total number of apneas and hypopneas per hour of sleep
2. *Respiratory disturbance index (RDI):* Sum of apneas, hypopneas, and RERAs per hour of sleep

Among these, *RDI is often preferred* for its inclusion of subthreshold events and can be used to classify **(Figs. 5A to D)** disease severity as:
- *Mild:* 5–14 events/hour
- *Moderate:* 15–29 events/hour
- *Severe:* ≥30 events/hour

DIFFERENTIAL DIAGNOSIS

In clinical practice, a physician must distinguish OSA from other conditions that present with similar features, such as excessive daytime sleepiness, fatigue, or disrupted sleep. The following differentials should be carefully evaluated:
- *Primary snoring:* While most individuals with OSA do snore, not all patients who snore suffer from OSA. Primary snoring occurs without apneic or hypopneic events and lacks the associated daytime symptoms.
- *Pulmonary disorders:* Conditions like *asthma* and *chronic obstructive pulmonary disease (COPD)* can cause nocturnal symptoms, including wheezing and breathlessness, which may overlap with OSA manifestations.
- *Sleep deprivation:* Chronic insufficient sleep may mimic the daytime fatigue and sleepiness seen in OSA, necessitating a thorough sleep history.

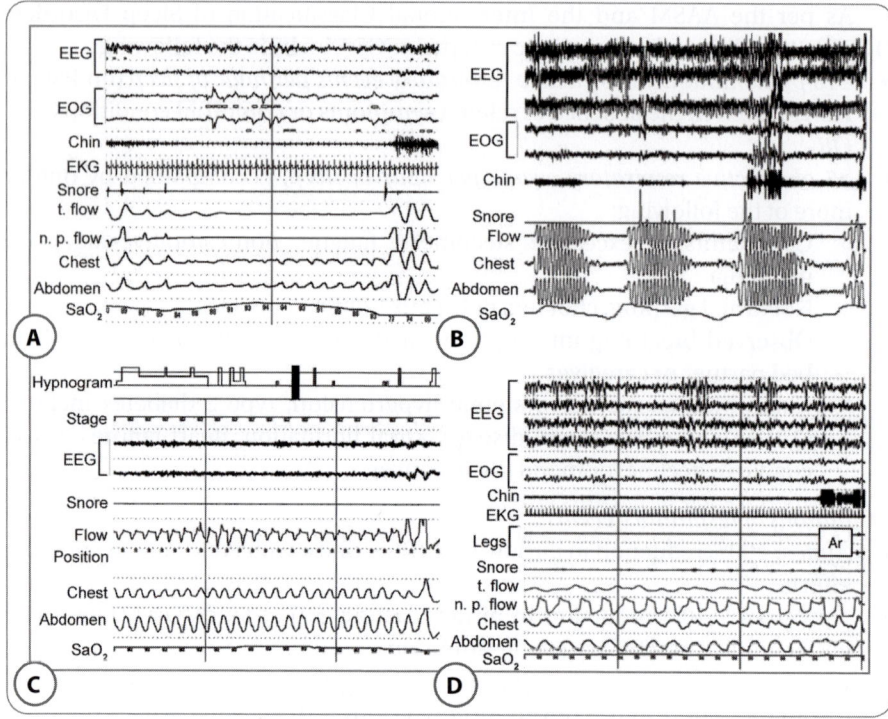

FIGS. 5A TO D: Obstructive apnea.

- *Other sleep disorders:* These include *central sleep apnea, narcolepsy, periodic limb movement disorder, restless legs syndrome*, and other non-OSA sleep-disordered breathing syndromes. Polysomnography is essential for differentiation.
- *Neurological conditions:* Disorders such as *Parkinson's disease, stroke*, or other central nervous system pathologies can result in hypersomnolence or fragmented sleep, mimicking OSA.
- *Neuromuscular disorders:* Diseases affecting respiratory muscle strength or coordination can contribute to hypoventilation and sleep-related breathing abnormalities.
- *Medical illnesses: Hypothyroidism, end-stage renal disease,* and *hepatic encephalopathy* may present with similar clinical profiles and should be ruled out through appropriate testing.
- *Pharmacological agents:* Use of *sedatives* (benzodiazepines, barbiturates, and Z-drugs), *antihistamines, antidepressants,* and *opioids* can depress the central nervous system and contribute to symptoms resembling OSA.
- *Psychiatric disorders:* Conditions such as *depression* and *anxiety* are frequently associated with non-restorative sleep and daytime fatigue and may coexist with or mimic OSA.
- *Substance abuse:* Chronic use of *alcohol, narcotics,* and other depressants can disrupt sleep architecture and promote airway collapse.

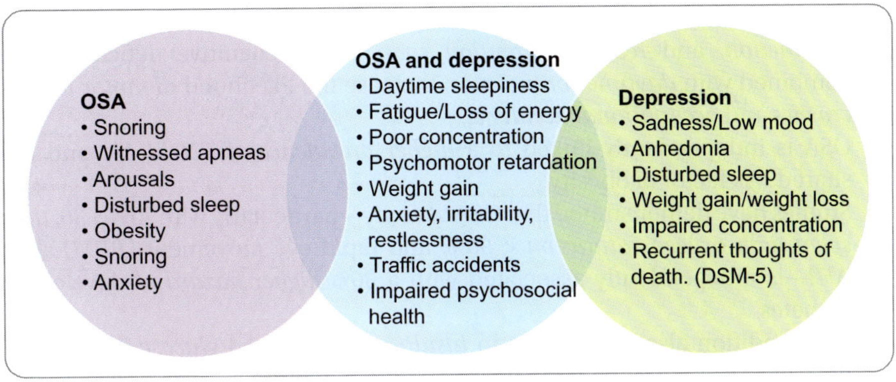

FIG. 6: Symptom overlap in obstructive sleep apnea and depression.
(DSM-5: Diagnostic and Statistical Manual of Mental Disorders, 5th Edition; OSA: obstructive sleep apnea)

- *Gastroesophageal reflux disease:* Nocturnal reflux may provoke arousals, coughing, or choking sensations during sleep, mimicking OSA-related awakenings **(Fig. 6)**.

COMPLICATIONS

Understanding the systemic impact of OSA is essential for physicians, as the condition is associated with multiple cardiovascular, cerebrovascular, metabolic, and neuropsychiatric complications. These adverse outcomes not only affect quality of life but also contribute to increased morbidity and premature mortality.

- OSA-induced *intermittent hypoxia* and *repeated sleep arousals* activate the sympathetic nervous system, resulting in *hemodynamic instability, endothelial dysfunction, inflammatory responses,* and *metabolic derangements.*
- Physicians should be aware of the significantly higher incidence of cardiovascular complications in OSA patients, including *myocardial infarction, heart failure, systemic hypertension, atrial fibrillation, coronary artery disease, QT interval prolongation, pulmonary hypertension,* and *venous thromboembolism.*
- Notably, OSA patients often exhibit a *"non-dipping" blood pressure pattern*—a failure to show the expected nocturnal decline in blood pressure—which has prognostic implications in hypertension management.
- A meta-analysis of 31 studies has shown that *CPAP therapy* provides a modest but statistically significant *reduction in blood pressure*, highlighting its therapeutic value in cardiovascular risk reduction.
- *Stroke risk* is elevated in OSA, particularly among *male patients*, underscoring the importance of early detection and risk stratification in this group.
- *Pulmonary hypertension*, classified under *Group 3* pulmonary hypertension in the World Health Organization (WHO) classification, is reported in *17–70%* of OSA patients, with most cases being *mild.*
- *Depression* occurs twice as frequently in individuals with OSA, with a higher burden noted in women. Physicians should consider mental health screening as part of routine OSA evaluation.

- Other *neuropsychiatric manifestations* include *memory impairment, executive dysfunction,* and *reduced attention span*. These cognitive deficits, when combined with *daytime somnolence,* increase the likelihood of *motor vehicle crashes* and *occupational accidents*.
- OSA is independently linked to a *higher prevalence of T2DM,* beyond the shared risk factor of obesity.
- Studies have demonstrated that OSA severity—particularly with *AHI > 30, time spent with oxygen saturation < 90%,* and rapid eye movement *(REM)-sleep AHI*—is independently associated with a *30% higher hazard* of developing diabetes.
- The condition also contributes to *insulin resistance* and *glucose intolerance,* both of which correlate strongly with the *RDI* and the extent of *sleep-related hypoxemia*.
- Up to *60%* of individuals with *metabolic syndrome* have *moderate-to-severe OSA,* and the coexistence of both conditions has been termed *"Syndrome Z."*
- OSA is independently associated with elevated *triglycerides, proinflammatory markers,* and accelerated *atherosclerosis*. Treatment with *CPAP* has been shown to improve several of these metabolic parameters.
- The chronic intermittent hypoxia characteristic of OSA may also *exacerbate nonalcoholic fatty liver disease (NAFLD),* especially in obese individuals, increasing its prevalence *two- to threefold*.
- Lastly, physicians should note that OSA has also been linked to an *increased risk of developing gout,* possibly due to intermittent nocturnal hypoxia affecting uric acid metabolism.

MANAGEMENT

- The cornerstone of OSA management begins with *comprehensive patient education and behavior modification*. Physicians must inform patients about the *natural course* of the disorder, *modifiable risk factors, potential long-term complications,* and the *heightened risk of accidents,* particularly those related to daytime somnolence.
- *Weight reduction* is essential for overweight or obese individuals. Physicians should advocate for *structured lifestyle interventions,* including dietary changes, physical activity, pharmacologic agents, or bariatric surgery when appropriate.
- Patients whose *OSA is predominantly positional,* as identified on PSG (i.e., more frequent apneas in the supine position), may benefit from *positional therapy*. This includes the use of specialized devices and, in some cases, *objective monitoring systems*.
- All patients must be counseled to *avoid alcohol and sedative medications,* especially those that depress central nervous system activity or contribute to weight gain, as these can exacerbate upper airway collapse during sleep.
- The *mainstay of treatment* for adults with OSA is *positive airway pressure (PAP) therapy,* primarily in the form of *CPAP* or *auto-titrating PAP (APAP)*. These modalities maintain airway patency and are effective across all severities of OSA.

- *CPAP therapy* significantly reduces the AHI, mitigates excessive daytime sleepiness, improves blood pressure control, and enhances overall quality of life. Physicians should emphasize *compliance and proper mask fitting* to maximize benefit.
- In patients unable to tolerate CPAP or with mild-to-moderate OSA, *oral appliances* may be considered. Devices such as *mandibular repositioning appliances* or *tongue-retaining devices* function by enlarging the upper airway. Though less effective than CPAP, they often have *higher patient adherence*.
- In cases where OSA is secondary to identifiable and correctable upper airway lesions (e.g., *adenoid or tonsillar hypertrophy, craniofacial abnormalities*), *surgical intervention* may be appropriate as a *first-line option*.
- Surgery may also serve as a *second-line therapy* in patients with documented CPAP or oral appliance failure or intolerance.
- In carefully selected patients who have *failed CPAP*, possess a *BMI <32 kg/m²*, and meet anatomical eligibility criteria, *hypoglossal nerve stimulation* has shown promising results. A meta-analysis demonstrated *significant reductions in AHI and daytime sleepiness* at 12-month follow-up.
- *Tracheostomy*, although definitive in bypassing upper airway obstruction and eliminating OSA, is *reserved for refractory cases* due to its *impact on quality of life*.
- As of now, *no pharmacologic agent has demonstrated long-term efficacy* comparable to PAP therapies. Physicians should be cautious in offering medical therapy as a standalone treatment.
- A *Cochrane review* of 25 pharmacological agents identified only 10 with potential short-term benefit. However, their *long-term safety and efficacy remain unestablished*.
- *Dronabinol*, a synthetic cannabinoid, has demonstrated reductions in AHI in moderate-to-severe OSA, but further *phase III trials are needed*, and it is *not currently recommended for routine use*.
- For patients who continue to experience *residual daytime sleepiness despite optimal PAP adherence*, the addition of *central nervous system stimulants* such as *modafinil or armodafinil* may be considered, following *exclusion of other reversible causes* **(Fig. 7)**.

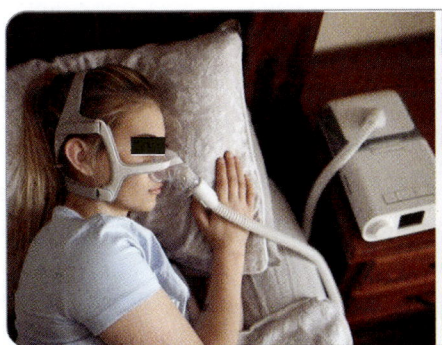
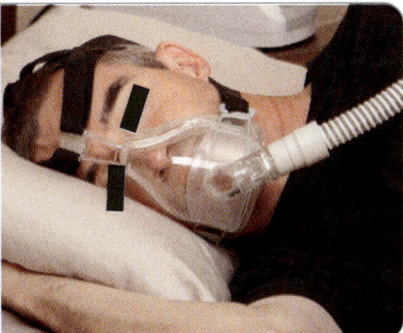

FIG. 7: Sleep patterns.

CONCLUSION

Obstructive sleep apnea is no longer a niche concern confined to sleep specialists—it is a pervasive, multisystem disorder with far-reaching implications across cardiovascular, metabolic, and neuropsychiatric health. For physicians, recognizing OSA as a common yet underdiagnosed condition is vital, given its strong associations with hypertension, diabetes, coronary artery disease, stroke, and impaired quality of life.

A comprehensive understanding of its epidemiology, pathophysiology, clinical manifestations, and diagnostic criteria enables timely identification of at-risk individuals. The use of polysomnography or validated home-based sleep studies remains the gold standard for diagnosis, while positive airway pressure (PAP) therapy continues to be the cornerstone of management.

Equally important is the physician's role in patient education, weight optimization, lifestyle modification, and management of comorbidities. Collaboration among primary care physicians, pulmonologists, endocrinologists, cardiologists, and sleep specialists ensures holistic and sustained care.

Early detection and effective treatment of OSA not only alleviate daytime symptoms and improve sleep quality but also mitigate long-term morbidity and mortality. With growing awareness and multidisciplinary engagement, physicians can play a transformative role in addressing this silent epidemic of modern medicine.

FURTHER READINGS

1. Peppard PE, Young T, Barnet JH, Palta M, Hagen EW, Hla KM. Increased prevalence of sleep-disordered breathing in adults. Am J Epidemiol. 2013;177(9):1006-14.
2. Benjafield AV, Ayas NT, Eastwood PR, Heinzer R, Ip MSM, Morrell MJ, et al. Estimation of the global prevalence and burden of obstructive sleep apnoea: a literature-based analysis. Lancet Respir Med. 2019;7(8):687-98.
3. Young T, Palta M, Dempsey J, Peppard PE, Nieto FJ, Hla KM. Burden of sleep apnea: rationale, design, and major findings of the Wisconsin Sleep Cohort study. WMJ. 2009;108(5):246-9.
4. Young T, Palta M, Dempsey J, Skatrud J, Weber S, Badr S. The occurrence of sleep-disordered breathing among middle-aged adults. N Engl J Med. 1993;328(17):1230-5.
5. Reddy EV, Kadhiravan T, Mishra HK, Sreenivas V, Handa KK, Sinha S, et al. Prevalence and risk factors of obstructive sleep apnea among middle-aged urban Indians: a community-based study. Sleep Med. 2009;10(8):913-8.

CHAPTER 41

Bronchial Asthma: Newer Therapies

Paramita Bhattacharya, Subhro Jyoti Mukherjee

INTRODUCTION

Bronchial asthma is a heterogeneous disorder of chronic inflammation of the airways, marked by bronchial hyperresponsiveness, reversible airflow obstruction, and symptoms like wheezing, breathlessness, chest tightness, and coughing, that vary over time and intensity, along with variable expiratory airflow limitation.

Although inhaled corticosteroids (ICS) and long-acting β_2-agonists (LABA) remain the foundation stone of asthma management, a substantial proportion of patients—especially those with severe or treatment-refractory asthma—require advanced therapies. Recent advances have enabled us to subclassify asthma into distinct phenotypes and endotypes (T2-high and T2-low inflammatory pathways), which have led to the emergence of newer therapies.

Breakthroughs have emerged in biologic treatments, procedural interventions, precision diagnostics, repurposed drugs, and digital tools. This chapter explores these novel therapies, their mechanisms, clinical evidence, and future prospects.

BRIEF PATHOPHYSIOLOGY

Earlier, bronchial asthma was thought to be mediated by excessive T-helper-2 (Th2) cell responses and immunoglobulin-E (IgE) hyper-responsiveness. But this only conveys to us the mechanism of allergic asthma. Present pathophysiology is based on clusters of clinical features, lung function, and level of inflammation—known as *"asthma phenotypes."* On the other hand, there are certain biological mechanisms linking the molecular pathway with the clinical features within each phenotype—known as *"asthma endotypes"* **(Table 1)**.

- *Type 2-high asthma*:
    - Majority (40–50%) of patients
    - Excessive Th2 cells' activation—release of inflammatory mediators—interleukins (ILs)—IL-4, IL-5, and IL-13
    - More common in severe asthma
    - Associated with—high eosinophil count, high FeNO (fractional excretion of nitric oxide), high serum periostin (surrogate marker for Th2 response)

TABLE 1: Major differences between T2-high and T2-low asthma.	
T2-high asthma	**T2-low asthma**
More severe	Less severe
Atopic/IgE-associated	Associated with neutrophilia
Eosinophilic	Absence of eosinophilia
Good response to T2 inhibition	Poor response to T2 inhibition
Good response to steroids	Poor response to steroids
(IgE: immunoglobulin E)	

- *Type 2-low asthma*:
  - Less common (30–40%)
  - Fewer allergic symptoms, presentation at a late age
  - Neutrophilic, mixed, or paucigranulocytic asthma
  - Mediated by IL-25 and IL-33

STANDARD THERAPY

The 2024 Global Initiative for Asthma (GINA) guidelines clearly advise all adults and adolescents with bronchial asthma to be treated with ICS-containing medications and advise against treatment with short-acting beta agonist (SABA) alone. It divides treatment into two tracks, with track 1 being preferred **(Tables 2 and 3)**.

REQUIREMENT OF NEWER THERAPIES IN ASTHMA

We need novel molecular therapies to treat the following subgroups:
- *Difficult asthma*:
  - Poor symptom control—frequent symptoms, frequent usage of reliever therapy, night awakenings, and limitation of activities of daily living
  - Frequent exacerbations (≥2/year), frequent hospital admissions (≥1/year), using OCS (oral corticosteroids)
- *Difficult-to-treat asthma*: Uncontrolled asthma—despite medium- or high-dose ICS with a second controller therapy (usually LABA) or with maintenance OCS
- *Severe asthma*: Uncontrolled asthma—despite on maximally tolerated high-dose ICS with LABA and worsening on reducing drug dosing

As per a study in the Netherlands (reported by Hekking et al., 2015), around 24% of asthma patients need to undergo GINA step 4–5 treatment. In this subgroup, 17% of patients have difficult-to-treat asthma and 3.7% of patients have severe asthma **(Flowchart 1)**.

TABLE 2: Different phenotypes and endotypes of bronchial asthma.

Domain	Phenotype	Endotype	Pathways	Therapeutic implications
Onset and atopy	Early-onset allergic asthma	T2-high allergic	Th2 cell-driven: • IL-4/15: IgE switching • IL-5: Eosinophil recruitment	• ICS responsive • Omalizumab (anti-IgE)
Severity/Course	Late-onset eosinophilic asthma	T2-high nonallergic eosinophilic	Innate lymphoid cells (ILC-2) driven: IL-5 and IL-13-mediated — • Adult onset • Severe • Frequent exacerbation	• Mepolizumab • Reslizumab • Benralizumab • Dupilumab
Steroid response	Noneosinophilic steroid-resistant asthma	T2-low neutrophilic	Neutrophilic sputum: low FeNO— • Th1: IFN (interferon)-mediated • Th17: IL-17-mediated	• Poor ICS response • Macrolides
Trigger-related	Aspirin-exacerbated respiratory disease (AERD)	T2-high eosinophilic	Dysregulated eicosanoid metabolism: • LT (leukotriene overproduction) • Reduced PGE2 • Mast cell activation	• LTRA (leukotriene receptor antagonist) • Aspirin desensitization • Biologics
Systemic or comorbid condition	Obese asthma phenotype	Mixed, often T2-low with metabolic inflammation	• Adipokine imbalance • Low eosinophils • Low FeNO • Reduced steroid sensitivity	• Weight reduction • Bariatric surgery
Occupational, irritants	Occupational asthma	Mixed, often non-T2	• Direct epithelial injury • IgE-independent mechanisms • Neutrophil activation	• Avoidance of exposures • Immunomodulators
Structural remodeling	Frequent exacerbator type	Mixed	• Viral infections • Epithelial alarmins-driven inflammation: IL-25, IL-33, TSLP-driven	• Limited ICS response • Tezepelumab • Antivirals

(FeNO: fractional exhaled nitric oxide; IL: interleukin; ICS: inhaled corticosteroid; IFN: interferon; IgE: immunoglobulin E; PGE2: prostaglandin E2; TSLP: thymic stromal lymphopoietin)

TABLE 3: Standard therapy for bronchial asthma (GINA 2024).

Step	Patient subgroup	Track 1 (preferred) (ICS-formoterol reliever)	Track 2 (alternative) (SABA—reliever)	Notes
1	Infrequent symptoms (≤2/month), no risk factors	• As needed • Low dose • ICS-formoterol	Take ICS whenever SABA is taken	Avoid SABA-only therapy
2	Symptoms >2/month	• As needed • Low dose • ICS-formoterol	Daily low-dose ICS + SABA as needed	If daily ICS intake adherence is poor, use an "as needed" approach
3	Symptoms most days, night waking, poor lung function	Low-dose maintenance ICS-formoterol + as needed (MART)	Daily low-dose ICS-LABA + SABA as needed	MART
4	Uncontrolled asthma on step 3	Medium-dose maintenance ICS-formoterol + as needed	Daily medium-dose ICS-LABA + SABA as needed	Short course of oral steroid during exacerbation
5	Severe asthma, not controlled on step 4	High-dose maintenance ICS-formoterol ± LAMA (tiotropium) ± biologics	Daily high-dose ICS-LABA ± LAMA (tiotropium) ± biologics	

(ICS: inhaled corticosteroid; LABA: long-acting β2 agonist; MART: maintenance and reliever therapy; SABA: short-acting β2 agonist)

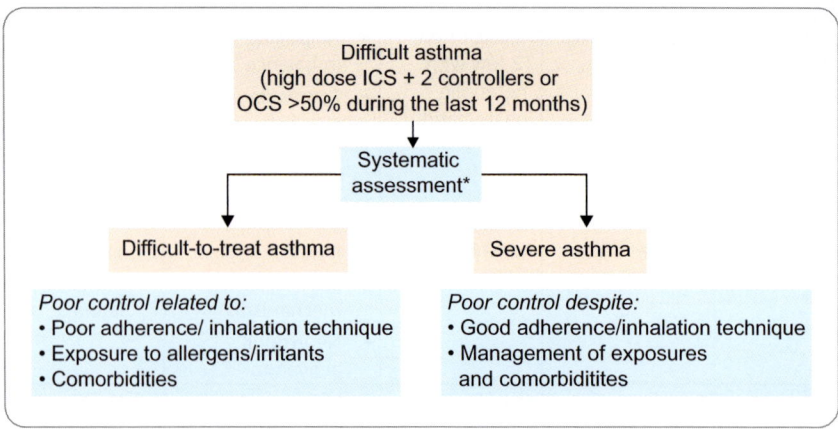

*Systematic assessment includes: inhaler technique check, treatment adherence evaluation, trigger/allergen exposure assessment, and comorbidity optimization (e.g., GERD, obesity, rhinosinusitis, anxiety, and smoking status).

FLOWCHART 1: Difficult asthma in cases.

(ICS: inhaled corticosteroid; OCS: oral corticosteroid)

Source: Porsbjerg C, Ulrik C, Skjold T, Backer V, Laerum B, Lehman S, et al. Nordic consensus statement on the systematic assessment and management of possible severe asthma in adults. Eur Clin Respir J. 2018;5(1):1440868.

BIOLOGICS IN ASTHMA

Targeted Biologic Therapies

Biologics have markedly transformed the management of severe asthma, especially in patients characterized by type 2 inflammation (e.g., elevated eosinophils, high FeNO). A robust meta-analysis (Kyriakopoulos et al.) shows that biologics reduce annual exacerbations by 44% and hospitalizations by 60%, improve lung function [mean forced expiratory volume in 1 second (FEV_1) increase of 0.11 L], and enhance quality of life with favorable safety profiles **(Table 4)**.

Newer Agents

Newer therapies surround the concept of "alarmin cytokines"—thymic stromal lymphopoietin (TSLP), IL-25, and IL-33. These are epithelial cell-derived mediators released on exposure to environmental triggers. They activate multiple effector cells and lead to the release of predominantly T2 cytokines. Their position in the upstream makes them an attractive target for future drug therapies **(Table 5)**.

Newer Approaches

In T2-low phenotypes, we have novel drugs attempting to target innate immunity pathways. These include the following **(Table 6)**:
- *Anti-IL-8, IL-17, IL-1, IL-6, IL-23, and tumor necrosis factor-alpha (TNF-α)*—investigational inhibition of neutrophilic mediators

TABLE 4: Targeted biologic therapies in bronchial asthma.

Agent	Mechanism of action	Patient selection
Omalizumab	Anti-IgE antibody	• Age ≥ 6 years • IgE level within reference range • Allergic sensitization on skin prick or serology
Reslizumab	Anti-IL-5 antibody	• Age ≥ 18 years • AEC ≥ 400/µL in the past 12 months
Mepolizumab	Anti-IL-5 antibody	• Age ≥ 12 years • AEC ≥ 300/µL in the past 12 months and ≥150/µL at the time of testing
Benralizumab	Anti-IL-5 receptor antibody—induces eosinophil apoptosis by antibody-dependent cytotoxicity	• Age ≥ 12 years • AEC ≥ 300/µL in the past 12 months
Dupilumab	Anti-IL-4 receptor antibody—inhibits both IL-4 and IL-13 pathways	• Age ≥ 12 years • AEC ≥ 300/µL in the past 12 months • FeNO > 25 ppb

(AEC: absolute eosinophil count; FeNO: fractional exhaled nitric oxide; IL: interleukin)

TABLE 5: Summary of alarmin cytokines.

Alarmin	Source	Action	Clinical significance
TSLP	• Airway epithelium • Mast cells	Activates dendritic cells • Th2 activation • Activates ILC2 • Enhances IgE class switching	Tezepelumab (anti-TSLP)—first alarmin biologic approved for severe asthma
IL-33	• Epithelial cells • Fibroblasts • Endothelial cells	Binds ST2 receptor—activation of: • Mast cells • ILC2 • Eosinophils Amplifies Th2 response	Blocked by investigational therapy • Itepekimab • Astegolimab
IL-25	• Epithelial cells • Eosinophils • Basophils	• Activates ILC2 and Th2 response • Also promotes eosinophilia	Under study

[ILC2: type 2 innate lymphoid cells; ST2: suppression of tumorigenicity 2 receptor (IL-33 receptor); TSLP: thymic stromal lymphopoietin]

TABLE 6: Novel agents targeting alarmin cytokines.

Agent	Mechanism	Trials	Regulatory status
Tezepelumab	Blocks TSLP—an epithelial alarmin upstream of both T2 and non-T2 pathways	NAVIGATOR—phase 3	FDA approved for add-on maintenance therapy in severe asthma (Dec 2021)
Astegolimab	Targets ST-2—the IL-33 receptor—blocks downstream signaling	Phase 2 RCT	Not yet approved
Itepekimab	Neutralizes IL-33 directly	Phase 2 RCT	Not yet approved

[FDA: Food and Drug Administration; IL: interleukin; RCT: randomized controlled trial; ST2: suppression of tumorigenicity 2 receptor (IL-33 receptor); TSLP: thymic stromal lymphopoietin]

- *Mitogen-activated protein (MAP) kinase, phosphoinositide 3 (PI3) kinase, and tyrosine kinase inhibitors*: Agents aimed at restoring corticosteroid sensitivity
- *Phosphodiesterase type 3 and type 4 (PDE3/PDE4) inhibitors*: Anti-inflammatory and bronchodilator potential are being explored in ongoing trials
- *Airway smooth muscle-targeted therapies*: In paucigranulocytic T2-low asthma **(Table 7)**

CONCLUSION

Bronchial asthma is a heterogeneous disease requiring a phenotype- and endotype-guided treatment approach. While inhaled corticosteroids remain

TABLE 7: Ongoing clinical trials.

Agent	Trial type	Mechanism	Phase/Status	Study Population
Tezepelumab	Structural/Airways function study	Anti-TSLP (alarmin)	Phase 3	Moderate-to-severe uncontrolled asthma
Tezepelumab	Maintenance step-down/remission study	Anti-TSLP (alarmin)	Phase 3b	Severe uncontrolled asthma
Itepekimab	Moderate-to-severe asthma	Anti-IL-33	Phase 2	Mild allergic asthma
Itepekimab	Long-term safety/tolerability study (COPD)	Anti-IL-33	Phase 3	COPD (safety cohort)
Dexpramipexole	EXHALE-2 (oral eosinophil lowering)	Oral eosinophil depletor	Phase 3	Severe eosinophilic asthma
Dexpramipexole	EXHALE-3	Oral eosinophil depletor	Phase 3	Severe eosinophilic asthma
Dexpramipexole	EXHALE-4	Oral eosinophil depletor	Phase 3	Eosinophilic asthma

(COPD: chronic obstructive pulmonary disease; IL: interleukin; TSLP: thymic stromal lymphopoietin)

the backbone of therapy, a significant proportion of patients need advanced treatments such as biologics, immunomodulators, and emerging alarmin-targeted therapies. Precision medicine has enabled improved outcomes in severe and treatment-refractory asthma. Future therapies focusing on upstream inflammatory pathways and steroid-resistant phenotypes hold the key to achieving disease remission and personalized care.

FURTHER READINGS

1. Seluk L, Davis AE, Rhoads S, Wechsler ME. Novel asthma treatments: advancing beyond approved novel step-up therapies for asthma. Ann Allergy Asthma Immunol. 2025;134(1):9-18.
2. Kyriakopoulos C, Gogali A, Markozannes G, Kostikas K. Biologic agents licensed for severe asthma: a systematic review and meta-analysis of randomised controlled trials. Eur Respir Rev. 2024;33(172):230238.
3. Gyawali B, Georas SN, Khurana S. Biologics in severe asthma: a state-of-the-art review. Eur Respir Rev. 2025;34(175):240088.
4. Faria N, Costa MI, Fernandes AL, Fernandes A, Fernandes B, Machado DC, et al. Biologic therapies for severe asthma: current insights and future directions. J Clin Med. 2025;14(9):3153.
5. Cazolla M, Hanania NA, Matera MG, Rogliani P. Biologics for severe asthma: deciphering what is best for the patient. Exper Rev Clin Immunol. 2025;21(8):1035-54.
6. Hekking PW, Wener RR, Amelink M, et al. The prevalence of severe refractory asthma. J Allergy Clin Immunol. 2015;135(4):896-902.

CHAPTER 42: 6-Minute Walk Test

Sonam Spalgais, Prashant Prakash

INTRODUCTION

The 6-minute walk test (6MWT) is a simple cardiopulmonary functional testing modality. It evaluates the global and integrated responses of all the systems involved during exercise, including the pulmonary and cardiovascular with other systems. It does not provide specific information on the function of different systems involved in exercise or exercise limitation, as is possible with maximal cardiopulmonary exercise testing. It is self-paced and assesses the submaximal level of functional capacity. Most patients do not achieve maximal exercise capacity during the 6MWT. However, because most activities of daily living are performed at submaximal levels of exertion, the 6-minute walk distance (6MWD) may better reflect the functional exercise level. It is a simple, practical test that requires a 100-ft hallway without equipment or advanced training. Walking is an activity performed daily by all but the most severely impaired patients. This test measures the distance that can be quickly walked on a flat surface in 6 minutes. The results can assist in ascertaining the degree of functional impairment and potentially lead to modifications in therapy.

CLINICAL EXERCISE TESTING

The commonly used walk tests are listed in **Box 1**. Despite so many walk tests, why we choose 6MWT over others is because of its relatively low complexity. The patient is asked to walk as far as possible for 6 minutes, with the primary outcome being 6MWD **(Box 2)**.

INDICATIONS AND CONTRAINDICATIONS

Box 3 summarizes the various indications.
Table 1 summarizes the list of absolute and relative contraindications.

TECHNICAL ASPECTS OF THE 6-MINUTE WALK TEST

Location: It is recommended that the test be performed along a long, flat, straight corridor. The walking course must have a length of 30 m. The length of the corridor should be marked every 3 m. The turnaround points should be marked with a cone.

BOX 1: Commonly used walk tests.

- Endurance walk test
- Oximetry
- 6MWT
- Endurance shuttle walk test
- Incremental shuttle walk test
- Stair climbing
- Upper extremity test
- Cardiopulmonary exercise testing

(6MWT: 6-minute walk test)

BOX 2: Why we chose 6MWT over others?

- Simplicity
- Reproducibility
- Delivers a consolidated image of the cardiopulmonary and musculoskeletal response to exercise
- Requires no special training
- Minimum equipment and items
- Safe and well tolerated
- Highly reflective of usual daily activity and exercise performance

(6MWT: 6-minute walk test)

BOX 3: Indications for 6MWT.

- *Pretreatment and post-treatment comparisons:*
  - Lung transplantation
  - Lung resection
  - Lung volume reduction surgery
  - Pulmonary rehabilitation
  - COPD
  - Pulmonary hypertension
  - Heart failure
- *Predictors of morbidity and mortality:*
  - Heart failure
  - COPD
  - Primary pulmonary hypertension
  - Idiopathic pulmonary fibrosis
- *Functional status (single measurement):*
  - COPD
  - Cystic fibrosis
  - Heart failure
  - Peripheral vascular disease
  - Fibromyalgia
  - Older patients

(6MWT: 6-minute walk test; COPD: chronic obstructive pulmonary disease)

TABLE 1: Contraindications for 6MWT.	
Absolute	**Relative**
• Acute myocardial infarction • Unstable angina • Uncontrolled arrhythmias • Syncope • Acute endocarditis/myocarditis/pericarditis • Severe aortic stenosis • Uncontrolled heart failure • Acute pulmonary embolism • Thrombosis of lower extremities • Suspected dissecting aneurysm • Uncontrolled asthma • Pulmonary edema • $SpO_2 < 85\%$ • Acute respiratory failure • Acute noncardiopulmonary disorder • Mental impairment	• Left main coronary stenosis • Moderate stenotic valvular disease • Untreated hypertension (>200/180 mm Hg) • High degree atrioventricular block • Hypertrophic cardiomyopathy • Pulmonary hypertension • Pregnancy • Electrolyte abnormalities • Orthopedic impairment

(6MWT: 6-minute walk test)

Rationale: A shorter corridor requires patients to take more time to reverse directions more often, reducing the 6MWD. Most studies have used a 30-m corridor, with a few studies using 20 or 50 m. The use of a treadmill for 6MWT is not recommended. One study comprising severe lung disease patients found that the mean distance walked on the treadmill was shorter by a mean of 14%.

Required equipment: The recommended equipment are as follows:
- Stopwatch
- Lap counter
- Cones
- Chair
- Worksheets
- Oxygen source
- Sphygmomanometer
- Mobile
- Automated electronic defibrillator

The person who performs the test must be knowledgeable in the standard protocol of the test, and the minimum requirement is training in basic life support.

Patient preparation: The guidelines recommended for the following:
- Comfortable clothing
- Appropriate shoes
- Should use usual walking aids
- Usual medicines should be continued
- Light meal is acceptable.
- Should not have exercised within 2 hours
- Rest for 10 minutes before testing

Technique:
- Measure the heart rate, blood pressure (BP), respiratory rate, and oxygen saturation (SpO_2).
- A "warm-up" period should not be performed.
- Baseline dyspnea and leg fatigue are then rated using the Borg scale.
- Set the lap counter and timer.
- Provide the detailed instructions on how to proceed.
- The patient is allowed to walk unassisted or with a walking aid.
- The technician should only address the patient during the test. As each minute passes, the patient should be informed of the time left to complete and encouraged.
- At the end of the test, record the Borg dyspnea and fatigue levels, check heart rate, BP, respiratory rate, and SpO_2, the number of laps from the counter or marks, and the total distance walked.

Instructions: Instruct the patient as follows during the test:
- "The object of the test is to walk for 6 minutes. You will walk back and forth in this hallway for 6 minutes, so you will be exerting yourself."
- "You will probably get out of breath or exhausted. You are permitted to slow down, to stop, and to rest as necessary. You may lean against the wall but resume walking as soon."
- "You should pivot briskly around the cones and continue back the other way without hesitation."
- "I will click it each time you turn around at this starting line. Remember that the object is to walk AS FAR AS POSSIBLE for 6 minutes."
- "Start now, or whenever you are ready."

The following standard encouragements are used during the test:
- After the end of each minute, inform him that he has so many minutes to go.
- When the timer shows only 1 minute remaining, tell the patient: "You are doing well. You have only 1 minute to go."

Do not use other words of encouragement.
- If the patient stops walking during the test and needs a rest, say this: "You can lean against the wall if you would like; then continue walking whenever you feel able." Do not stop the timer.
- If the patient stops before the 6 minutes are up and refuses to continue (or you decide that they should not continue), discontinue the walk and note the distance.
- When the timer is 15 seconds from completion, say this: "In a moment, I'm going to tell you to stop. When I do, just stop right."
- When the timer rings, say this: "Stop!"
- *After reporting*: Record the postwalk Borg dyspnea and fatigue levels.
- Calculate the total distance walked.

When to stop 6MWT: The test should stop if the patient complains of chest pain, intolerable dyspnea, leg cramps, staggering, diaphoresis, and pale or ashen appearance during the test.

Supplemental oxygen: If oxygen supplementation is needed during the walk, then do the test with oxygen supplementation. During all walks, oxygen should be delivered in the same way with the same flow. The type of oxygen delivery device should also be noted on the report.

Reporting: The report of 6MWT mainly consists of 6MWD and oxygen desaturation. Other parameters are heart rate, dyspnea, and leg fatigue. The 6MWD is the primary outcome, given its excellent reliability and validity, as well as a strong relationship to important clinical outcomes. The 6MWD should be reported for every test. Oxygen desaturation provides information regarding exercise-induced desaturation, disease severity, and disease progress. Constant monitoring of SpO_2 during the 6MWT is optional.

INTERPRETATION

Most 6MWTs will be done before and after intervention, and the primary question to be answered is whether the patient has experienced a clinically significant improvement. The interpretation is commonly done using the minimal clinically important difference (MCID) and responsiveness to 6MWD.

Minimal clinically important difference: Available evidence suggests a MCID of 30 minutes for the 6MWD in adults with chronic respiratory disease. There is currently little evidence to suggest that the MCID varies according to patient characteristics.

Responsiveness of the 6MWD: 6MWD appears to be responsive to treatment effects in patients with chronic obstructive pulmonary disease (COPD), interstitial lung disease (ILD), and pulmonary arterial hypertension (PAH).

SAFETY AND COMPLICATIONS

The 6MWT is a safe test with rare complications. The common adverse event was oxygen desaturation < 80% in 5% of testing. Patient symptoms prematurely terminated the test in 1%. Chest pain and tachycardia have been reported much less frequently. Testing should be performed in a location where a rapid, appropriate response to an emergency is possible. Supplies that must be available include oxygen, sublingual nitroglycerine, aspirin, and albuterol. If a patient is on chronic oxygen therapy, oxygen should be given at the standard rate.

CONCLUSION

The 6MWT is a useful functional capacity test. It is a submaximal test that is simple to perform and interpret. The test has been widely used for preoperative and postoperative evaluation and for measuring the response to therapeutic interventions for pulmonary and cardiac disease. A standardized approach is crucial as the test is extremely sensitive to methodology.

FURTHER READINGS

1. ATS Committee on Proficiency Standards for Clinical Pulmonary Function Laboratories. ATS statement: guidelines for the six-minute walk test. Am J Respir Crit Care Med. 20021;166(1):111-7.
2. Holland AE, Spruit MA, Troosters T, Puhan MA, Pepin V, Saey D, et al. An official European Respiratory Society/American Thoracic Society technical standard: field walking tests in chronic respiratory disease. Eur Respir J. 2014;44(6):1428-46.
3. Agarwala P, Salzman SH. Six-minute walk test: clinical role, technique, coding, and reimbursement. Chest. 2020;157(3):603-11.
4. Nixon PA, Joswiak ML, Fricker FJ. A six-minute walk test for assessing exercise tolerance in severely ill children. J Pediatr. 1996;129:362-6.
5. Stevens D, Elpern E, Sharma K, Szidon P, Ankin M, Kesten S. Comparison of hallway and treadmill six-minute walk tests. Am J Respir Crit Care Med. 1999;160:1540-3.
6. Jenkins S, Cecins N. Six-minute walk test: observed adverse events and oxygen desaturation in a large cohort of patients with chronic lung disease. Intern Med J. 2011;41(5):416-22.

CHAPTER 43: Interpretation of Spirometry

Prashant Prakash, Sonam Spalgais, Abhishek Raj

INTRODUCTION

The two foremost societies of respiratory medicine in India, namely the Indian Chest Society and the National College of Chest Physicians of India, have collaborated to develop evidence-based guidelines with an aim to assist physicians at all levels of healthcare in performing and interpreting spirometry in a scientific manner. The consensus statement was aimed at covering all important domains relevant to clinicians working under diverse settings in India.

In the preparation of these guidelines, major guidelines from American Thoracic Society (ATS), British Thoracic Society, European Respiratory Society (ERS), and other international professional bodies were also reviewed in detail.

GENERATING/STANDARDIZING NUMERICAL AND GRAPHICAL DATA, INTERPRETATIVE ALGORITHMS, AND TEST REPORTING

Standardizing Display of Numerical/Graphical Data

All flows should be reported in liters per second at BTPS conditions. FEV_1 and VC should be reported in liters, to 2 decimal places. Volume–time graph and flow–volume loop should be reported and displayed as per the standard recommendations **(Figs. 1 and 2)**. Flow-volume loops are essential as they provide an idea on the quality of the spirometry. In addition, they may yield valuable clues to the presence of obstructive airway disease **(Fig. 2)**. A small and concave or scooped curve suggests obstructive disorder. A small curve with steep slope suggests restriction.

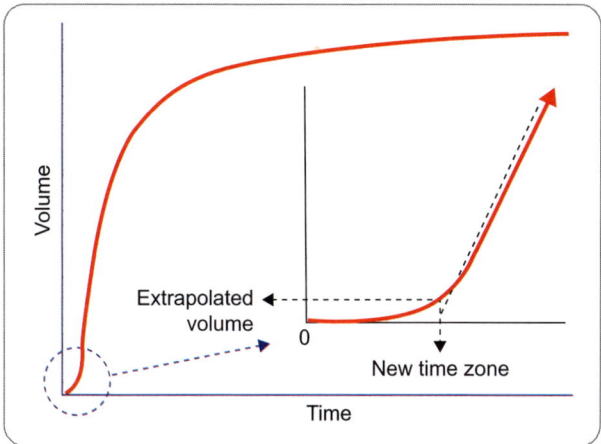

FIG. 1: A typical volume-time trace from spirometry. Note the smooth and rapid rise in expired volume and a volume plateau toward the end of exhalation. The graphical method to calculate time of start of test, as well as extrapolated volume, from the early portion of the curve is also illustrated.

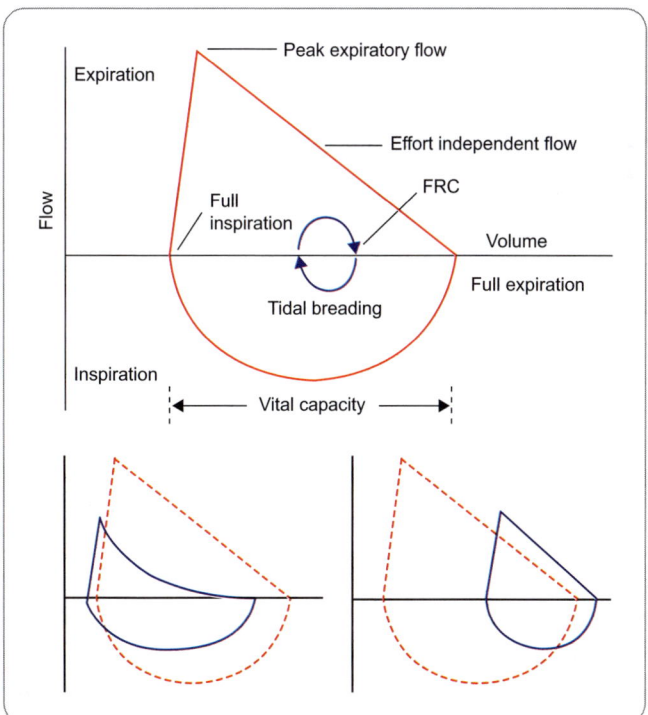

FIG. 2: Flow-volume loops. The upper panel shows a typical flow-volume loop and the various subdivisions of lung volume. The bottom panel shows changes in the shape of flow volume loop in obstructive (right) and restrictive (left) defects, with the dotted line representing the normal loop.
(FRC: functional residual capacity)

Variables to be Used for Spirometry Interpretation

According to the Joint Indian Chest Society–National College of Chest Physicians (India) guidelines for spirometry, the following recommendations were made for variables which should be used for spirometry interpretation:
- The primary variables for reporting spirometry should include FEV_1 (in liters), VC (FVC or SVC) (in liters), FEV_1/VC (%), and PEF (L/s).
- SVC may be additionally performed and reported if airflow limitation is suspected.
- If VC is determined by both slow and forced maneuvers, the larger of the two should be reported.
- A flow–volume loop and volume–time graphs should be included in the report.
- Reporting of additional variables (e.g., $FEF_{25-75\%}$ or $FEF_{75\%}$) is not recommended.

Defining Spirometric Variables as Normal or Abnormal

In practice, observed spirometric values below the predicted lower limit of normal (LLN) should be reported as abnormal. The practice of using a fixed ratio ($FEV_1/VC < 0.7$) or a fixed percentage of the predicted value (80% of the predicted value of FEV_1 or FVC or 60% of the predicted value of $FEF_{25-75\%}$) to differentiate normal from abnormal is discouraged and statistically derived LLN should be used.

Interpretation of Spirometry Data

Only a spirometry record with normal FEV_1, VC, and FEV_1/VC (i.e., all values above their respective predicted LLN values) should be interpreted as being normal.

Obstructive Ventilatory Defect

Any spirometry record with FEV_1/VC value below its predicted LLN should be interpreted as having an obstructive abnormality. Such a defect is commonly seen in disorders associated with airflow limitation, such as asthma and chronic obstructive pulmonary disease (COPD). It may also be observed in diseases with small airway obstruction (such as bronchiolitis), cystic fibrosis, bronchiectasis, airway tumors, and others. The typical flow volume loop in obstructive ventilatory defect is depicted in **Figures 2 and 3**.

Restrictive Ventilatory Defect

Restrictive defects are common in conditions with loss of functioning lung parenchyma (e.g., diffuse parenchymal lung diseases, lung collapse/atelectasis, pneumonia, and after lung resection). Such defects are also seen in patients with neuromuscular disorders (due to decrease in generation of force necessary for a good spirometric maneuver) and diseases of the chest wall and the pleura (e.g., obesity, kyphoscoliosis, large pleural effusion, and pleural fibrosis). The diagnosis of a restrictive ventilatory defect is made when the total lung capacity (TLC) is

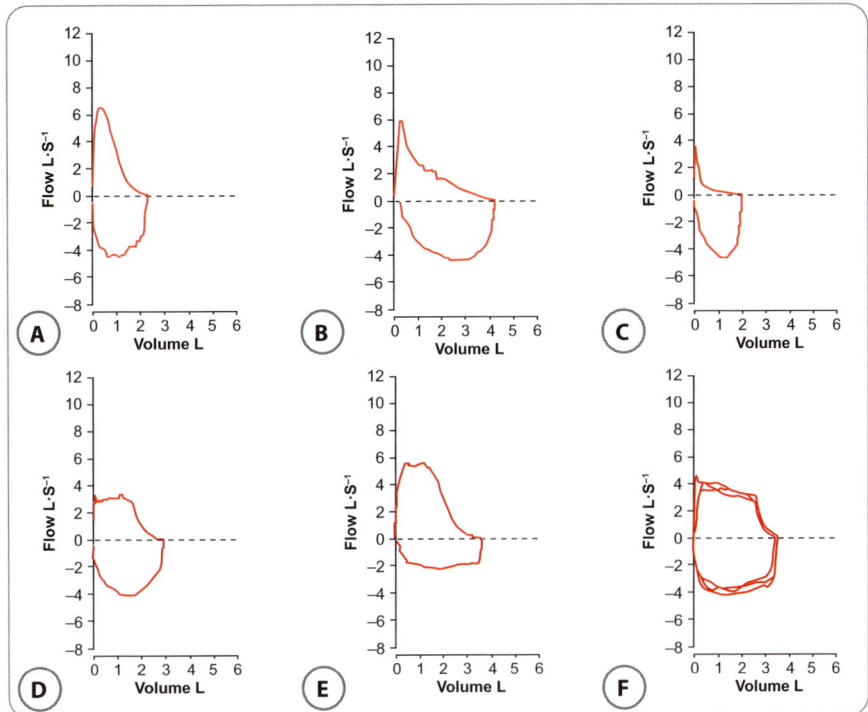

FIGS. 3A TO F: Representative flow-volume loops illustrating normal physiology and various patterns of airflow obstruction. This set of figures displays six flow-volume loop patterns: (A) A normal subject's loop with slight end expiratory curvilinearity; (B) Moderate airflow limitation characteristic of asthma; (C) Severe airflow limitation typically seen in chronic obstructive pulmonary disease (COPD); (D) Variable intrathoracic upper airway obstruction; (E) Variable extrathoracic upper airway obstruction; and (F) Fixed upper airway obstruction demonstrated across three separate maneuvers.

reduced. This requires measurement of lung volumes, and hence, restrictive lung defects cannot be diagnosed with the use of spirometry alone. However, a restrictive defect may be suspected on spirometry if the VC is reduced below the LLN, in the presence of normal or increased FEV_1/VC ratio (i.e., value above corresponding LLN). The ability of spirometry to suggest a restrictive defect is at best modest. The sensitivity of a reduced VC in predicting a decreased TLC varies from 59 to 88.6% in various studies. However, the negative predictive value of a low VC or a reduced VC along with a normal FEV_1/VC ratio is generally >90%. Hence, the presence of a normal VC may obviate the need for performing lung volume measurements to exclude restrictive lung disease. The typical flow volume loop in restrictive ventilatory defect is depicted in **Figure 2**.

Mixed Ventilatory Defect

Coexistence of a restrictive defect (low TLC) and an obstructive defect ($FEV_1/VC < LLN$) is termed as mixed ventilatory defect. Measurement of lung volume is essential to make this diagnosis. However, spirometry may suggest such a defect when both VC and FEV_1/VC are below the LLN.

Therefore, a normal FVC in the presence of an obstructive ventilatory defect practically rules out superimposed restrictive defect. On the other hand, a low FVC in the presence of an obstructive ventilatory defect is mostly a result of severe obstruction, but measurement of TLC is required to rule out a coexisting restrictive defect.

Other Abnormalities

A decrease in both FEV_1 and VC in the presence of a normal FEV_1/VC ratio and a normal TLC is a nonspecific pattern. A reduced VC and normal FEV_1/VC ratio would suggest restrictive defect, but a normal TLC rules it out. Similarly, a low FEV_1 and normal TLC would favor an obstructive defect, but a normal ratio of FEV_1/VC goes against it. This is common when the test is not properly performed, and the patient fails to inhale or exhale completely.

According to the Joint Indian Chest Society-National College of Chest Physicians (India) guidelines for spirometry, the following recommendations were made for spirometry interpretation:
- A spirometric variable is to be reported as abnormal when the values obtained are less than what is generally expected in apparently healthy individuals of similar age, gender, body habitus, and ethnicity.
- Statistically derived LLN should be used in preference to fixed cut-offs for identifying abnormal values.
- FEV_1/VC less than the LLN should be interpreted as diagnostic of obstructive ventilatory defect.
- VC below the LLN, with normal or increased FEV_1/VC, may suggest a restrictive defect.
- VC greater than the LLN usually rules out the presence of a true restrictive defect.
- Diagnosis of true restriction cannot be made using spirometry alone and requires a measurement of the TLC.
- Reduction of both VC and FEV_1/VC below LLN may suggest either obstructive or mixed defect, and estimation of TLC may be necessary to differentiate between these two patterns.

Use of Fixed Ratio versus Lower Limit of Normal During Interpretation

An obstructive spirometric defect should preferably be identified when the FEV_1/FVC ratio is less than the LLN for the reference population, and a fixed cut-off should not be used. However, in situations where data on statistically valid LLN figures are not available (or impractical to calculate, as in some field settings), FEV_1/VC ratio <70% may be employed to define airway obstruction in a high probability clinical setting.

Categorization of the Severity of an Abnormal Spirometry Report

FEV_1 is reduced in both obstructive and restrictive lung diseases, and a reduced FEV_1 can be considered an indicator for impaired lung function. FEV_1 expressed as a percentage of predicted normal value can be employed to categorize severity of impairment of lung function (both restrictive and obstructive). Although the correlation of lung function to morbidity and mortality is well established, there is no universally accepted scheme of categorization of severity of pulmonary function. Severity classification suggested by the GOLD (for COPD) and ERS/ATS (for obstructive airway diseases) includes five categories based on postbronchodilator $FEV_1\%$ predicted. VC is reduced in restrictive diseases, including parenchymal lung diseases and neuromuscular diseases. The classification of severity of restrictive defects was conventionally based on VC measurements. However, since the correlation between FEV_1 and VC is good when FEV_1/FVC is normal, the ATS/ERS endorsed $FEV_1\%$ to classify restrictive defect as well, thereby making the severity classification uniform (for both obstructive and restrictive defects). The correlation between the previous severity classification based on VC and the current FEV_1-based classification for restrictive defects is reasonably good. However, they cannot be used interchangeably since up to 31.3% were noted to have discordant categorization.

According to the Joint Indian Chest Society–National College of Chest Physicians (India) guidelines for spirometry, the following recommendations were made for categorization of an abnormal spirometry report:
- Severity assessment of both restrictive and obstructive defects on spirometry should be based on FEV_1 values.
- Impairment of pulmonary function (obstructive or restrictive) can be categorized as mild, moderate, and severe when FEV_1 is ≥70%, 50–69%, and <50% predicted, respectively.

Place of Forced Expiratory Volume in 6 Seconds in Spirometry Interpretation

Forced expiratory volume in 6 seconds (FEV_6) is the maximal volume of air that is expelled in the first 6 seconds of a FVC maneuver. 99% individuals can obtain their FVC in 6.64 seconds or less.

FEV_1/FEV_6 ratio has been evaluated as an alternative to FEV_1/FVC in interpreting spirometry, and both have been shown to be comparable in diagnosing airway obstruction. However, similar to FEV_1/FVC, employing a fixed cut-off to diagnose obstruction is not preferred and wherever feasible, FEV_1/FEV_6 lower than the statistically derived LLN for the reference population is to be used.

The role of FEV_1/FEV_6 as an alternative to FEV_1/FVC for suspecting restrictive defects has been studied, and both indices are comparable in predicting reduction in TLC. Apart from its role in diagnosing obstructive and restrictive defects, FEV_6 has also been shown to be equivalent to FVC in the assessment of bronchodilator response. A definite end-of-test criteria, shorter time for completing a test, lesser chances of syncope, lesser exertion, and diagnostic capability comparable to FVC are the potential advantages favoring the use of FEV_6.

In conclusion, there are sufficient data suggesting that FEV_6 may be a reasonable surrogate for FVC. However, there are little data from India, and reference equations need to be generated before the routine use of FEV_6.

Is Spirometry Helpful in Detecting Central/Upper Airway Obstruction

Miller and Hyatt evaluated the utility of flow–volume loops in central/upper airway obstruction and identified four patterns: (1) Flattening of inspiratory loop in extrathoracic airway obstruction **(Fig. 3E)**, (2) flattening of expiratory loop in intrathoracic airway obstruction **(Fig. 3D)**, (3) flattening of both loops in fixed airway obstruction **(Fig. 3F)**, and (4) unclassifiable or atypical flow–volume loop.

Central/upper airway obstruction is associated with a significantly reduced PEF, but usually, FEV_1 and VC are unaffected. Hence, FEV_1/PEF ratio >8 can suggest central/upper airway obstruction. Since poor patient effort could result in similar findings, it has been suggested that at least three acceptable and evaluable flow–volume loops are essential to assess central/upper airway obstruction by spirometry.

Spirometry is not the preferred test for the diagnosis of central/upper airway obstruction due to its poor diagnostic capability as well as the easy availability of better alternate investigations. In the modern era where imaging, bronchoscopy, and laryngosocopy are widely available, the utility of spriometry in the diagnosis of upper airway obstruction is modest at best.

ROLE OF ADDITIONAL PARAMETERS IN INTERPRETING SPIROMETRY

According to the Joint Indian Chest Society–National College of Chest Physicians (India) guidelines for spirometry, the following recommendations were made for the use of additional parameters in interpreting spirometry:
- The measurement of additional spirometric values, $FEF_{25\%-75\%}$ and $FEF_{75\%}$, do not have an additional advantage to the routinely measured parameters namely, FEV_1, VC, and FEV_1/VC. They can be misleading and are not recommended for the interpretation of spirometry.

CONCLUSION

Spirometry interpretation, as guided by the Joint Indian Chest Society–National College of Chest Physicians (India) guidelines, fundamentally relies on comparing *observed values* to the *predicted Lower Limit of Normal (LLN)*. A spirometric variable is considered *abnormal* if the value obtained is less than what is expected in healthy individuals of similar demographics.

FURTHER READINGS

1. Aggarwal AN, Agarwal R, Dhooria S, Prasad KT, Sehgal IS, Muthu V, et al. Joint Indian Chest Society-National College of Chest Physicians (India) guidelines for spirometry. Lung India. 2019;36:S1-35.
2. Miller MR, Hankinson J, Brusasco V, Burgos F, Casaburi R, Coates A, et al. Standardisation of spirometry. Eur Respir J. 2005;26:319-38.
3. Pellegrino R, Viegi G, Brusasco V, Crapo RO, Burgos F, Casaburi R, et al. Interpretative strategies for lung function tests. Eur Respir J. 2005;26:948-68.

SECTION 16

Rheumatology

CHAPTER 44

When should We Escalate the Treatment in Rheumatoid Arthritis from the Traditional DMARDS to Biologics?

SS Dariya, Aradhana Sharma

INTRODUCTION

Rheumatoid arthritis (RA) is a chronic autoimmune disease that primarily affects the joints, causing pain, swelling, and stiffness because of inflammation of the synovium of the joints and finally leads to joint damage and deformity.

The 2010 ACR/EULAR (American College of Rheumatology/European League Against Rheumatism) criteria are used to classify patients with definite RA, requiring a score of 6 or more based on joint involvement, serology [rheumatoid factor (RF)/anticyclic citrullinated peptide (anti-CCP)], acute-phase reactants, and symptom duration.

Disease-modifying antirheumatic drugs (DMARDs) are a class of medications used to treat RA and other autoimmune diseases. DMARDs work by suppressing the immune system and reducing inflammation, thus improving symptoms like pain, stiffness, and swelling and helping to prevent long-term damage and preserve joint function.

Biological medications, or biologics, are a type of DMARD (bDMARD) used to treat RA. They are target-specific parts of the immune system that cause inflammation and help to reduce the signs and symptoms of RA and potentially slow disease progression.

The approach to adopt before starting the treatment of RA patients is as follows:
- Aimed at the best care which must be based on a shared decision between the patient and the rheumatologist.
- Decisions are based on disease activity, safety issues, and other patient factors, such as comorbidities and progression of structural damage.
- Require access to multiple drugs with different modes of action to address the heterogeneity of RA
- Incurs high individual, medical, and societal costs, all of which should be considered in its management by the treating rheumatologist
- Aimed at reaching a target of sustained remission or low disease activity in every patient

In RA treatment, bDMARDs and conventional DMARDs can be accelerated or switched to different strategies when disease activity is not adequately controlled. Acceleration means intensifying treatment, either by switching to a more potent DMARD or combination therapy or by initiating bDMARDs earlier than initially planned.

Acceleration should be considered when:
- *Failure to achieve treatment goals:* If a patient does not achieve remission or low disease activity with conventional DMARDs either as monotherapy or in combination, acceleration is often necessary.

  Moreover, a synthetic DMARD combination is preferred over DMARD monotherapy, as there is increasing evidence of a window of opportunity in patients with early RA in which the antirheumatic therapy should be as intense as possible, also indicating a need for early identification of these patients. When low disease activity is not reached, treatment should be switched to another strategy.

  It is relevant to realize that nowadays, disease remission, rather than low disease activity, should be the treatment target.
- *Early aggressive RA:* Some patients, especially those with early, aggressive RA, may benefit from more intensive therapy from the start, potentially including a combination of conventional DMARDs or early introduction of bDMARDs.
- *Radiographic progression*: If imaging studies show signs of joint damage despite treatment, it is crucial to accelerate treatment to prevent further progression.

  Considering that stopping progression of joint damage is one of the most important objectives of treatment in RA, a recent systematic review concluded that only swollen joint count (SJC) and acute phase reactants, but not patient global assessment (PGA), were independent predictors of radiographic progression.
- *Symptom severity and impact on function*: If a patient's symptoms are severe and significantly impacting daily life, treatment may be accelerated even if they are not experiencing radiographic progression.
- *Comorbidities*: The presence of comorbidities can influence the choice of DMARDs and the need for acceleration.
- *Immunogenicity of bDMARDs*: In some cases, the body may develop antibodies [antidrug antibodies (ADAs)] against bDMARDs, reducing their effectiveness. If this occurs, treatment may need to be accelerated or switched to a different bDMARD or combined with other therapies to mitigate the immunogenicity.

Biologics and DMARD: Points to be considered–
- Biologics have a more precise treatment target than conventional DMARDs. Some studies have shown biologics to result in less radiological deterioration (joint damage seen on X-rays) in patients with severe disease. Most biologics start working faster than DMARDs. However, there is no strong evidence that biologic drugs have superior efficacy or result in better clinical and radiographic outcomes compared to traditional DMARDs.
- Biologics can work well for some people who need more than the initial combination therapy of traditional DMARDs and/or nonsteroidal anti-inflammatory drugs (NSAIDs) and steroids. However, bDMARDs carry high

risks of side effects, and also they are more costly. Nonetheless, experts recommend using biologic drugs sooner rather than later if they are needed. Hence, it is worth to remember that every person reacts differently to different drugs. So, a biologic drug that works very well for one person may not work for someone else.
- Like most medications, biologics can cause side effects. Minor side effects of biologic drugs include nausea, abdominal pain, and injection site reactions like redness and itching. Biologic agents interfere with the body's ability to fight bacterial, viral, and fungal infections and may cause serious infections like herpes zoster and tuberculosis and other side effects like severe life-threatening allergic reactions and lymphoma.
- There are mixed levels of evidence about the long-term safety and efficacy of biologic medications. However, for the most part, bDMARDs appear to be safe for long-term use.

Treatment decisions in case of RA should be individualized based on the patient's specific situation, including disease activity, severity, comorbidities, and patient preferences.

CONCLUSION

Acceleration of RA treatment is a complex decision, often involving a balance between efficacy, safety, and individual patient factors. It is crucial to monitor disease activity and response to treatment closely and adjust the treatment plan accordingly.

FURTHER READINGS

1. Aletaha D, Neogi T, Silman AJ, Funovits J, Felson DT, Bingham CO 3rd, et al. 2010 Rheumatoid arthritis classification criteria: an American College of Rheumatology/European League Against Rheumatism collaborative initiative. Ann Rheum Dis. 2010;69(9):1580-8.
2. Grigor C, Capell H, Stirling A, McMahon AD, Lock P, Vallance R, et al. Effect of a treatment strategy of tight control for rheumatoid arthritis (the TICORA study): a single-blind randomised controlled trial. Lancet. 2004;364:263-9.
3. Navarro-Compan V, Gherghe AM, Smolen JS, Aletaha D, Landewe R, van der Heijde D. Relationship between disease activity indices and their individual components and radiographic progression in RA: a systematic literature review. Rheumatology (Oxford). 2015;54:994-1007.

CHAPTER 45

Diabetes Mellitus–Rheumatology Interface

Priyanka Saha, Sumit Sarkar, Sandipan Banik, Sandipan Mondal, Amit Chakraborty, Smarajit Banik

■ INTRODUCTION

The interface between diabetes mellitus and rheumatology involves a complex relationship where diabetes mellitus can manifest with various rheumatic and musculoskeletal complications, and inflammatory rheumatic diseases like rheumatoid arthritis (RA) share common inflammatory pathways with diabetes mellitus, particularly type 2 diabetes mellitus (T2DM). Patients with RA have an increased risk of developing T2DM, likely due to chronic systemic inflammation mediated by proinflammatory cytokines such as tumor necrosis factor alpha (TNF-α) and interleukin-6 (IL-6), which are implicated in both diseases.

■ RHEUMATIC MANIFESTATIONS IN DIABETES MELLITUS

Diabetes mellitus is associated with several rheumatic musculoskeletal manifestations, including:
- Limited joint mobility syndromes like diabetic cheiroarthropathy
- Adhesive capsulitis (frozen shoulder)
- Trigger finger (stenosing tenosynovitis)
- Dupuytren's contractures
- Diabetic amyotrophy and muscle infarction

These conditions cause pain, disability, and functional limitations, reducing quality of life for diabetic patients and impacting glycemic control.

■ DIABETIC CHEIROARTHROPATHY

Diabetic cheiroarthropathy (DCA), also called diabetic stiff hand syndrome or limited joint mobility syndrome, is a complication of both type 1 diabetes mellitus (T1DM) and T2DM characterized by limited movement and stiffness of the small joints of the hands along with thickening and tightening of the skin over the fingers and hands.

Diabetic cheiroarthropathy is associated with microvascular complications of diabetes mellitus, such as retinopathy and nephropathy. It typically affects patients with long-standing or poorly controlled diabetes mellitus, and prevalence rates vary from 8 to 50% depending on the study population **(Fig. 1)**.

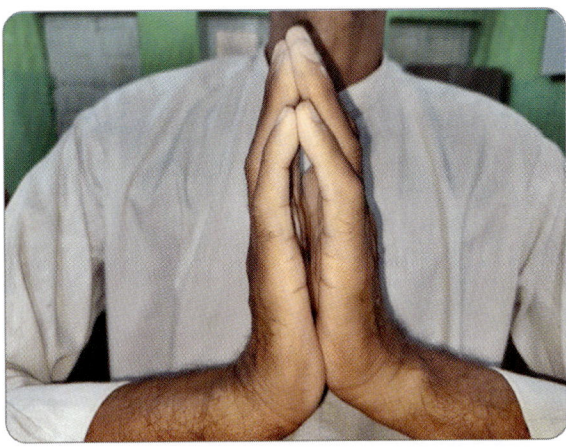

FIG. 1: Limited extension and flexion of proximal and distal finger joints.

Clinical Features
- Limited extension and flexion of proximal and distal finger joints
- Thickened, tight, waxy skin over hands
- Positive "prayer sign" and "tabletop sign"
- Sometimes associated with Dupuytren's contracture

Pathophysiology
- Hyperglycemia causes glycosylation and crosslinking of collagen.
- Collagen proliferation and decreased degradation in skin, tendons, and periarticular tissues
- Microangiopathy leading to low-grade ischemia and fibrosis

Diagnosis and Management
- Clinical examination (prayer sign and joint mobility)
- Physiotherapy is the mainstay of treatment.

ADHESIVE CAPSULITIS

Adhesive capsulitis, also known as frozen shoulder, is a painful and debilitating condition characterized by progressive stiffness and loss of motion in the shoulder joint. It mainly affects middle-aged adults and is marked by inflammation and fibrosis of the shoulder capsule, leading to significant limitation in both active and passive movements **(Fig. 2)**.

Key Features
- Progressive loss of shoulder range of motion
- Pain, particularly at night
- Stiffness and fibrosis of the joint capsule, especially affecting the rotator interval and coracohumeral ligament

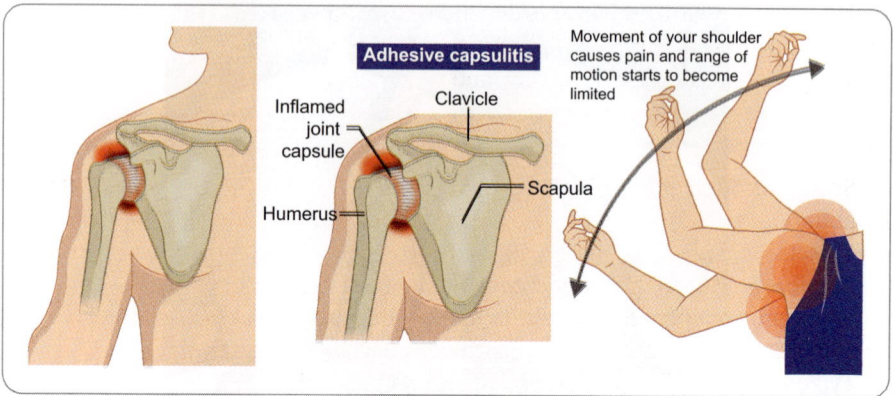

FIG. 2: Frozen shoulder.

- Can involve thickening and contraction of the joint capsule
- Often bilateral and more common in women aged 40–60 years
- Associated with diabetes mellitus and thyroid disease

Pathophysiology

- Initial inflammation of the synovium lining the shoulder joint
- Followed by fibrotic changes and thickening, leading to restricted movement
- Elevated inflammatory cytokines and fibroblast proliferation contribute to fibrosis
- *Histological stages mirror clinical phases*: Inflammation, fibrosis, and thawing

Natural History

- Typically progresses through stages of pain, stiffness, and eventual improvement
- Duration ranges from months to years.
- Approximately 20–50% of patients may have persistent symptoms beyond 3 years.

Treatment

- Physical therapy and pain management
- Corticosteroid injections may relieve inflammation.
- Surgery (capsular release or manipulation under anesthesia) in refractory cases
- Management of underlying conditions, such as diabetes mellitus, is important.

■ DIABETIC AMYOTROPHY

Diabetic amyotrophy is also known as diabetic lumbosacral radiculoplexus neuropathy or Bruns–Garland syndrome. It is a rare form of diabetic neuropathy characterized by severe, often unilateral pain in the hips, thighs, or buttocks, followed by muscle weakness and atrophy in the proximal lower extremities.

Diabetic amyotrophy primarily affects people with T2DM, usually older adults, and presents with symptoms such as intense, deep aching or burning pain, asymmetrical muscle wasting, and weakness **(Fig. 3)**.

Key Features
- Severe, sudden aching/burning pain in the hip, thigh, buttock, or sometimes abdomen and chest
- Muscle weakness and wasting, mostly proximal and often asymmetric
- Possible foot drop due to nerve involvement in the legs
- Symptoms mainly affect one side initially but can spread to the other.
- Unexplained weight loss and possible mood/sleep disturbances
- Typically occurs in middle-aged or older adults with T2DM

Causes and Pathophysiology
- High blood sugar damages nerves, but diabetic amyotrophy also involves an immune-mediated inflammation (microvasculitis) of small blood vessels supplying nerves.
- This leads to ischemic nerve injury and inflammation, causing pain and weakness.

Diagnosis
- Clinical symptoms and history
- Blood tests for diabetes mellitus management
- Electromyography and nerve conduction studies
- Imaging, like magnetic resonance imaging (MRI) or computed tomography (CT), to exclude other nerve-related causes
- Sometimes, spinal fluid analysis is used to detect inflammation.

Treatment
- Tight glycemic control to prevent further nerve damage
- Pain management with medications such as gabapentin, pregabalin, or antidepressants

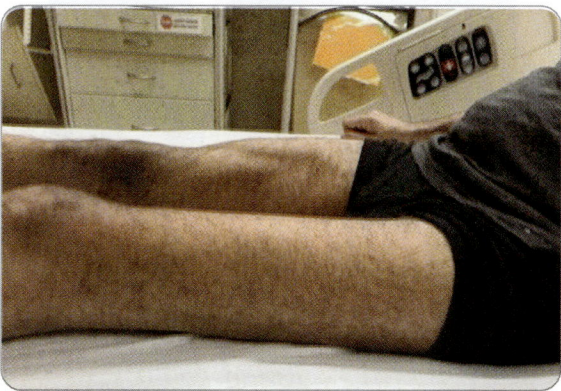

FIG. 3: Diabetic lumbosacral radiculoplexus neuropathy.

- Physical therapy to maintain muscle strength and mobility
- Symptoms often improve over months, though full recovery is variable.

DUPUYTREN'S CONTRACTURE

Dupuytren's contracture is a condition where one or more fingers become permanently bent toward the palm due to thickening and tightening of the tissue under the skin of the palm (the palmar fascia) **(Fig. 4)**.

Key Features
- Begins as small nodules in the palm
- Progresses to thick cords, causing finger contraction
- Most commonly affects the ring and little fingers
- Results in the inability to fully straighten fingers
- Usually not painful, but may cause discomfort or itching
- Can affect one or both hands
- Causes and risk factors
- Predisposing factors
- Associated with alcoholism, smoking, diabetes mellitus, thyroid problems, and liver disease
- Possibly triggered by previous hand trauma or epilepsy

Symptoms
- Palmar nodules and thickened tissue
- Skin puckering and tightening
- Flexed fingers that cannot be straightened
- Loss of hand function in severe cases

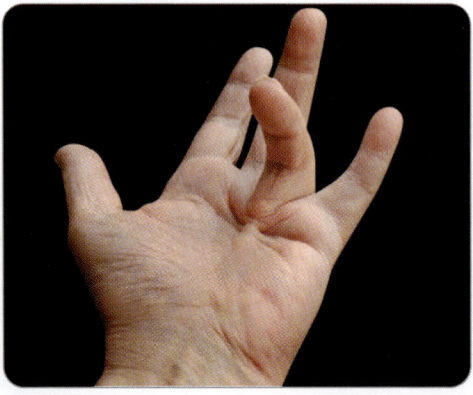

FIG. 4: Dupuytren's contracture.

Treatment
- Observation for mild cases
- Nonsurgical options like injections
- Surgery to remove thickened tissue or release contracture in advanced cases

This condition is chronic and progressive but can be managed to improve hand function and quality of life.

SHARED PATHOPHYSIOLOGY OF DIABETES MELLITUS AND RHEUMATOID ARTHRITIS

The shared pathophysiology of diabetes mellitus (mostly type 2) and RA involves common inflammatory mechanisms. Furthermore, traditional risk factors like physical inactivity and metabolic syndrome, more common in RA patients, also increase diabetes mellitus risk.

Key shared features include:
- Overproduction of inflammatory cytokines (TNF-α and IL-6) that impair insulin sensitivity and promote insulin resistance
- IL-1β causing beta-cell dysfunction and apoptosis in the pancreas
- Chronic systemic inflammation underlying both RA and diabetes mellitus pathogenesis
- Increased risk of T2DM incidence in RA patients due to inflammation and related metabolic factors
- Thus, inflammation and immune system dysregulation constitute the core shared pathophysiology connecting RA and diabetes mellitus.

GENETIC CONNECTION BETWEEN TYPE 1 DIABETES MELLITUS AND RHEUMATOID ARTHRITIS

The shared susceptibility loci between RA and T1DM include both major histocompatibility complex (MHC) and non-MHC regions:

The *HLA-DRB1* gene in the MHC class II region is a major shared genetic locus between RA and T1DM, playing a key role in autoimmune susceptibility.

Several non-MHC loci are also shared risk loci for both diseases. These include PTPN22, AFF3, CTLA4, TNFAIP3, and TAGAP.

A specific study identified seven single-nucleotide polymorphisms (SNPs) initially associated with T1DM that also showed association with RA:
- SKAP2/rs7804356
- GLIS3/rs7020673
- GSDMB/rs2290400
- BACH2/rs11755527
- C6orf173/rs9388489
- PRKCQ/rs947474
- DLK1/rs941576

These shared loci primarily affect immune regulation, contributing to the risk of autoimmunity in both diseases.

DISEASE-MODIFYING ANTIRHEUMATIC DRUG AND DIABETES MELLITUS

Disease-modifying antirheumatic drugs (DMARDs) have varying effects on diabetes mellitus risk and glucose control, particularly in patients with RA and other systemic inflammatory conditions.

Key points include the following: Use of biologic DMARDs (bDMARDs) like TNF-α inhibitors and abatacept is associated with a significantly reduced risk of developing T2DM. IL-1 receptor antagonists also improve β-cell function and glucose sensitivity.
- Long-term use of synthetic DMARDs such as hydroxychloroquine (HCQ) and methotrexate (MTX) is associated with a reduction in the incidence of diabetes mellitus, while tacrolimus increases diabetes mellitus risk.
- Combination therapies with bDMARDs or MTX combinations show lower diabetes mellitus risk compared to MTX monotherapy. HCQ alone significantly reduces diabetes mellitus risk and TNF-α inhibitors tend to be protective.
- A large study found that TNF inhibitors and HCQ reduced the risk of new-onset diabetes mellitus compared to other nonbiologic DMARDs. MTX did not show as strong an effect alone.

Disease-modifying antirheumatic drugs may exert antihyperglycemic effects via anti-inflammatory, insulin-sensitizing, and insulinotropic mechanisms, potentially benefiting patients with inflammatory rheumatic diseases who also have or are at risk for diabetes mellitus.

CORTICOSTEROID USAGE AND DIABETES MELLITUS

Although many people's blood sugar levels return to normal after discontinuation of corticosteroids, some individuals, especially those with higher risk factors like obesity, family history, or pre-existing glucose intolerance, may continue to have diabetes mellitus or develop T2DM later.

Risk and Development

The risk of developing diabetes mellitus is dose-dependent, with higher doses and prolonged use of glucocorticoids increasing the likelihood.

Studies show that at 1 year, the cumulative risk of diabetes mellitus increases significantly with higher daily doses of prednisolone equivalents, reaching up to 5% or more with a ≥25 mg daily dose.

This risk persists despite controlling for inflammation and disease activity, indicating a direct impact of glucocorticoids on glucose metabolism.

Mechanism and Persistence

Glucocorticoids induce hyperglycemia by causing peripheral insulin resistance, increased hepatic glucose production, and pancreatic beta-cell dysfunction.

While some recovery of beta-cell function can occur after stopping glucocorticoids, the metabolic changes can become permanent or unmask latent diabetes mellitus.

CONCLUSION

The diabetes mellitus–rheumatology interface involves shared inflammatory and metabolic pathways, bidirectional risk of comorbid conditions, and overlapping clinical presentations that require integrated management approaches.

FURTHER READINGS

1. Tian Z, Mclaughlin J, Verma A, Chinoy H, Heald AH. The relationship between rheumatoid arthritis and diabetes mellitus: a systematic review and meta-analysis. Cardiovasc Endocrinol Metab. 2021;10(2):125-31.
2. Arthritis Foundation, Linda R. Rheumatoid arthritis and type 2 diabetes. [online] Available from https://www.arthritis.org/health-wellness/about-arthritis/related-conditions/other-diseases/rheumatoid-arthritis-and-type-2-diabetes [Last accessed October, 2025].
3. Gupta V, Santhi SSE, Ravi S, Ramanan EA. Rheumatological and Musculoskeletal Complications in Diabetes Patients. [online] Available from https://jofem.org/index.php/jofem/article/view/811/284284593 [Last accessed October, 2025].

CHAPTER 46

Antiphospholipid Syndrome: A Brief Review

Partha Sarkar, Poulami Das, Chandrapaul Gupta

INTRODUCTION

Antiphospholipid syndrome (APS) is a systemic autoimmune disorder characterized by vascular and obstetric manifestations due to antiphospholipid (aPL) antibodies. The word itself is a misnomer because the antibodies are not against phospholipids but instead target the plasma proteins that bind to anionic phospholipids. The major aPL antibodies detected are lupus anticoagulant (LA), anticardiolipin (aCL) antibody, and anti-β_2 glycoprotein I (anti-β_2 GPI) antibody. The prevalence of APS in the general population is estimated to be 40–50 per 100,000.

Antiphospholipid syndrome can exist in isolation without any definable associated disease (primary APS) or occur in association with systemic lupus erythematosus (SLE) or other autoimmune diseases (secondary APS). One-third of the patients with SLE possess aPL antibodies and 10–15% develop APS.

PATHOGENESIS

The initiating events for the induction of aPL antibodies seem to be endothelial injury induced by infections, trauma, and oxidative stress in an appropriate genetic background [primary APS is associated with human leukocyte antigen (HLA) DRw53 and DR4]. The binding of the aPL antibodies to the disrupted endothelial cells leads to a proinflammatory and prothrombotic state. There is complement activation, platelet and neutrophil activation, cytokine production, neutrophil extracellular trap (NET) formation, decreased protein C activity, and interference with trophoblasts and decidual cells (trophoblast apoptosis). All these processes cause inflammation, vasculopathy, thrombosis, and pregnancy complications.

CLINICAL FEATURES AND DIAGNOSIS

Antiphospholipid syndrome, being a rare disease, its clinical spectrum, classification, and management are continuously advancing and thus its identification and suspicion are challenging.

Majority of the patients develop deep vein thrombosis (primarily in the lower limb) and often cause pulmonary emboli. Thrombosis of pulmonary arteries leads to pulmonary hypertension and that of hepatic veins leads to Budd–Chiari syndrome. Other venous thrombosis manifestations include cerebral venous thrombosis (causes intracranial hypertension and focal neurological deficits) and renal, retinal, mesenteric, or splanchnic vein thrombosis. Arterial thrombosis in the brain can manifest as a transient ischemic attack, stroke, migraine, or cognitive dysfunction. Cardiac involvement includes myocardial ischemia, cardiac valve thickening/dysfunction, and Libman–Sacks endocarditis. Patients can also present with peripheral artery thrombosis such as acute limb ischemia, ischemic leg ulcer, or digital gangrene. Premature atherosclerosis has also been recognized as a feature of APS. Some of the microvascular complications include livedo reticularis, livedo racemosa, and livedoid vasculopathy. Another microvascular feature is aPL nephropathy, which is characterized by hypertension, proteinuria (mild to nephrotic range), hematuria, and mild renal insufficiency. The main hematological manifestations are thrombocytopenia and autoimmune hemolytic anemia. Obstetric complications manifest as placental insufficiency with intrauterine fetal growth restriction, prefetal (<10 weeks of gestation) or fetal death, pre-eclampsia, or eclampsia. Arthralgia, arthritis, osteoporosis, or nontraumatic fractures may also occur in APS.

The diagnosis of APS should always be considered in cases of thrombosis, cerebral vascular accidents in individuals <55 years of age, or pregnancy morbidity, in the presence of livedo reticularis or thrombocytopenia.

According to the 2023 American College of Rheumatology/European Alliance of Associations for Rheumatology (ACR/EULAR) classification criteria for APS, the presence of at least three points from clinical domains and three points from laboratory domains is required to classify APS. The clinical domains include: (1) venous thromboembolism, (2) arterial thrombosis, (3) microvascular events, (4) cardiac valve disease (thickening or vegetation), (5) obstetric complications, and (6) hematologic manifestations (thrombocytopenia). The laboratory domains are: (1) LA and (2) aCL and/or anti-β_2 GPI antibodies.

A three-step procedure (screening–mixing study–confirmation) with two screening test systems [diluted Russell's viper venom time and a sensitive activated partial thromboplastin time (low phospholipids and silica as activator)] is necessary to confirm the presence of LAC. The LAC test should be considered positive if at least one of the two test systems yields a positive result following all three steps (phospholipid-dependent correction of the prolonged screening tests). If the patient is on heparin, the test should be done 12 hours after halting heparin. If the patient is on vitamin K antagonists (VKAs), it is recommended to do the test after 2 weeks of discontinuing it. aCL antibody [immunoglobulin G (IgG), immunoglobulin M (IgM), and immunoglobulin A (IgA)] is tested by enzyme-linked immunosorbent assay (ELISA), and a moderate-to-high positivity of two readings at least 12 weeks apart confirms the laboratory diagnosis of aCL antibody. If the patients have clinical features of APS, but aCL antibody and LA are negative, detecting anti-β_2 GPI IgG/IgM antibodies by ELISA is of clinical importance.

Catastrophic aPL syndrome (CAPS), a rare, fulminant, life-threatening form of APS, is characterized by (1) thrombosis in three or more organ systems,

(2) developing within a week, (3) histologic evidence of small-vessel thrombosis in at least one organ, and (4) presence of aPL antibody. The most common organ involvement is acute renal failure. It is often precipitated by infection, trauma, pregnancy, SLE flare, or drugs like thiazides or oral contraceptive pills (OCPs).

DIFFERENTIAL DIAGNOSES

The differential diagnoses of APS include inherited thrombophilia (factor V Leiden mutation, protein C or S deficiency, and hyperhomocysteinemia), acquired prothrombotic states (malignancy, OCPs, and hormone replacement therapy), thrombotic thrombocytopenic purpura (TTP), hemolytic uremic syndrome (HUS), heparin-induced thrombocytopenia (HIT), disseminated intravascular coagulation (DIC), paroxysmal nocturnal hemoglobinuria (PNH), atherosclerotic vascular disease, and cholesterol emboli syndrome. Factor V Leiden mutation and protein C or S deficiency mainly present with venous thrombosis, and pregnancy morbidity is rarely seen. TTP classically presents as an acute emergency with features of platelet-rich microvascular thrombosis, thrombocytopenia, microangiopathic hemolytic anemia (MAHA), and neurological and renal impairment, whereas APS has a recurrent chronic course. HUS is characterized by MAHA, thrombocytopenia, and acute kidney injury. HUS usually affects children, and laboratories reveal increased lactate dehydrogenase (LDH), schistocytes, and a normal coagulation profile, whereas APS shows a paradoxical prolonged activated partial thromboplastin time (aPTT). Disseminated intravascular coagulation (DIC) (consumptive coagulopathy) often occurs secondary to sepsis, trauma, malignancy, or obstetric complications, and laboratory reports show increased prothrombin time (PT), aPTT, D-dimer, and schistocytes. Atherosclerotic vascular disease presents with angina, claudication, ischemic stroke, or myocardial infarction (MI) but not typically with fetal loss. Though the presentation of cholesterol emboli syndrome is very similar to APS (livedo reticularis, renal failure, and peripheral gangrene), it often develops post angiography or anticoagulation, and laboratory reports reveal eosinophilia, hypocomplementemia, and raised C-reactive protein (CRP).

PROGNOSIS

Overall, morbidity is high in patients with APS, with more than 30% of them developing permanent organ damage and more than 20% developing severe disability at a 10-year follow-up. Poor outcome is usually seen in CAPS, pulmonary hypertension, central nervous system involvement, and gangrene. The mortality despite treatment is high in CAPS. Some European studies have observed 90–94% survival over 10 years.

TREATMENT

For asymptomatic or SLE patients with a high-risk aPL profile and no evidence of previous thrombotic episode or any pregnancy morbidity, prophylactic treatment with low-dose aspirin (LDA) (75–100 mg daily) is recommended (primary thromboprophylaxis).

After the first thrombotic event, APS patients should be started on VKA for life, with an aim to achieve an international normalized ratio (INR) ranging between 2.0 and 3.0 in case of an unprovoked venous thrombosis. For those with arterial thrombosis, the INR target should be 3.0–4.0 or 2.0–3.0 with or without LDA, depending on the thrombotic/hemorrhagic patient profile. Treatment duration is generally lifelong.

In a nonpregnant woman with a history of APS-related obstetric complications (with or without SLE), prophylactic treatment with LDA seems to reduce the risk of subsequent thrombotic events. In a pregnant lady with a history of obstetric APS, combination therapy with LDA and prophylactic dose of low molecular weight heparin (LMWH) (enoxaparin 20–40 mg SC every 24 hours) is recommended, whereas in case of thrombotic APS, LDA along with therapeutic LMWH (enoxaparin 1 mg/kg body weight SC every 12 hours or 1.5 mg/kg body weight every 24 hours) should be administered. When recurrent obstetric complications occur, despite the ongoing standard treatment, the LMWH should be increased from prophylactic to therapeutic dose, and alternative options like oral hydroxychloroquine 400 mg/day or low-dose prednisolone should be considered. The heparin should be continued throughout the pregnancy and 6 weeks postpartum. Warfarin is contraindicated in pregnancy but is compatible with breastfeeding.

Catastrophic aPL syndrome requires high-intensity anticoagulation with heparin, pulse methyl prednisolone, and intravenous immunoglobulin or plasmapheresis along with appropriate management for triggering events such as infections. For refractory CAPS, B-cell depletion (e.g., with rituximab) or complement inhibition (e.g., with eculizumab) therapies are alternative options. Sirolimus (mTOR inhibitor) may be used in APS nephropathy.

One should also minimize the other risks such as smoking, hypertension, diabetes mellitus, obesity, immobilization, OCPs, etc. Low vitamin D level in serum is associated with thrombotic manifestations. Also, vitamin D has immunomodulatory action and inhibits anti-β_2 GPI-mediated tissue factor expression. Statins should be used in case of dyslipidemia and for their additional anti-inflammatory and antiplatelet action.

Direct oral anticoagulants (DOACs) are not recommended in APS, especially those with triple aPL positivity. The use of rivaroxaban in high-risk patients with APS was associated with an increased rate of thromboembolic events compared to warfarin.

Patients who are tolerating anticoagulation well and have no other systemic autoimmune diseases should undergo routine checkups twice a year. Coagulation studies are done before initiating anticoagulation and during therapy to guide dosing. Additionally, complete blood count, renal function test, and biochemistry panel should be done to monitor the patients.

CONCLUSION

Antiphospholipid syndrome, being a rare disease, its clinical spectrum, classification, and management are continuously advancing and thus its identification and suspicion are challenging. The diagnosis of APS should always be considered in cases of thrombosis, cerebral vascular accidents in individuals <55 years of age, or pregnancy morbidity, in the presence of livedo reticularis or thrombocytopenia. Prompt recognition and sustained anticoagulation are vital to prevent recurrent thrombosis and obstetric complications.

FURTHER READINGS

1. Longo D, Fauci AS, Kasper DL, Hauser S, Jameson JL. Harrison's Principles of Internal Medicine, 22nd edition. New York: McGraw-Hill; 2025.
2. Paul BJ. Essentials of Clinical Rheumatology, 1st edition. Delhi: Evangel Publishing (P) Ltd; 2021.
3. Handa R. Clinical Rheumatology, 1st edition. Singapore: Springer Verlag; 2021.
4. Barbhaiya M, Zuily S, Naden R, Hendry A, Manneville F, Amigo MC. The 2023 ACR/EULAR antiphospholipid syndrome classification criteria. Arthritis Rheumatol. 2023;75(10):1687-702.
5. Garcia D, Erka D. Diagnosis and Management of the Antiphospholipid Syndrome. N Engl J Med. 2018;378(21):2010-21.
6. Singhal M, Goyal A, Rout P. Antiphospholipid syndrome. In: StatPearls [Internet]. Treasure Island (FL): StatPearls Publishing; 2025. Available from https://www.ncbi.nlm.nih.gov/books/NBK430980/ [Last accessed October, 2025].

Immunoglobulin 4-related Disease

S Chandrasekar, S Krupha

INTRODUCTION

Immunoglobulin 4-related disease (IgG4-RD) is a multiorgan immune-mediated condition. Awareness of this disease is essential due to its tendency to mimic malignancies and other autoimmune conditions such as Sjögren's syndrome, idiopathic membranous nephropathy, and granulomatosis with polyangiitis.

EPIDEMIOLOGY

Unlike other autoimmune conditions, this disease has a male predilection (3:2 to 3:1 male-to-female ratio), with almost equal severity in both genders. It predominantly affects older men, mostly in their sixth decade. IgG4-RD was first recognized in the pancreas, initially described in cases of AIP. Subsequently, other organs such as the orbit, meninges, major salivary glands, lymph nodes, retroperitoneum, thyroid gland, lungs, aorta, kidneys, and bile ducts have been identified as involved. The true prevalence of the disease remains undetermined due to insufficient data. Most available data include cases of AIP in the Japanese population.

ETIOLOGY AND PATHOGENESIS

It is still unclear whether IgG4 is directly involved in the disease pathogenesis. Substantial elevations of both IgG4 and plasmablasts have been reported in IgG4-RD and appear to mirror disease activity. Despite this, more than half of biopsy-proven cases of IgG4-RD have normal IgG4 levels before treatment initiation. Among patients with elevated IgG4 levels, the range of values is extremely broad. An approximately six- to eightfold increase in IgG4 strongly suggests the diagnosis. Occasionally, IgG4 levels can exceed 4 mg/dL. Unlike other IgG subclasses, IgG4 has the property of suppressing inflammation. Its response develops after chronic exposure to an antigen as part of a tolerogenic mechanism. IgG4 forms half-antibodies through a process called Fab arm exchange, resulting in IgG4 molecules with two different binding specificities. These subsequently form asymmetric antibodies by recombination of dissociated arms. The purpose of this process is to mop up antigens through monovalent binding, which tends to downregulate inflammation.

Role of B cells and T cells

Plasma cells and plasmablasts produce most of the IgG4; in most cases, plasmablasts are found in high concentrations. Both plasmablasts and IgG4 serve as good biomarkers to assess disease activity. These circulating plasmablasts exhibit high levels of somatic hypermutation, a hallmark of interaction with T cells at the germinal centers of lymph nodes. Recent studies have identified clonal expansion of CD4+ cytotoxic T lymphocytes in the peripheral blood and fibrotic lesions of patients with IgG4-RD.

CLINICAL MANIFESTATIONS

Immunoglobulin 4-related disease often has a subacute presentation involving multiple organ systems. It frequently presents with vague symptoms such as fatigue, weight loss, arthralgias, enthesopathy, and other musculoskeletal symptoms in the context of atopy or allergy.

Nervous and Ophthalmic Manifestations

It is the most common cause of idiopathic hypertrophic pachymeningitis and hypophysitis, which can lead to hormone deficiencies from both the anterior and posterior pituitary. Perineural thickening of the peripheral nerves of the orbit, especially the trigeminal and infraorbital nerves, is present. The most common ophthalmic presentation includes dacryoadenitis. It can also cause scleritis, nasolacrimal duct obstructions, and pseudotumors. The triad of dacryoadenitis with enlargement of the parotid and submandibular glands is a classic presentation of IgG4-RD, historically known as Mikulicz's disease. These are usually painless, asymptomatic enlargements that are highly responsive to steroids.

Ear, Nose, Throat, and Lymph Nodes

An allergic inflammatory response is triggered in these organs, leading to allergic rhinitis, nasal polyps, and chronic rhinosinusitis. Destructive mass lesions can form in the sinuses, pharynx, hypopharynx, and Waldeyer's ring. IgG4-RD is typically associated with generalized lymphadenopathy and can mimic Castleman's disease. Although Riedel's thyroiditis has been convincingly linked to IgG4-RD, fibrosing Hashimoto's thyroiditis requires further study to establish a connection.

Blood Vessels

Immunoglobulin 4-related disease can cause aortitis, which may lead to aneurysms and dissections in the thoracic aorta. Microscopic findings include obliterative arteritis and obliterative phlebitis. It can also cause chronic periaortitis, characterized by a triad of IgG4-related retroperitoneal fibrosis, abdominal aortitis, and perianeurysmal fibrosis, causing flank, lower back, and thigh pain.

Lung

Manifestations can range from thickening of the bronchovascular bundle to pleural thickening, pulmonary nodules, and interstitial lung disease.

Kidney

Tubulointerstitial nephritis is the most characteristic form of IgG4-RD, often associated with profound hypocomplementemia and subnephrotic proteinuria. Kidneys can undergo atrophy despite treatment. Membranous glomerulonephropathy can also occur in IgG4-RD.

Pancreas

Two subtypes of autoimmune pancreatitis (AIP) exist; type 1 is associated with IgG4-RD. These commonly present with obstructive jaundice due to sclerosing cholangitis. IgG4-related cholangitis can occur alongside IgG4-related cholecystitis. Sclerosing lesions of both the mesentery and mediastinum are also described. Biopsy-proven prostatic disease has been reported, often resulting in abrupt symptomatic relief of benign prostatic hypertrophy once treatment is initiated.

PATHOLOGICAL FEATURES

Hallmarks

- Dense lymphoplasmacytic infiltrate rich in IgG4 plasma cells
- Storiform fibrosis
- Obliterative phlebitis
  Obliterative venulitis is difficult to identify using eosin and hematoxylin stains; special connective tissue stains such as elastin Van Gieson are useful.

Pathological Mimics

- Multicentric Castleman disease and IgG4-RD show considerable overlap, given the high frequency of lymphadenopathy.
- Histiocytic disorders like Rosai–Dorfman–Destombes disease and Erdheim–Chester disease cause inflammatory mass lesions that can mimic IgG4-RD.
- Extrapulmonary sarcoidosis may share clinical features similar to those of IgG4-RD, including polyclonal hypergammaglobulinemia, lymphadenopathy, pulmonary nodules, sclerosing mesenteritis, and pachymeningitis.

Immunostaining

No number of IgG4-positive cells alone in a biopsy is sufficient to support the diagnosis of IgG4-RD. Among patients with serum IgG4 testing in a healthcare system, the positive predictive value of a level > 135 mg/dL was 34%. Among patients with pancreatic disease, the positive predictive value of a level > 140 mg/dL was 36%. Whereas for a plasmablast count of 900/mL, a sensitivity of 95%, specificity of 82%, positive predictive value of 86%, and negative predictive value of 97% have been calculated. A finding of more than 30 IgG4 plasma cells per high-power field (HPF) has good specificity for type 1 AIP and more than 10 for IgG4-related tubulointerstitial nephritis. Most cases show an IgG4/IgG+ plasma cell ratio > 40%.

RADIOLOGICAL CHARACTERISTICS

Radiological images cannot differentiate between malignancy and benign disease in the affected organs; however, they are helpful for monitoring. A combination of computed tomography (CT) and magnetic resonance imaging (MRI) can identify affected organs and monitor disease activity, remission, or relapse. Patients with the following findings have a high probability of AIP:
- A diffusely enlarged pancreas with delayed enhancement and border irregularity
- Presence or absence of a capsule-like rim on contrast-enhanced CT or MRI
- Serum IgG4 levels more than twice the upper limit of normal

Endoscopic retrograde cholangiopancreatography (ERCP) and endoscopic ultrasound (EUS) can help obtain tissue samples for diagnosis. In renal lesions, lesions are commonly bilateral and multiple and involve the cortex. Radiological findings are classified as:
- Large, solitary masses
- Small, peripheral cortical nodules
- Round or wedge-shaped lesions
- Diffuse, patchy involvement

Utility of positron emission tomography (PET) CT: 18F-fluorodeoxyglucose positron emission tomography (FDG PET)/CT may be an effective diagnostic tool in IgG4-RD, as it can highlight active inflammatory lesions and thus enable estimation of the extent of disease. Furthermore, FDG PET/CT is a useful tool for staging and monitoring of disease activity, for assessing response to treatment, and also for guiding biopsies.

Mayo Clinic HISORT Criteria for the Diagnosis of Autoimmune Pancreatitis

- *Histopathology (one or both criteria required)*:
  i. Characteristic appearances within biopsy or resection material
  ii. At least 10 IgG4-positive plasma cells per HPF within areas of lymphoplasmacytic infiltrate
- *Imaging and serology (three criteria required)*:
  i. Diffusely enlarged pancreas with delayed and "rim" enhancement
  ii. Irregular pancreatic duct
  iii. Increased serum IgG4 concentration
- *Response to steroid therapy (three criteria required)*:
  i. Unexplained pancreatic disease after a full clinical workup, including exclusion of cancer
  ii. Raised serum IgG4 concentration and/or extrapancreatic organ involvement with increased numbers of tissue IgG4-positive plasma cells
  iii. Resolution or marked improvement in the disease with steroid therapy

Japanese Comprehensive Clinical Diagnostic Criteria for Immunoglobulin 4-related Disease

- *Clinical examination:* Characteristic diffuse or localized swelling or masses in single or multiple organs
- *Hematological examination:* Elevated serum IgG4 concentrations (>135 mg/dL)
- *Histopathological examination:*
  - Marked lymphocyte and plasmacytic infiltration and fibrosis
  - *Infiltration of IgG4+ plasma cells*: Ratio of IgG4+/IgG+ cells > 40% and > 10 IgG4+ plasma cells per HPF

Diagnostic categories:
- *Definite*: 1 + 2 + 3
- *Probable*: 1 + 3
- *Possible*: 1 + 2

Biomarkers for Monitoring Immunoglobulin 4-related Disease

Several biomarkers are useful for monitoring disease activity and response to treatment in IgG4-RD. These systemic markers, including IgG4, IgE, and plasmablast count, show changes reflecting disease activity **(Table 1)**. Furthermore, specific organ involvement can be assessed using localized laboratory tests, as outlined in **Table 2**.

TABLE 1: Biomarkers used for monitoring immunoglobulin G4-related disease (IgG4-RD) activity.

Biomarker	Change
Immunoglobulin G4	↑
Immunoglobulin E	↑
Eosinophil count	↑
Complement components 3 and 4	↓
Erythrocyte sedimentation rate (ESR)	↑
Plasmablast count	↑
Memory B cell count	↑

Organ-specific Laboratory Tests

TABLE 2: Organ-specific laboratory changes observed in immunoglobulin G4-related disease (IgG4-RD).

Test	Change
Lipase	↑
Alanine transaminase (ALT), aspartate transaminase (AST)	↑
Alkaline phosphatase, gamma-glutamyl transferase, bilirubin	↑
Creatinine	↑
Total urine protein to creatinine ratio	↑

TREATMENT

The optimal treatment for IgG4-RD remains unknown. Glucocorticoids are currently the first-line therapy. The usual initial dose is *0.5–1.0 mg/kg* of prednisone, adjusted according to the severity of presentation. The initial dose is typically continued for 2–4 weeks and then tapered over 2–3 months.

Some studies indicate that a majority of patients relapse after corticosteroid withdrawal. Since this disease primarily affects middle-aged to elderly individuals—who are at a higher risk of osteoporosis, diabetes, and infections—steroid-sparing agents such as *azathioprine* and *mycophenolate mofetil* are being explored.

Clinical response to *rituximab* has shown significant improvement in disease activity, as demonstrated in two prospective, open-label single-arm trials. Patients are usually treated with 1 g twice over 14 days, and many achieve remission without a concomitant oral corticosteroid course.

T-cell-targeted therapies are being studied; however, *abatacept*, an inhibitor of T-cell co-stimulation and activation, did not show promising results.

Inebilizumab has been shown to reduce the risk of flares and increase the likelihood of flare-free complete remission at 1 year, potentially confirming the role of CD19-targeted B-cell depletion as a treatment for IgG4-RD.

Approximately 60% of patients have exocrine or endocrine damage at diagnosis and should be managed with pancreatic enzyme replacement therapy at doses of ≥1,000 units/kg/meal and 500 units/kg/meal with snacks. Vitamin levels should be replenished and monitored annually.

Furthermore, FDG PET/CT is useful for staging and monitoring disease activity, assessing response to treatment, and guiding biopsies.

CONCLUSION

Immunoglobulin G4-related disease is a multiorgan immune-mediated condition that can mimic both malignancies and other autoimmune disorders. Its clinical manifestations are diverse, frequently affecting the pancreas (Type 1 AIP), kidneys, orbits, and blood vessels. Diagnosis relies on a constellation of findings, including characteristic histopathological hallmarks—dense IgG4-rich lymphoplasmacytic infiltrate, storiform fibrosis, and obliterative phlebitis—often alongside elevated serum IgG4. Glucocorticoids are the first-line treatment, but relapse is common. Therefore, rituximab, a B-cell depleting agent, has emerged as an effective, steroid-sparing alternative for achieving and maintaining remission. Awareness and early diagnosis are critical for initiating prompt therapy and preventing irreversible organ damage.

FURTHER READINGS

1. Wallace ZS, Katz G, Hernandez-Barco YG, Baker MC. Current and future advances in practice: IgG4-related disease. Rheumatol Adv Pract. 2024;8(2):rkae020.
2. Wong AJ, Planck SR, Choi D, Harrington CA, Troxell ML, Houghton DC, et al. IgG4 immunostaining and its implications in orbital inflammatory disease. PLoS One. 2014;9(10):e109847.
3. Stone JH, Khosroshahi A, Zhang W, Della Torre E, Okazaki K, Tanaka Y, et al. Inebilizumab for treatment of IgG4-related disease. N Engl J Med. 2025;392(12):1168-77.
4. Lang D, Zwerina J, Pieringer H. IgG4-related disease: current challenges and future prospects. Ther Clin Risk Manag. 2016;12:189-99.
5. Chen LYC, Mattman A, Seidman MA, Carruthers MN. IgG4-related disease: what a hematologist needs to know. Haematologica. 2019;104(3):444-55.

CHAPTER 48

Red Flags in Rheumatology

Ritu

INTRODUCTION

Clinicians can distinguish between common or benign musculoskeletal symptoms and those brought on by systemic autoimmune, infectious, vasculitis, neoplastic, or drug-induced causes by using red flags, which are warning signs. These can be broadly categorized into *systemic* and *localized* red flags depending on whether they indicate widespread multiorgan involvement or isolated joint/tissue pathology.

They serve as "clinical alarms," indicating that a seemingly benign rheumatologic manifestation could potentially be hiding the following:

- Inflammation that could endanger life or organs
- Arthritis that is rapidly destructive
- Severe connective tissue disease or vasculitis
- Covert illness or cancer
- A side effect of immunosuppressive treatment

Rheumatic diseases can cause irreversible damage to the joints and other systems, making it more difficult to manage symptoms and maintain mobility. Moreover, complications including infections, organ damage, and cardiovascular disease are more likely to arise the longer a condition is left untreated. Therefore, it is crucial to comprehend the significance of red flag signs.

GENERAL APPROACH TO RED FLAGS IN RHEUMATOLOGY

In rheumatology, a general approach to red flags is recognizing symptoms and indicators that point to potential complication that need immediate attention. According to the 2019 consensus recommendation for spondylarthritis and inflammatory bowel disease (IBD), serious warning signs such as perianal abscesses, dactylitis, chronic low back pain, and rectal bleeding should be considered. The 2020 worldwide framework calls for detailed clinical reasoning beyond isolated indications and stresses the use of comprehensive histories and coupled red flags for the detection of significant rheumatic diseases. Additionally, in managing rheumatoid arthritis (RA), the American College of Rheumatology emphasizes identifying red signals to strike a balance between infection risks and treatment aggressiveness.

SYSTEMIC RED FLAGS

Serious underlying pathology that requires immediate assessment is indicated by systemic red flags. Fever, unexplainable weight loss, chronic lethargy, night sweats, and overall malaise are examples of constitutional symptoms that can indicate systemic inflammation. Symmetric polyarthritis with RA-like morning stiffness, joint swelling, and soreness, vasculitis skin lesions, neurological impairments, and organomegaly or lymphadenopathy suggestive of systemic autoimmune illness are other warning signs. In order to rule out potentially fatal illnesses like vasculitis, a flare-up of connective tissue disease, or cancer, it is also important to promptly investigate the presence of nocturnal pain that is not alleviated by analgesics, rapid functional decline, or systemic upset.

LOCALIZED RED FLAG SIGNS

Musculoskeletal

Acute monoarticular inflammatory arthritis is a "red flag" presentation (e.g., septic arthritis, gout, pseudogout) that may require arthrocentesis or hospitalization if infection is suspected. New-onset inflammatory polyarthritis has a wide differential diagnosis [e.g., RA, hepatitis-related arthritis, chikungunya arthritis, serum sickness, drug-induced lupus, systemic lupus erythematosus (SLE), polyarticular septic arthritis] and may require targeted laboratory investigations more so than synovial fluid analyses. Certain conditions, such as acute gout, can be precipitated in hospitalized patients by surgery, dehydration, or medications and should be considered when hospitalized patients are evaluated for the acute onset of a musculoskeletal condition **(Table 1)**.

Dermatological and Mucocutaneous

Refer to **Table 1**.

Ocular

Refer to **Table 2**.

TABLE 1: Dermatological and mucocutaneous clues in rheumatological disorder.

Rheumatological disorder	Dermatological warning signs/cutaneous clues	Clinical significance
Systemic lupus erythematosus (SLE)	Malar (butterfly) rash, discoid lesions, photosensitive rash, vasculitis ulcers, alopecia	Suggests systemic disease activity; risk of nephritis or vasculitis

Continued

Continued

Rheumatological disorder	Dermatological warning signs/cutaneous clues	Clinical significance
Dermatomyositis	Heliotrope rash, Gottron's papules, periungual telangiectasia, "shawl sign", mechanic's hands	May indicate underlying malignancy or rapidly progressive ILD
Systemic sclerosis (scleroderma)	Sclerodactyly, digital ulcers, telangiectasia, salt-and-pepper pigmentation, calcinosis cutis	Digital ulcers vascular crisis; rapidly progressive skin thickening internal organ involvement
Rheumatoid arthritis (RA)	Rheumatoid nodules, vasculitis ulcers, palmar erythema	Nodules/ulcers suggest severe, seropositive, extra-articular disease
Vasculitis (e.g., PAN, GPA, MPA)	Palpable purpura, livedo reticularis, ulcers, digital gangrene	Cutaneous vasculitis may indicate systemic vessel involvement; emergency red flag
Psoriatic arthritis	Erythematous plaques with silvery scales, nail pitting, onycholysis	Nail involvement predicts distal interphalangeal arthritis; skin flare precedes joint disease
Behçet's disease	Recurrent oral and genital ulcers, erythema nodosum-like lesions, pathergy	Frequent flares suggest high systemic inflammatory burden; risk of ocular/CNS disease
Reactive arthritis	Keratoderma blennorrhagicum, circinate balanitis	Indicates ongoing infection-triggered immune response
Mixed connective tissue disease (MCTD)	Puffy hands, scleroderma changes, malar rash, Raynaud's phenomenon	May herald overlap features with SLE or systemic sclerosis
Adult-onset still's disease (AOSD)	Evanescent salmon-pink rash (fever associated)	Rash during fever spikes indicates systemic inflammatory activity

TABLE 2: Ocular disorders associated with disease need urgent ophthalmological consultation.

Sign and symptoms	Ophthalmologic diagnosis	Rheumatic disease
Sens of burning and foreign body, itching, photophobia, corneal ulceration	Dry eye	Sjögren's syndrome, rheumatoid arthritis, systemic lupus erythematosus, scleroderma
Pain, redness, photophobia, blurred vision		Ankylosing spondylitis, psoriatic arthritis, reactive arthritis, juvenile idiopathic arthritis, Behçet's disease.
Deep pain, sclera redness, photophobia epiphora	Scleritis	Rheumatoid arthritis, systemic lupus erythematosus, ANCA-related vasculits, Behçet's disease
Decreased vision, pain, photophobia	Keratitis	Sjögren's syndrome, rheumatoid arthritis. ANCA-related vasculitis, systemic lupus erythematosus, Behçet's disease
Loss of vision	Retinal vasculitis	Systemic lupus erythematosus, ANCA-related vasculitis, Behçet's disease, sarcoidosis, rheumatoid arthritis

Neurological
Refer to **Table 3**.

Cardiopulmonary
In rheumatological disorders, cardiopulmonary involvement frequently denotes serious systemic activity with potentially fatal consequences. Indicators of interstitial lung disease, pulmonary hypertension, myocarditis, pericarditis, or vasculitis-related pulmonary hemorrhage include unexplained dyspnea, chest pain, cough, hemoptysis, orthopnea, and palpitations. Pleuritis and pericardial effusion are early warning signs for SLE, while growing exertional dyspnea in SLE indicates pulmonary fibrosis or pulmonary arterial hypertension (PAH). Even in cases with mild joint illness, RA patients should be closely monitored for silent interstitial lung disease or pericardial effusion. Hemoptysis or respiratory difficulty in antineutrophil cytoplasmic antibody (ANCA)-associated vasculitis may indicate diffuse alveolar hemorrhage, a life-threatening condition. To avoid morbidity and death, early detection and focused assessment using biomarkers [e.g., NT-pro-B-type natriuretic peptide (BNP), troponin], high-resolution computed tomography (HRCT) chest, and echocardiography are crucial **(Tables 2 and 3)**.

TABLE 3: Neurological involvement in rheumatic diseases.	
Condition	**Neurological syndromes**
Antiphospholipid syndrome	Transverse myelopathy, stroke, migraine, memory loss, demyelination, movement disorders
Temporal arteritis/giant cell arteritis and Takayasu's arteritis	Headache, visual loss, papilledema, amaurosis fugax, stroke
Systemic vasculitis	Peripheral neuropathy, mononeuritis multiplex, stroke, polymyositis, meningoencephalitis
Eosinophilic granulomatosis with polyangiitis	Peripheral or cranial neuropathy, mononeuritis multiplex, encephalopathy
Dermatomyositis and polymyositis	Proximal myopathy
Mixed connective tissue disease	Proximal myopathy
Rheumatoid arthritis	Rheumatoid vasculitis causing stroke and/or neuropathy, atlantoaxial subluxation, polymyositis; mononeuritis multiplex, peripheral neuropathy
Systemic lupus erythematosus	Aseptic meningitis, demyelinating syndrome, chorea, myelopathy, seizures, anxiety/mood disorders; psychosis, Guillain–Barré syndrome, plexopathy; cranial and/or peripheral neuropathy, myasthenia gravis, autonomic disorder, stroke, migraine, headache
Behçet's disease	Meningitis, encephalitis, seizure, stroke, headache
Scleroderma	Proximal myopathy, plexopathy, intracerebral inflammation
Sjögren's syndrome	Myelopathy, polyneuropathy, motor neurone syndromes, cognitive dysfunction

LABORATORY AND IMAGING RED FLAGS

Serological and proteomic biomarkers are useful in confirming clinically suspected preliminary diagnosis, monitoring the treatment response and prognosis of autoimmune diseases. In nearly 70% of RA patients RA factor is positive and may be an indicator of worse prognosis. High RF levels may show aggressive joint disease, rheumatoid nodules, and accompanying extra-articular involvement. In the early stages of disease the groups show similar characteristics, but with time the anti-CCP antibodies positive group are observed to have more erosion and the disease progresses more severely **(Table 4)**.

Imaging: Early bone erosion correlates with poor long-term radiographic and functional outcome, and early progression in radiographic erosion is related to future impairment in physical function. In early undifferentiated arthritis, the presence of radiographic erosion increases the risk of developing persistent arthritis. MRI bone edema is a strong independent predictor of subsequent radiographic progression in early RA and should be considered as a prognostic indicator. Joint inflammation (synovitis) detected by magnetic resonance imaging (MRI) or ultrasonography, as well as joint damage detected by conventional radiographs, MRI, or ultrasonography, can also be considered for the prediction of further joint damage.

TABLE 4: ANA patterns and prognostic implications in rheumatological disorders.

Disorder	ANA pattern/specific autoantibody	Prognostic implication
Systemic lupus erythematosus (SLE)	• Homogeneous (anti-dsDNA, anti-histone) • Speckled (anti-Smith, anti-RNP) • Anti-C1q	• High anti-dsDNA—renal involvement and flares • Anti-C1q—lupus nephritis risk • Anti-Smith—severe systemic disease
Systemic sclerosis (SSc)	• Nucleolar (anti-fibrillarin/U3 RNP) • Centromere • Anti-topoisomerase I (Scl-70)	• Anti-Scl-70—diffuse cutaneous SSc, interstitial lung disease • Anticentromere—limited SSc, pulmonary hypertension risk • Antifibrillarin—severe organ involvement
Mixed connective tissue disease (MCTD)	Speckled ANA (anti-U1-RNP)	Pulmonary hypertension, cardiac, and renal complications
Sjögren's Syndrome (SJS)	Speckled (anti-Ro/SSA, anti-La/SSB)	Extra glandular involvement, lymphoma risk with persistent high titters
Idiopathic inflammatory myopathies (IIMs)	Speckled or cytoplasmic (anti-Mi-2, anti-MDA5, anti-TIF1-γ)	• Anti-MDA5—rapidly progressive ILD, poor survival • Anti-TIF1-γ—malignancy association
Drug-induced lupus	Homogeneous (anti-histone)	Usually resolves after drug withdrawal; rarely severe organ involvement

(ANA: anti-nuclear antibody; dsDNA: double-stranded DNA; ILD: interstitial lung disease; RNP: ribonucleoprotein; TIF1: transcription intermediary factor 1)

RED FLAGS SUGGESTING ALTERNATIVE AND COEXISTING DIAGNOSIS

Lymphadenopathy is common clinical finding and diagnostic challenge. Given that lymph node enlargement is a prevalent finding within the clinical spectrum of several well-known rheumatologic illnesses, including RA, SLE, and SS, evaluating lymphadenopathy is very pertinent in the field of rheumatology. Furthermore, because successful targeted therapy can now affect the prognosis of rare immunological disorders such as Castleman disease and IgG4-related disease, lymphadenopathy is a defining feature of these conditions that must be taken into account in the differential diagnosis. In the case of paraneoplastic rheumatic syndromes, rheumatic symptoms can coincide, precede, or follow the diagnosis of cancer or herald its recurrence, generally at no longer than 2 years before the diagnosis of associated cancers. Fevers, weight loss, fatigue, and night sweats, otherwise known as "B symptoms" must initially prompt a search for "red flag" pathologies such as malignancy and infection. Certain rheumatological conditions (e.g., dermatomyositis) can be associated with malignancy. Most medications used in rheumatology are also immunosuppressive and therefore put patients at higher risk of infections, including with atypical pathogens.

CONCLUSION

- Red flags are early indicators of serious or systemic rheumatologic illness.
- In order to prevent organ damage and death, prompt identification and intervention are essential.
- Red flags unique to a particular organ, such as hematuria, lung symptoms, skin ulcers, or neurological abnormalities, should be evaluated right away.
- A worse prognosis is indicated by certain laboratory abnormalities, such as high-titer ANA, anti-dsDNA, anti-Scl-70, ANCA positive, and cryoglobulins.
- The most precise diagnostic and prognostic information is obtained by combining clinical, serological, and imaging data.
- Results are improved and the right immunosuppressive or targeted therapy is guided by early detection and referral.
- Red flag detection in routine rheumatology practice still depends on clinician education and attentiveness.

FURTHER READINGS

1. Felice C, Leccese P, Scudeller L, Lubrano E, Cantini F, Castiglione F, et al. Red flags for appropriate referral to the gastroenterologist and the rheumatologist of patients with inflammatory bowel disease and spondyloarthritis. Clin Exp Immunol. 2019;196(1):123-38.
2. PMM. Red Flags. [Online] Available from https://www.pmmonline.org/doctor/clinical-assessment/red-flags/ [Last accessed October, 2025].
3. Hauser S, Loscalzo J, Fauci AS, Kasper DL. Harrison's principles of internal medicine, 21st edition. New York: McGraw Hill; 2022.
4. Habibullah T, Habibullah A, Simsim R. Skin Manifestations of Rheumatological Diseases. In: Almoallim H, Cheikh M, (Eds). Skills in Rheumatology. Singapore: Springer; 2021.
5. Dankiewicz-Fares I, Jeka D, Barczyńska T. Ocular involvement in rheumatic diseases. Reumatologia. 2023;61(5):389-94.

CHAPTER 49

The Adventure of Systemic Vasculitis: Care and Clinical Research

Aman Sharma

■ INTRODUCTION

Systemic vasculitis is characterized by the inflammation of the blood vessel wall resulting in organ dysfunction due to ischemia, hemorrhage, or necrosis. These are a group of complex and mostly multisystem disorders with each subtype having a unique pattern of clinical presentation. Once a physician is able to do that pattern recognition, the diagnosis is not difficult.

■ EPIDEMIOLOGY

Takayasu's arteritis (TA) is most commonly described and giant cell arteritis (GCA) is rare. Granulomatosis with polyangiitis (GPA) has been reported more commonly from North India. A rare monogenic disease called deficiency of adenosine deaminase 2 (DADA2) seen more commonly in Aggarwal/Jain community is being recognized in India.

■ CLASSIFICATION

The first effort to classify was done by Zeek in 1950s. The American College of Rheumatology (ACR) gave its criteria in 1990. Subsequently, a new entity of microscopic polyangiitis (MPA) was proposed in the definitions given in Chapel Hill consensus conference (CHCC) nomenclature system. Consensus methodology algorithm incorporating various soft pointers and antineutrophil cytoplasmic antibodies (ANCA) has been validated by us. Subsequently the revised CHCC nomenclature system was proposed. It is important to understand that these are all classification criteria or nomenclature systems and not "diagnostic criteria" and patient may still have vasculitis even if he does not fulfill any classification criteria and these disorders may manifest with lesser known or unknown presentations. ACR European Alliance of Associations for Rheumatology (EULAR) criteria for GPA, MPA, eosinophilic granulomatosis with polyangiitis (EGPA), TAK, and GCA based upon on the Diagnostic and Classification Criteria for Vasculitis (DCVAS) study have been published recently.

IMPORTANT INDIVIDUAL VASCULITIC DISORDERS

Large Vessel Vasculitis

Takayasu arteritis and GCA are types of large vessel vasculitis.

- *Takayasu's arteritis:* There is inflammation of the aorta and its branches. Acute stage (preocclusive stage) is characterized by fever, musculoskeletal symptoms, and weight loss. Diagnosis is rarely made at this stage during imaging for pyrexia of unknown origin (PUO) evaluation. Most patients diagnosed at a later stage of narrowing/stenosis of vessels present with symptoms of ischemia of ocular, cerebral, renovascular, cardiopulmonary, and peripheral vascular systems. There may be absence of upper limb pulses ("pulseless disease"). Computed tomography (CT) and magnetic resonance (MR) angiography can delineate the extent of involvement. Steroids and immunosuppression are the backbone of management.

- *Giant cell arteritis:* This should be considered in elderly patients with recent headache, jaw claudication, features of polymyalgia rheumatica, and visual impairment. There is tenderness over the superficial temporal artery and scalp. These may be carotid artery tenderness (carotidynia). Erythrocyte sedimentation rate (ESR) and C-reactive protein (CRP) are elevated. "Halo sign" on the ultrasound examination of superficial temporal arteries is very sensitive with high specificity. Temporal artery biopsy may be negative due to patchy involvement. Treatment should be started immediately to prevent vision loss. Corticosteroids are the mainstay. Other drugs like methotrexate may be required in some patients. Anti-interleukin-6 (IL-6) monoclonal antibodies (tocilizumab) and abatacept (blocks T-cell function) have been shown to be effective.

Medium Vessel Vasculitis

Classical polyarteritis nodosa (cPAN) and Kawasaki disease are the two medium vessel vasculitides. Kawasaki disease is a vasculitis of childhood.

Classical polyarteritis nodosa (cPAN): The patients present with fever constitutional symptoms, weight loss, hypertension, mononeuritis multiplex, gastrointestinal involvement as abdominal angina, testicular pain, and cardiac involvement in the form of cardiomyopathy. There may be hepatic, renal or splenic infarction, and angiography may show microaneurysms. A new variant of polyarteritis nodosa (PAN) due to DADA2 caused by mutations in *ADA2* gene was described in the New England Journal of Medicine (NEJM) in 2014. Various mutations including two novel mutations described by us have been reported in *CECR1* gene. One of largest cohorts of DADA2 in the world has been reported from India. The patients have livedoid rash, stroke, peripheral neuropathy, and digital gangrene, and respond only to high dose steroids and antitumor necrosis factor (TNFs). They do not respond to other drugs such as cyclophosphamide, azathioprine, mycophenolate, or methotrexate, etc.

Small Vessel Vasculitis

There are two subgroups: (1) ANCA associated vasculitis (AAV) and (2) immune complex vasculitis.

The subtypes of AAV are GPA, previously Wegener's granulomatosis, MPA, and EGPA, previously Churg Strauss syndrome.

Granulomatosis with Polyangiitis

Common clinical presentation is in the form of upper airways, lungs, and kidney involvement. Upper airway involvement and granulomatous inflammation differentiate it from MPA. The upper airway involvement is in the form of nasal crusting, nasal bleed, nasal ulcers, recurrent sinusitis, saddle nose deformity, and occasionally bony destruction with sinus formation. Lung involvement may vary from asymptomatic lung nodules with or without cavitation to life threatening diffuse alveolar hemorrhage. The kidney involvement is in the form of pauci-immune crescentic glomerulonephritis presenting as rapidly progressive renal failure. The presentation based upon ANCA positivity and negativity are also being compared these days. There can be necrotizing scleritis, scleromalacia perforans, peripheral ulcerative keratitis, corneal melt, and orbital pseudotumor. Variety of skin lesions are also seen and these may vary from palpable purpura, nodules, ulcers, and cutaneous infarcts. Neurological involvement usually in the form of mononeuritis multiplex and central nervous system (CNS) involvement is rare. In our experience of 105 GPA patients, Indian patients were noted to be younger and with less arthritis, renal, and peripheral nerve involvement as compared to Western cohorts.

The diagnosis is largely based upon clinical setting supported by histopathology and ANCA positivity. Recent international consensus statement recommends that high-quality immunoassays can be used as the primary screening method for AVV without the categorical need for indirect immunofluorescence (IIF). The CT paranasal sinuses (PNS) may show bone destruction and sinusitis. HRCT may show nodules, ground-glass opacities (GGOs), and small fibrotic bands.

The approach to treatment is largely same for all AAVs. There is an initial phase of remission induction followed by remission maintenance. Drug of choice for remission induction are cyclophosphamide or rituximab. If the disease is very mild then methotrexate may be used. Remission can be maintained with drugs such as rituximab, azathioprine, methotrexate, and mycophenolate mofetil. Plasma exchange can be used in patients with rapidly progressive renal failure (RPRF) and serum creatinine > 5.6 mg/dL, and diffuse alveolar hemorrhage. Treatment of relapsing and refractory disease is a challenge and should be planned in consultation with vasculitis experts.

Microscopic Polyangiitis

MPA is characterized by necrotizing vasculitis, with no immune deposits and no granuloma formation. The clinical presentation is in the form of constitutional symptoms and renal involvement. The renal involvement is in the form of rapidly progressive glomerulonephritis (RPGN). There is microscopic hematuria and proteinuria. Kidney biopsy shows pauci-immune glomerulonephritis. There may be oliguria/anuria and need for dialysis at presentation. There can be renal and pulmonary presenting as reno-pulmonary syndrome. Pulmonary involvement may be in the form of alveolar hemorrhage. Pulmonary fibrosis may be seen in about one-third of the patients. There is no upper airway involvement. Mononeuritis multiplex is the dominant neurological manifestation and is seen commonly. The other manifestations may be in the form of skin rash and eye involvement. Heart and gastrointestinal tract are involved rarely.

Dominant ANCA pattern seen in these patients is p-ANCA and myeloperoxidase (MPO). C-ANCA and PR3 positivity is uncommon. The treatment is on the lines of other AAVs as described earlier in description of GPA.

Eosinophilic Granulomatosis with Polyangiitis

This is one of the rarest forms of AAV. ANCA positivity is seen in only 30–40% patients. There are three prototype clinical phases. First is prodromal phase of allergic manifestations and asthma. Second phase is characterized by blood eosinophilia (> $1,500/mm^3$), and tissue eosinophilia. Third phase is of vasculitis. The three phases may not occur sequentially and may overlap. The common clinical manifestations are in the form of constitutional symptoms, rhinitis, polyposis, and asthma. There are lung infiltrates. Nodules and alveolar hemorrhage are rare. Skin and peripheral nervous system involvement is also common. The skin manifestations may vary from palpable purpura, cutaneous nodules, livedo reticularis, ulcerations, and infarcts. Peripheral nervous system involvement is common. Cardiomyopathy has been associated with increased mortality in these patients. Other uncommon manifestations can be gastrointestinal involvement in form of pain abdomen, diarrhea, and vomiting. The diagnosis is based upon suggestive clinical findings supported by histopathology wherever possible. The treatment depends upon type and severity of the disease. Immunosuppression and antiasthma measures are the mainstay of treatment.

There are various other subgroups of vasculitides but description of all of those subtypes is outside the preview of this chapter and these would only be in numerated below.

- *Immune complex small vessel vasculitis:* Antiglomerular basement membrane (GBM) disease, cryoglobulinemic vasculitis, immunoglobulin A (IgA) vasculitis (previously Henoch–Schönlein purpura), hypocomplementemic urticarial vasculitis.
- *Variable vessel vasculitis:* Behçet's disease and Cogan syndrome.
- *Single organ vasculitis:* Cutaneous leukocytoclastic angiitis, primary angiitis of CNS, isolated arteritis, and other single organ vasculitides.
- *Vasculitis associated with systemic disease:* Lupus vasculitis, rheumatoid vasculitis, sarcoid vasculitis, and vasculitis associated with other connective tissue diseases.
- *Vasculitis associated with probable etiology:* Hepatitis C virus (HCV)-associated cryoglobulinemic vasculitis, hepatitis B virus (HBV) associated PAN, syphilis associated aortitis, drug associated immune complex vasculitis, drug associated ANCA associated vasculitis, and cancer associated vasculitis.

CONCLUSION

Systemic vasculitis is a diverse group of disorders defined by blood vessel inflammation, leading to organ damage via ischemia or necrosis. Accurate diagnosis relies on pattern recognition, supported by classification systems like the CHCC nomenclature, and key serological markers such as ANCA. Treatment strategies, spanning from immunosuppressive therapy (glucocorticoids and cyclophosphamide/rituximab) to targeted therapies, must be aggressive yet tailored to the specific subtype. Given the complexity and potential for severe morbidity, the ultimate goal remains the induction of durable drug-free remission achieved through early diagnosis, personalized care, and continuous clinical research.

FURTHER READINGS

1. Sharma A. Textbook of systemic vasculitis, 2nd edition. New Delhi: Jaypee Brothers Medical publishers private limited; 2023.
2. Hoffman GS, Weyand CM, Langford CA, Goronzy JJ. Inflammatory diseases of blood vessels, 2nd edition. USA: Wiley-Blackwell; 2012.
3. Sharma A, Sharma K, Dogra S. Granulomatous vasculitis. Dermatology Clinics. 2015;33(3):475-87.
4. Sharma A, Sagar V, Parkash M, Gupta V, Khaire N, Pinto B, et al. Giant cell arteritis in India: Report from a tertiary care center along with total published experience from India. Neurology India. 2015;63(5):681-6.
5. Sharma A, Naidu G, Sharma V, Jha S, Dhooria A, Dhir V, et al. Deficiency of Adenosine Deaminase 2 in Adults and Children: Experience from India. Arthritis Rheumatol. 2021;73(2):276-85.

SECTION 17

Urology

CHAPTER 50

Erectile Dysfunction Decoded: Diagnosis to Therapy

Deepak K Jumani

INTRODUCTION

Erectile dysfunction (ED), also known as impotence, is the inability to get or keep an erection firm enough for satisfying sexual intercourse. While transient ED is relatively common, persistent ED lasting for six months or more—especially when accompanied by interpersonal distress and occurring with all partners—can significantly affect both the individual and their partner, creating strain in the relationship. Many men may begin to avoid sexual activity out of fear of failure or of being judged for their performance in the bedroom. This tragedy in the bedroom today has also been identified convincingly to be a subclinical cardiovascular disease. However, ED is a manageable condition, and treatment options range from lifestyle changes to medication and medical devices. It is no longer a myth or mystery but surely can be corrected and hence ED is a correctible dysfunction. Since few years medical research has shown proven results with wide variety of options and hence ED is totally decoded.

Erectile dysfunction is a complex process involving the brain, hormones, nerves, emotions, muscles, and blood vessels. ED can result from problems in any of these systems. Causes are often categorized as organic, psychological, situational, or a combination of all. Researchers have also identified a genetic link to ED. Scientists have identified a single locus (rs17185536-T) on chromosome 6 near the single-minded family basic helix-loop-helix transcription factor 1 (*SIM1*) gene that was *significantly associated with the risk of ED*. Hence, it is important to identify the causes of ED which enable us to manage the symptom of ED the most important point to ponder here is should ED be considered as a symptom or a disease. Well, if it is a symptom, then some pharmacotherapy is the answer, but if it is considered to be a disease, which mandates an approach to give a substantial cure, which included nutritional intervention, reversal of metabolic syndrome, regenerative medicine, and lifestyle modification for lifetime. Very little importance is given to pharmacotherapy which till date has not been able to correct the etiopathology of ED.

Organic causes mainly include vasculogenic causes viz diabetes, hypertension, dyslipidemia, obesity cardiovascular diseases, which result in clogging of the penile arteries and reducing the blood flow required for optimum erections. Neurogenic causes which include multiple sclerosis, Parkinson's disease, or spinal cord injuries can interfere with signals from the brain to the penis. Hormonal causes include low testosterone, thyroid issues, prolactin issues, etc., certain medications, viz., antidepressants, antihypertensives such as betablockers, diuretics, antihistamines, and prostate cancer drugs. Medicines prescribed for alopecia include Finasteride are common culprits. Excess of alcohol, tobacco, smoking, *gutka, bidi, charas*, etc., and illicit drugs can all cause or worsen ED. Sleep disorders, chronic kidney disease, chronic liver diseases, and Peyronie's disease can also be linked to ED.

Compelling evidence exists to prove that ED today first is an endothelial dysfunction as in individuals with normal endothelium the endothelium derived nitric oxide (NO), which is a signaling molecule and initiator of erectogenic process is adequate and results in an optimum erection required for a satisfying sexual act. However, as we age NO decreases as we age, and at 60 years, only 15% NO is present which is not sufficient for desired erection.

Secondly in diabetics, ED is also due to mitochondrial dysfunction. At the islet B-cell level, acute insulin release is regulated by mitochondrial ATP production, and mitochondrial ROS may contribute to the long-term deterioration of insulin secretory capacity seen in type 2 diabetes. Diabetes being an inflammaging disease, ROS contribute to defects in both insulin secretion and insulin action and to the long-term complications of diabetes. Inflammatory damage that characterizes type 1 and type 2 diabetes is mediated at least in part through islet ROS.

Psychological causes include stress and anxiety, like worrying about sexual performance or other life stressors of career, family disputes, and finances, which can interfere with sexual arousal. Depression—mental health conditions such as depression can reduce libido and contribute to ED. Relationship problems—issues with a partner can affect sexual function.

One undeniable fact is that, regardless of the underlying cause, a psychological component is almost always present in ED. Thus, ED is not the result of a single factor—it is multifactorial, involving both organic and psychogenic elements.

Having understood the major etiology of ED, it is important to rule out pure psychogenic causes because if the cause of ED is purely psychogenic, these patients do not need any pharmacotherapy, they just need counseling because if they are prescribed pharmacotherapy, they become dependent on these medications which lower the individual's self-esteem and confidence.

To rule out psychogenic causes, one needs to ask in the history taking the onset of ED as its acute onset and after some relationship mishap or some stressful situations. Organic ED is always gradual and due to some vasculogenic, neurogenic, Homonogenic, or iatrogenic etiology.

The two very important validated questionnaires which help us in identifying the severity of ED are:
1. International Index of Erectile function (IIEF) is a 15-questionnaire document, which gives us the severity over a period of 4 weeks.
2. Sexual Health inventory of Men (SHIM) is a 5-questionnaire document, which gives us the severity over a period of 6 months.

STRATEGIES TO MANAGE ERECTILE DYSFUNCTION

- *Advice:* Smoking, diet, and exercise
- *Blood pressure:* <130/80 mm Hg
- *Cholesterol:* TC <150, LDL <100, and HDL >40
- *Diabetes control:* HbA1c ≤ 7%
- *Eye examination:* Annual examination
- *Oral cavity examination:* Monthly examination
- *Feet examination:* Monthly examination
- *Guardian drugs:* Aspirin, ACEI, and statins
- *Heart risk score:* UKPDS, Framingham, and hormones
- *Impotence Rx:* Drugs, injectables, etc.
- Cremasteric reflex and bulbocavernosus reflex to be checked.
- *Office sildenafil test:* Sildenafil 50 mg tablet or a mouth dissolving film is given to the patient, and patient is made to think erotic and stimulate himself and called back after an hour, and if he has obvious change in diameter and length of his penis, it proves that ED is purely psychological or situational. Trained physicians can also give extracavernous injections of vasoactive drugs such as papaverine and observed after half an hour to see obvious change in the penile architecture.

Additional tests in adults we do are as follows:
- Serum testosterone free and total
- Sex hormone binding globulin
- Free T3, T4, and TSH
- Serum FSH and LH prolactin
- Estimation of serum estradiol
- Estimation of vitamin D, vitamin B12, and uric acid
- USG of scrotum and Doppler studies
- Serum PSA free and total
- Digital rectal examination (DRE) for changes in the prostate
- Rigi scan [A Rigi scan is a noninvasive diagnostic device used to evaluate ED by measuring changes in penile rigidity and circumference during sleep. It is considered a gold standard for differentiating between psychological and organic causes of ED by monitoring nocturnal penile tumescence (NPT) and rigidity.]
- Stamp test (To perform the stamp test, a man applies a ring of postage stamps around his penis before bed and checks in the morning to see if the stamps have broken, indicating an erection occurred.) **(Table 1)**.

Pharmacotherapy is the first line of treatment preferred, but the consensus of management of ED suggests that all the modalities of treatment with side effects, costs, etc., should be explained to the patient, and he should be asked for his preferred choice **(Table 2)**.

MEDICATION-BASED THERAPY MAINLY PDE5 INHIBITORS

- *Side effects of PDE5 inhibits include*: Facial flushing, headache, nasal congestion, dizziness, dyspepsia, visual disturbance (blue halo rarely priapism and some cases of malignant melanoma).

TABLE 1: Once ED is diagnosed, treatment is as follows.

First line	Oral pharmacotherapy	Counseling	Lifestyle modifications
Second line	• Injection of ICVAD • Vacuum erection device • Intraurethral prostaglandins	Counseling	Lifestyle modifications
Third line	• List (low intensity shockwave therapy) • Penile implants • Regenerative medicine (PRP, stem cell therapy, and gene therapy) • Nanotechnology	Counseling	Lifestyle modifications

TABLE 2: PDE5 inhibitors.

Parameters	Sildenafil	Tadalafil	Vardenafil	Denial	Avanafil
Dose	25 mg, 50 mg, and 100 mg	2.5 mg, 5 mg, 10 mg, and 20 mg	20 mg	100 mg	100 mg and 200 mg
Onset of action	45 minutes	45–120 minutes	30–45 minutes	30–45 minutes	15–20 minutes
Duration of action	5–7 hours	36 hours	5–6 hours	10–12 hours	5 hours

- *Contraindications of PDE5 inhibitors include*: Nitrates, recent CV event, hypotension, anatomical penile defect, retinal injuries, sickle cell anemias, multiple myeloma, leukemias.
- *Drug interactions include*: Nitrates (glyceryl trinitrate, isosorbide mono, or dinitrate) if chest pain after taking sildenafil/vardenafil no nitrates 24 hours, tadalafil no nitrates 48 hours, recreational amyl nitrate (poppers).
- Cytochrome P450 inhibitors, protease inhibitors, especially ritonavir use very small dose, cimetidine, ketoconazole, erythromycin, and α-blockers

Low-dose PDE5 inhibitor as tadalafil in the dose of 2.5 mg or 5 mg once a day given for period of 4-6 weeks is a valid choice to avoid adverse side effects.

Avanafil among all is shown to have lesser side effects, and this is the only PDE5 inhibitor, which has been studied in patients who are also on nitrates. The idea is that we advise the patients who is on nitrates to skip the nitrate on the day he wants to have sexual act, take avanafil. This drug is washed out from his body in next 5 hours, and the next day again he can take his nitrate.

It is observed that there are limitations to prescribing PDE5 inhibitors as 40–50% patients do not respond to these medications and available technically with prescription only. Typically, these medications start effective only after 45 minutes to 2 hours, so sex has to be planned, and this lacks the pleasure of spontaneity. Moreover, today we see these medications are used by all as recreational drug.

Other modalities include—extracavernous injections of papaverine and chlorpromazine, but we need to be cautious as priapism is very common, vacuum erectile devise is cumbersome, and patients develop numbness at the base of penis, intraurethral prostaglandins do work in some patients, surgical treatments like penile implants are costly and unavoidable complications of mechanical failure and infections. Regenerative therapies like PRP, stem cell and gene therapy and nanotechnology we lack robust evidence.

Large studies have shown great promising results with low intensity shock wave therapy as it is noninvasive but expensive and also needs concomitant pharmacotherapy along with it.

Lastly, I believe after proven research from Cleveland clinic and discoveries of Nobel Laureate Dr Linus Pauling, that nutrition intervention is of prime importance, as nutrition intervention not only halts but even reverses coronary artery disease. So, the art and science of sexual fitness depend upon what you put in your body and what you do for your body.

Erectile dysfunction at any age is not an option, not for anyone. It is how gracefully we handle the process and how lucky we are as the process handles us. It is really nice to know that ED if diagnosed earlier, it is a blessing in disguise. Remission/reversal of diabetes, counseling, lifestyle modification use of L-arginine with fenugreek safest for arousal and desire, PDE5 inhibitors, statins and realistic expectations are the key to the decode this menace in the bedroom and the fact thus is that ED is a correctile dysfunction.

CONCLUSION

Erectile dysfunction at any age is neither inevitable nor acceptable—it is a condition that calls for understanding, timely action, and compassionate care. What truly matters is how gracefully we navigate this process and how wisely we allow it to guide us toward better health. When recognized early, ED can, in fact, be a blessing in disguise—an opportunity to uncover underlying issues such as diabetes or cardiovascular risk and initiate meaningful change.

Through lifestyle modification, counseling, metabolic control, and the judicious use of therapies such as L-arginine with fenugreek, PDE5 inhibitors, and statins, we can restore not only sexual function but also confidence and connection. Ultimately, erectile dysfunction is not a "defect" but a correctile dysfunction—a condition that, when addressed holistically, can lead to profound healing for both body and relationship.

FURTHER READINGS

1. Jumani DK. Sex has no expiry Date. New Delhi, India; 2018.
2. Masters WH, Johnson VE, Kolodny RC. Masters and Johnson on sex and human loving. Kinsey Institute: USA; 1986.
3. Mulhall J, Hsaio W. Mens Sexual Health and Fertility. 2014. ResearchGate UK.
4. Burnett AL. The Manhood Rx. Bloomsbury Publishing: USA; 2022. bloombury.com